BASIC ORAL SURGERY

Andreas Filippi | Fabio Saccardin | Sebastian Kühl (eds)

BASIC
ORAL SURGERY

With contributions by:
Stephan Acham, Zeynab Ahmed, Korbinian Benz, Constantin Berli, Michael M. Bornstein, Dorothea Dagassan-Berndt, Cornelia Filippi, Irène Hitz Lindenmüller, Jochen Jackowski, Norbert Jakse, Marc Joos, Petra Rugani, Bernd Stadlinger, Frank Peter Strietzel, Silvio Valdec, Hendrik Zeiß, Andrea Zürcher

QUINTESSENCE PUBLISHING

Berlin | Chicago | Tokyo
Barcelona | London | Milan | Mexico City | Paris | Prague | Seoul | Warsaw

One book, one tree: In support of reforestation worldwide and to address the climate crisis, for every book sold Quintessence Publishing will plant a tree (https://onetreeplanted.org/).

A video shows more than many photographs
Numerous videos are included in this book that illustrate the content and enrich the reading experience. These can easily be played via QR code using a smartphone or tablet.

Alternatively, the videos can also be accessed via this link:
https://video.qvnet.de/b23070/

A CIP record for this book is available from the British Library.
ISBN: 978-1-78698-118-9

QUINTESSENCE PUBLISHING DEUTSCHLAND

Quintessenz Verlags-GmbH
Ifenpfad 2–4
12107 Berlin, Germany
www.quintessence-publishing.com

Quintessence Publishing Co Ltd
Grafton Road, New Malden
Surrey KT3 3AB, United Kingdom
www.quintessence-publishing.com

Editing, production, and reproductions:
Quintessenz Verlags-GmbH, Berlin

Printed and bound in Croatia by Grafički zavod Hrvatske d.o.o

Preface

Only a few decades ago, German university dentistry consisted of four core subjects: Operative Dentistry and Endodontics, Prosthetics, Orthodontics, and Oral Surgery. Since then, beginning with a detachment of orthodontics from general dentistry, specialization within dentistry has increased. Such specialization is the result of an enormous increase in knowledge and scientific evidence within dentistry. However, it also means that, nowadays, professionals practicing general dentistry prefer to refer complex anamneses, cases, and/or patients to specialists for treatment due to a lack of equipment or know-how or for financial reasons. Furthermore, there is also a group of (self-paying or privately insured) patients who prefer to be treated by a specialist than by a general practitioner – a trend that has existed in the medical field for quite some time. Particularly in and around larger cities, there are now specialist practices for endodontology, periodontology, pediatric dentistry, implantology, craniomandibular function, sports dentistry, and even oral surgery or oral and maxillofacial surgery.

There are also dental professionals who do not wish to perform oral surgery in their daily practice. On the one hand, this is understandable if experience, skills or confidence are lacking, and thus the time and expenditure invested are disproportional to the turnover and success rates. On the other hand, however, it is inconvenient to constantly refer tooth extractions to a specialist dentist. After all, it is not only older patients who greatly appreciate it when most treatments can be performed at their family dentist.

Practical oral surgery training within dental education has not improved in recent decades. There are understandable reasons for this: Especially at universities with very high student numbers, it can be difficult to find a sufficient number of patients who require surgical procedures (implants, apicoectomies, wisdom tooth removals, etc) that can be performed by students. Also, there is a high level of supervision required because a dentist must be available in the immediate vicinity to assist the student for the entire duration of the procedure. Another reason is that one can complete a postgraduate degree in oral surgery and specialize in this way. This reduces the pressure on universities to teach all practical oral surgery skills during undergraduate dental education: from tooth extraction to plastic surgery to surgical tooth removal, tooth-preserving surgery, soft tissue surgery, and implant surgery. It is therefore not surprising that postgraduate practical training courses on basic oral surgery are attended by younger colleagues, in particular.

The same phenomenon has been experienced for many years in orthodontics: Theoretical training during undergraduate education is good, while practical training de facto does not exist and must be acquired after graduation. Postgraduate training centers and master's degree programs in this field are in high demand, and thus the chances of obtaining a specialist dental degree are rather slim.

This book deals exclusively with the basics of oral surgery, which is often not taught sustainably enough during undergraduate dental education. It is therefore simply missing after graduation and is often covered too briefly and in too text-heavy a manner in textbooks. However, it is precisely these fundamentals of oral surgery that are required in order to be able to perform the many basic procedures that occur in general dental practice without raising blood pressure and causing a sweat to break out.

This book is not designed as a textbook, but rather as an atlas: The clinical chapters in particular all map their theoretical content in an identically structured manner: indications, contraindications, specific risks, local anesthesia, step-by-step clinical procedure, wound care and closure, postoperative controls and course, and only a few relevant literature references. The strength of these chapters is the series of images and the videos embedded with links, which can be viewed via a smartphone or tablet. This combination is not only beautiful but also, and more importantly, it is timely, and significantly expands the scope and value of a reference book. This combination of images and videos means that the book should increase the practitioner's confidence before, during, and after oral surgical interventions. Some repetition in the content and also a few contradictory statements by the expert team of authors are intentional on the part of the editors.

Our special thanks go to all those who contributed to the creation of this book: our coauthors Stephan Acham, Zeynab Ahmed, Korbinian Benz, Constantin Berli, Michael Bornstein, Dorothea Dagassan-Berndt, Cornelia Filippi, Irène Hitz Lindenmüller, Norbert Jakse, Jochen Jackowski, Marc Joos, Petra Rugani, Bernd Stadlinger, Frank Striezel, Silvio Valdec, Hendrik Zeiß, and Andrea Zürcher.

Our thanks also go to Sabrina Peterer for the cover image, which continues the style of the now iconic covers of Andreas Filippi's books; to Anita Hattenbach of Quintessence Publishing for the always trusting, incredibly pleasant, and highly professional editing; and to all the staff involved at Quintessence Publishing in Berlin. Thank you also for allowing us to link some screenshots and videos from the excellent app by Giulio Rasperini entitled "The Oral Surgery Suture Trainer."

Thank you too for allowing us to use surgical videos from the large collection of Sebastian Kühl, who films each of his treatments using a magnifier camera, and compresses them into short video clips.

And thank you to all our colleagues at our excellent and efficient Department of Oral Surgery at the University Center for Dental Medicine in Basel for your support. You are like family to us.

Basel, 31.08.2020
Andreas Filippi, Fabio Saccardin, Sebastian Kühl

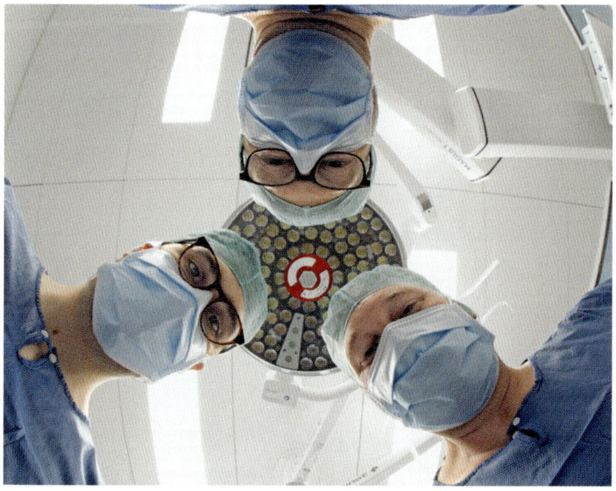

Editors' contact details

Prof. Dr. Andreas Filippi
Dr. Fabio Saccardin
Prof. Dr. Sebastian Kühl
Department of Oral Surgery
University Center for Dental Medicine Basel UZB
University of Basel
Mattenstr. 40
CH – 4058 Basel, Switzerland

Prof. Dr. Michael M. Bornstein
Department of Oral Health & Medicine
University Center for Dental Medicine Basel UZB
University of Basel
Mattenstr. 40
CH – 4058 Basel, Switzerland
and
Faculty of Dentistry
The University of Hong Kong
Hong Kong SAR, China

Authors' contact details

Priv.-Doz. Dr. Stephan Acham
Department of Dental Medicine and Oral Health
Division of Oral Surgery and Orthodontics
Medical University of Graz
Billrothgasse 4
A – 8010 Graz, Austria

Zeynab Ahmed
Department of Oral Surgery
University Center for Dental Medicine Basel UZB
University of Basel
Mattenstr. 40
CH – 4058 Basel, Switzerland

Dr. Korbinian Benz
Department of Oral Surgery and
Polyclinic Outpatient Clinic
Faculty of Health
Witten/Herdecke University
Alfred-Herrhausen-Str. 45
D – 58455 Witten, Germany

Dr. Constantin Berli
Department of Oral Surgery
University Center for Dental Medicine Basel UZB
University of Basel
Mattenstr. 40
CH – 4058 Basel, Switzerland

Dr. Dorothea Dagassan-Berndt
Center for Dental Imaging
University Center for Dental Medicine Basel UZB
University of Basel
Mattenstr. 40
CH – 4058 Basel, Switzerland

Dr. Cornelia Filippi
Department of General Pediatric and
Adolescent Dentistry
University Center for Dental Medicine Basel UZB
University of Basel
Mattenstr. 40
CH – 4058 Basel, Switzerland

Dr. Irène Hitz Lindenmüller
Department of Oral Surgery
University Center for Dental Medicine Basel UZB
University of Basel
Mattenstr. 40
CH – 4058 Basel, Switzerland

Prof. Dr. Jochen Jackowski
Department of Oral Surgery and
Polyclinic Outpatient Clinic
Faculty of Health
Witten/Herdecke University
Alfred-Herrhausen-Str. 45
D – 58455 Witten, Germany

Authors' contact details

Prof. Dr. Dr. Norbert Jakse
Department of Dental Medicine and Oral Health
Division of Oral Surgery and Orthodontics
Medical University of Graz
Billrothgasse 4
A – 8010 Graz, Austria

Dr. Marc Joos
Department of Oral Surgery
University Center for Dental Medicine Basel UZB
University of Basel
Mattenstr. 40
CH – 4058 Basel, Switzerland

Dr. Petra Rugani
Department of Dental Medicine and Oral Health
Division of Oral Surgery and Orthodontics
Medical University of Graz
Billrothgasse 4
A – 8010 Graz, Austria

Prof. Dr. Dr. Bernd Stadlinger
Clinic of Oral Surgery –
Clinic of Cranio-Maxillofacial Surgery
Center of Dental Medicine
University of Zurich
Plattenstr. 11
CH – 8032 Zurich, Switzerland

Priv.-Doz. Dr. Frank Peter Strietzel
Charité – Universitätsmedizin Berlin
Department of Periodontology, Oral Medicine
and Oral Surgery
Aßmannshauserstraße 4–6
D – 14197 Berlin, Germany

Dr. Silvio Valdec
Clinic of Oral Surgery –
Clinic of Cranio-Maxillofacial Surgery
Center of Dental Medicine
University of Zurich
Plattenstr. 11
CH – 8032 Zurich, Switzerland

Dr. Hendrik Zeiß
Ehlers & Feldmeier
Lawyers Notaries Specialized Attorneys
D – 44139 Dortmund, Germany

Dr. Andrea Zürcher
Department of Oral Surgery
University Center for Dental Medicine Basel UZB
University of Basel
Mattenstr. 40
CH – 4058 Basel, Switzerland

Contents

Anamnesis

1

Michael M. Bornstein

1 Anamnesis

Before any (dental) medical therapy and follow-up care, a case history (anamnesis) must be taken. Since few dentists have had their own experience with serious incidents in the dental office, there is unfortunately little awareness of such risks. However, it is well known from the field of medicine that a large proportion of medical errors are due to an inadequate medical history taking. Dentists can therefore only fulfill their responsibility for a complication-free treatment of their patients by observing the anamnesis. If the anamnesis is well organized and the patient is involved, it can be easily integrated into the daily practice, prevent complications, and optimize patient loyalty by building trust. A well-founded anamnesis thus forms the basis of every diagnosis, is central to therapy planning, and makes it possible to initiate targeted adjustments to the progress controls or even further therapeutic measures during follow-up care.

The term 'anamnesis' comes from Greek and means memory or recollection. In dental practice, anamnesis is usually performed with standardized questionnaires (Fig 1-1), which are completed by the patient, either in printed form or digitally (online). The patient's medical/dental history should always be asked for or checked in a specific discussion between the dentist and the patient. It is not uncommon for relevant information on existing diseases or current medication to be missed because the patient does not understand the questions in the medical history form correctly, does not know the names of the medications or has simply forgotten them. Thanks to the case history, a relationship of trust is also established between the dentist and the patient, which forms an important foundation for the further diagnostic and therapeutic steps. Anamnesis is not a static or one-time process. On the contrary, it should be understood as an opportunity in diagnostics, therapy (planning), and follow-up in dentistry, and especially in oral surgery. This means that an anamnesis should be taken extensively and in detail during the initial diagnosis, which may take some time. Thereafter, the history should be briefly reviewed at every available opportunity and adjusted if necessary, which underscores the nature of the history as being an opportunity. Thus, the anamnesis should be understood as a dynamic process in oral surgical therapy.

A case history is structured according to the following sub-aspects:

- the medical or general anamnesis,
- the social and family history, and
- the specific dental history, which should record the current complaints and also the reason for the visit to the doctor/dentist (subjective patient request).

For patients with dementia, the medical history should ideally be taken with the involvement of a person responsible for the patient. If there are communication problems (e.g. in the case of migrants/asylum seekers), an interpreter should be organized. In the case of minors, a person with parental authority should be involved. In the following, the individual aspects of the medical history will be discussed in detail and their importance presented and discussed for diagnosis, therapy planning, and aftercare in order to avoid complications.

Medical history questionnaire

Your state of health can have an influence on dental treatment. We therefore ask you to complete this questionnaire. Your information will be treated in strict confidence and is subject to confidentiality.

Patient	O Mr	O Mrs	Email	______________
Surname	______________________________		Tel (private)	______________
First name	______________________________		Tel (business)	______________
Street and no.	______________________________		Mobile	______________
Postal code, City	______________________________		Nationality	______________
Date of birth	______________________________		Occupation	______________
Insurance No.: ______________	O Health ______________________________		O Dental ______________	O Accident ______________
Additional support	O Supplementary benefit/s		O Social welfare	O No support?
Legal representative	O Mr	O Mrs		
First name, Surname	______________________________		Tel (private)	______________
Street and no.	______________________________		Tel (business)	______________
Postal code, City	______________________________		Mobile	______________

O **General practitioner/** O **attending physician/** O **pediatrician**

	O Mr	O Mrs		
First name, Surname	______________________________		Tel (business)	______________
Street and no.	______________________________		Mobile	______________
Postal code, City	______________________________			
O **Private dentist**	O Mr	O Mrs		
First name, Surname	______________________________		Tel (business)	______________
Street and no.	______________________________		Mobile	______________
Postal code, City	______________________________			

Reason for clinic visit: ____

Referring physician or dentist	First name ______________________	Street and no. __________________
	Surname ______________________	Postal code, City ________________

Questions about health status of patient

01. Are/were you recently treated by a doctor? If yes, due to which **disease**? ________________________	O Yes	O No
02. Have you had any **operations**? If yes, for what reason? ________________________	O Yes	O No
03. Do you have/have you ever had **hepatitis** (jaundice, liver inflammation)?	O Yes	O No
04. Are you currently taking any **medications** on a regular basis? If yes, which ones?________________________	O Yes	O No
Do you take bisphosphonates (e.g. for osteoporosis)?	O Yes	O No

a

Fig 1-1 In dental practice and also at university clinics, the case history is usually taken by means of standardized questionnaires before the actual consultation. The anamnesis form shown here (a and b) is used at the University Center for Dental Medicine Basel UZB.

1 Anamnesis

05. Do you suffer from **cardiovascular diseases**? If yes, please tick O Too high/too low blood pressure Value:	O Yes	O No
	O Angina pectoris	O Heart attack
O Heart valve defect/artificial heart valve	O Stroke	O Endocarditis
06. Are you **HIV positive**?	O Yes	O No
07. Do you suffer from a **blood disease**? If yes, please tick O Blood disorder (hemophilia) O Blood anemia (anemia)	O Yes	O No
Do you take **blood thinning medication**?	O Yes	O No
08. Do you suffer from a **metabolic disease**? If yes, please tick O Thyroid disease O Diabetes O Other ______________________________________	O Yes	O No
09. Do you suffer from any **allergies**? If yes, please tick O Hay fever O Asthma O Other___________ Are you hypersensitive to:	O Yes	O No
O Mouth rinses? O Medications? O Foodstuffs?	O Injections?	
10. Have you ever had: O A sinus infection? O Rheumatism/joint swelling? O Digestive disorders? O Hormonal disorders? O Tuberculosis? O Organ diseases (lungs, liver, kidney, etc)?	O Chemotherapy? For what reason? ______________________________ O Radiation? Where?_____________ O Any other serious illnesses? If yes, which? _________________ ______________________________	
11. Are you currently **pregnant**? How many weeks?__________	O Yes	O No
12. Do you have **prosthetic joint/s**, a **pacemaker** or any **other implants**? Which?___________________________________	O Yes	O No
13. Are you a smoker? What? ________ How many?________	O Yes	O No
14. Do you suffer from **bad breath**?	O Yes	O No
15. Do you own a **mouthguard** that you wear regularly when you play sport?	O Yes	O No
Have you recently had a **dental accident**?	O Yes	O No

I **acknowledge** that the data or findings of my medical history, including radiographs and photographs, copies or printouts thereof, will be exchanged with my physician or other persons subject to medical confidentiality such as insurance companies, etc, for the purpose of any necessary clarifications or information, and that the data necessary for billing, collection, and accounting will be forwarded to the institutions involved.

Date: ______________ Signature:

I **agree** that, if necessary, local anesthesia will be given to me. I am aware that in very rare cases irritation may occur in the lower jaw and tongue (persistent numbness, tingling), which will usually disappear. I acknowledge that after dental surgical procedures under local anesthesia there is an increased risk for several hours of road traffic accidents.

Date: ______________ Signature:

I **agree** that all data collected about me, tissue samples, and extracted teeth may be used for scientific purposes in medical research, anonymously, and in strict compliance with confidentiality. Data may also be consulted, in strict confidentiality, for testing and control purposes by the competent authorities and the Cantonal Ethics Committee. In this regard, the treating dentists are released from patient confidentiality. I may revoke this consent at any time (right of veto) without incurring any disadvantages.

Date: ______________ Signature:

b

The general anamnesis: recording of medically relevant diagnoses and medication

The general medical history is usually taken primarily in the form of standardized questionnaires in order to record important points of general health and subsequently to enable a targeted discussion with the patient or follow-up questions. All relevant diseases and diagnoses of the cardiovascular system, gastrointestinal tract, metabolic system, nervous system, blood and coagulation system, and musculoskeletal system as well as any infectious diseases that have been experienced in the past or are currently in progress are recorded. Due to the demographic change in our society toward an increasingly older population structure, the recognition of patients under polypharmacy and those with multimorbidity is becoming more and more relevant.

Unfortunately, there is no uniform definition at present of polypharmacy (synonyms: polymedication, polypharmacotherapy). Usually, the number of drugs that are taken simultaneously is the criterion for the definition, although the actual number varies in the literature – five or more drugs taken simultaneously is most frequently mentioned. Multimorbidity is defined as the simultaneous occurrence of two or more chronic diseases. In Switzerland today, about 30% of the entire population is multimorbid by definition, and this trend is increasing. Multimorbidity and age are to be regarded as the main risk factors for polypharmacy. This is exemplified by the following impressive figures: in Switzerland, 80% of people older than 70 years of age take medication daily, and 50% of them take five or more medications per day. Therefore, if patients are aged 60 to 70 and describe themselves as completely healthy and also deny taking medication, it is worth asking to double-check about this (Fig 1-2).

In addition, the patient's general practitioner can be consulted specifically, providing the patient's consent has been gained. Particularly before planned invasive oral surgical procedures, it can be extremely important that the knowledge gained from the patient as well as the medical history are interdisciplinarily networked, and that reports, diagnoses, and medication lists are requested from the general practitioner and

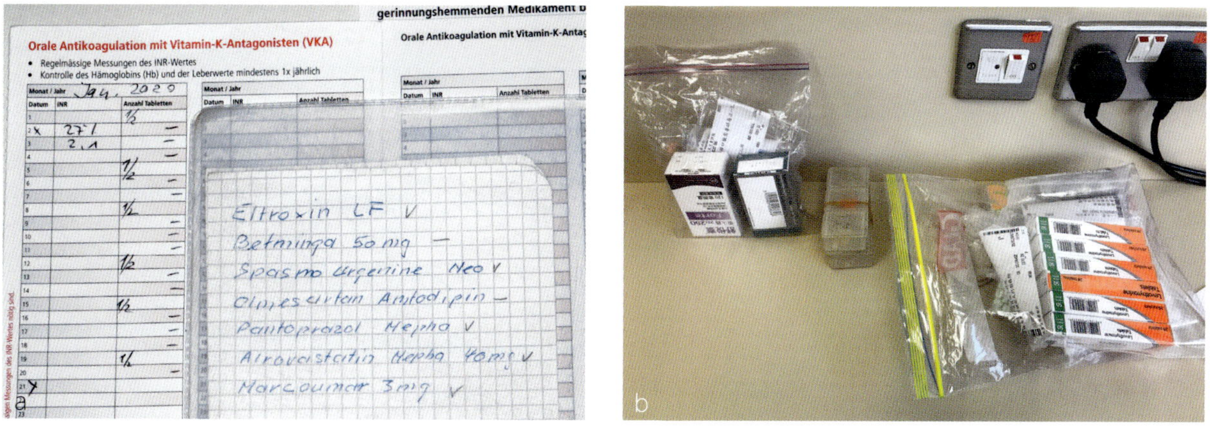

Fig 1-2 Two examples of how patients react when asked about medication intake: (a) A 75-year-old patient shows the card indicating the regular checking of the INR value (including Quick) as well as her self-administered list of medications, with ticks indicating the medications currently taken. At the moment, there are five medications, including an anticoagulation drug; thus, polypharmacy is present in this case. (b) An almost 80-year-old patient from Hong Kong does not keep a separate medication list but has brought along to the initial consultation all the medications she takes, including the dosage regimen.

the specialist. This information must be updated regularly. The following section will briefly highlight some important problem areas and potential risk factors.

Infectious diseases

It is important for the dentist and the dental practice staff to know whether an infectious disease such as human immunodeficiency virus (HIV) or hepatitis is present so that appropriate protective measures can be taken. In addition, attention can then be paid to any typical cutaneous or oral efflorescences that may be present during the course of the extra- and intraoral examination.

Cardiovascular diseases

According to the World Health Organization (WHO), cardiovascular diseases are the most common group of chronic diseases in people over 50 years of age. It is particularly important to record whether the patient is taking anticoagulants because this results in an increased tendency to bleed during procedures. Ideally, the various groups of anticoagulants (vitamin K antagonists, new direct oral anticoagulants, platelet aggregation inhibitors) should be identified before therapy is initiated, and their effects or risks associated with surgery should be understood. If there is a risk of endocarditis (e.g. patients with heart valve replacements or congenital cardiac conditions), antibiotic prophylaxis is indicated before oral surgery or even periodontal procedures.

Bone metabolism (especially antiresorptive medication)

In older patients, it is advisable to specifically inquire about osteoporosis (caveat: also in men, although this often becomes relevant a decade later in life) or an underlying oncologic disease, especially with regard to the current or previous use of antiresorptive medications such as bisphosphonates or monoclonal antibodies (denosumab). Bisphosphonates, in particular, have a long half-life and continue to influence bone metabolism even years after therapeutic use. In the case of denosumab, on the other hand, the rebound effect is particularly problematic when the drug is discontinued, as there is then a marked loss of bone density that can be associated with fractures.

In patients undergoing therapy with antiresorptive drugs, it is particularly important to pay attention to an increased risk of osteonecrosis of the jawbone during oral surgery. Here, patients with malignant bone diseases (metastatic breast, prostate or lung carcinomas) belong to the high-risk group (Fig 1-3), and osteoporosis patients belong to the low-risk group (Fig 1-4), which, however, also depends on the dose, the duration of drug intake, and the possibly of existing additional systemic diseases or their pharmacologic therapy.

Diabetes mellitus

If diabetes mellitus is known, it should be ascertained whether it is well controlled before the start of invasive treatment. A good reference value is the long-term glucose level (HbA1c), which should ideally be below 7%. If diabetes is not adequately controlled, delayed wound healing can be expected after oral surgery.

Medications that affect oral health

From a preventive dentistry perspective, general medical factors and medications that have an impact on oral health – especially saliva production and the gingiva (gingival hyperplasia) – should be considered. There are numerous medications such as antihypertensives or antidepressants that significantly impair saliva production quantitatively and qualitatively, which then manifests clinically as hyposalivation (xerostomia). On the other hand, immunosuppressants in organ transplant patients, antiepileptic drugs in epileptics or the use of calcium

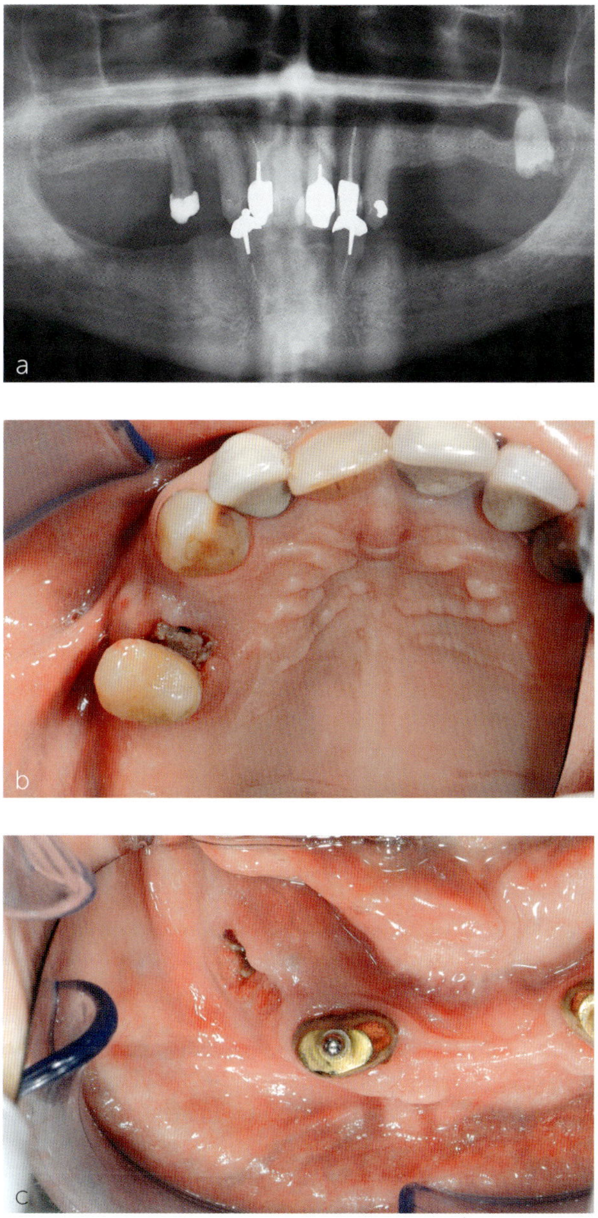

Fig 1-3 The panoramic radiograph (a) of a 77-year-old patient with metastatic prostate carcinoma and on zoledronate therapy (i.v.) shows the condition after various tooth extractions in the maxilla and mandible. In the maxillary region 14 (b) and the mandibular region 44 (c), impaired wound healing with partially exposed bone has occurred. Thus, drug-associated osteonecrosis under high-dose bisphosphonate therapy is suspected.

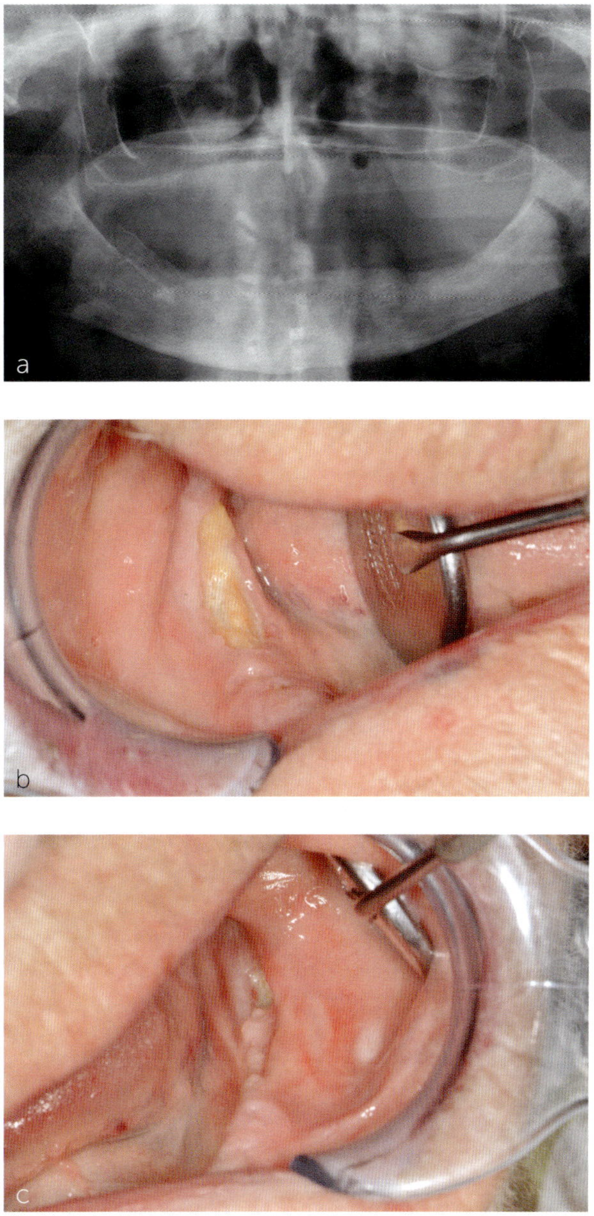

Fig 1-4 Panoramic view (a) of an 84-year-old female patient with osteoporosis and under long-term oral bisphosphonate therapy (alendronate) shows the condition after removal of the remaining mandibular teeth. In regions 47/48 (b) and 37/38 (c) there is clearly impaired wound healing with exposed bone. Thus, drug-associated osteonecrosis under low-dose bisphosphonate therapy is suspected.

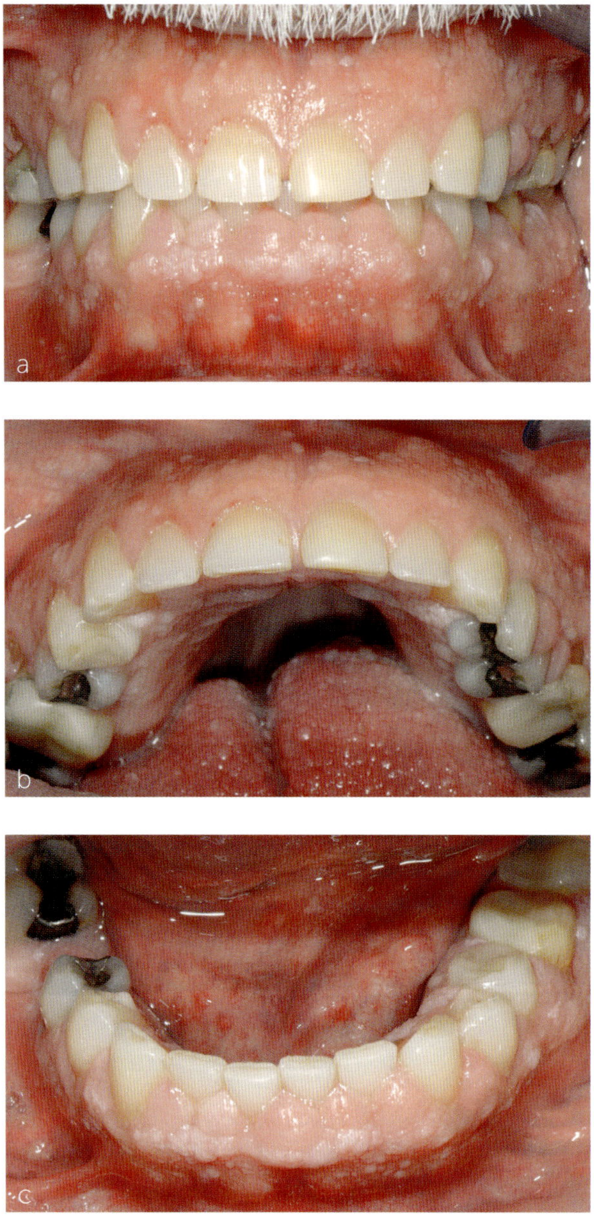

Fig 1-5 Generalized growths on the gingiva in the maxilla and mandible (a) in a 59-year-old patient on amlodipine therapy for hypertension. In particular, the papillae in the maxillary posterior (b) and mandibular anterior (c) regions show pronounced bulbous growths.

antagonists (nifedipine, amlodipine) in patients with hypertension must be taken into account, which can lead to gingival overgrowth (Fig 1-5).

Allergies

Specific questions should also be asked about any existing allergy to commonly used dental materials or medications. Of particular importance in oral surgery are any penicillin, latex or iodine allergies.

Social and family history

In the social history section, questions are asked about living conditions, occupation, and alcohol and tobacco consumption, and, in the case of women, about an existing pregnancy. Often, this part of the anamnesis is integrated into the general part, i.e. into the corresponding questionnaire, so that a clear distinction between these two is no longer possible. Knowledge of the patient's socioeconomic circumstances is important to be able to plan adequate therapy from this point of view.

A family history makes sense if hereditary anomalies, diseases, and malocclusions are present such as anomalies in the number of teeth, tooth shape, and tooth structure. In addition, a family history should also be taken if dysgnathia and syndromes are present in direct relatives, i.e. the patient's parents, siblings, and/or children.

The specific dental anamnesis

The specific dental anamnesis contains the patient's account of the current dentoalveolar disease or problem and should include the onset, course, subjective symptoms, and previous treatments. The complaints in the area of the masticatory organ should be specifically recorded. Is it a dental problem? Or does the problem seem to originate more from the bone (maxilla or mandible) or the temporomandibular joint? Is the problem acute or chronic? In the case of complaints and pain, specific questions are asked about the duration, intensity, trigger, and character as well as the quality, time, place, and measures taken thus far. With regard to the urgency of therapy, it is also helpful to ask how much the patient is affected by the current condition in everyday life. Pain can be indicated on a visual analog scale (VAS) from 1 to 10 and can thus also be quantified objectively. In the general dental context, the specific dental anamnesis also includes a preventive dental anamnesis, which involves a specific enquiry about oral hygiene habits and the use of dental care products and brushing techniques. Questions are also asked about the frequency, duration, and timing of dental care. A detailed dietary history with a special dietary questionnaire may be useful if an increased risk of caries and/or erosion is suspected. It is not uncommon for patients to be unaware of their high sugar and acid consumption.

Conclusion

A detailed medical history forms the basis for the findings, diagnosis, targeted treatment planning with subsequent therapy, and follow-up care. In the case of planned oral surgery, this detailed medical history should help to minimize complications during treatment. Complications can lead to a failure of the treatment itself (e.g. loss of teeth or implants) or, on the other hand, to serious wound healing disorders or infections, which then necessitate costly and lengthy follow-up treatments. It is the responsibility of the dentist to obtain the most comprehensive information possible by asking specific and precise questions and, if necessary, in consultation with the general practitioner or specialist. This is essential for diagnosis and treatment planning. In view of the above, it can be emphasized that a good and comprehensive medical history is the key to successful therapy. In addition, the medical history should be updated and supplemented at the regular follow-up appointments. Thus, history taking is not a one-time or static event but a dynamic process.

Recommended literature

1. Breil D. Arzneimittelcocktail im Alter: Was macht Sinn? Sometimes less is more. Primary and Hospital Care – Allgemeine Innere Medizin 2016;16:17–20.
2. Eremenko M. Anamnese als Herausforderung für das Praxisteam. Ein Beispiel anhand parodontaler Erkrankungen. Prophylaxe Journal 2018;2:12–15.
3. Gutwald R, Gellrich NC, Schmelzeisen R. Einführung in die zahnärztliche Chirurgie. 1. Auflage. München: Urban und Fischer, 2003:102–103.
4. Reichart PA, Hausamen JE, Becker J, Neukam FW, Schliephake H, Schmelzeisen R. Curriculum. Zahn-, Mund- und Kieferkrankheiten. 2. Band. 2. Auflage. Berlin: Quintessenz, 2002:25–26.
5. Schriber M, Suter VGA, Bornstein MM. Anamnese – weshalb sie so wichtig ist. Dimensions/ Swiss Dental Hygenists 2015;14:6–9/26–29.
6. Schwenzer N, Ehrenfeld M. Chirurgische Grundlagen, 4. Auflage, Stuttgart: Georg Thieme 2008:2–5.
7. Wieland TM, Rychter O. Risiken und praktische Aspekte im Umgang mit mehreren Medikamenten. Hausarzt Praxis 2015;10:2–5.
8. World Health Organization (WHO). World Report on Ageing and Health. WHO Press, Geneva, 2015.

Hygiene, instruments, and suture materials

2

Fabio Saccardin, Constantin Berli, Andreas Filippi

Aspects of hygiene in oral surgical procedures

The hygiene guidelines include measures to prevent nosocomial infections. However, this presupposes that all staff in the treatment room or operating room are aware of the guidelines for asepsis and comply with them. Both the surgeon and the assisting surgical staff are equally responsible for asepsis in the sterile area. If the hygiene guidelines cannot be observed, this must be reported to the responsible surgeon. Any violation or disregard of asepsis must be corrected immediately.

For major surgical procedures beyond tooth removals, instead of their everyday professional clothing all staff in the treatment room must wear specific surgical clothing or shirt and trousers (usually disposable), washable and front-closed shoes, and a surgical cap to fully cover their hair. The protective mouth-nose mask covers the nose as well as the chin area and should be adequately fastened and sealed. It is worn during patient preparation as well as during the surgical procedure. Once the protective mouth-nose mask is soaked, it must be changed.

Hands should be washed with a gentle soap solution only upon entering the work site, when they are visibly soiled, after each toilet use, and before and after eating (Figs 2-1 to 2-15). Hand washing should be limited to these indications and should not routinely occur between all treatments. Hand disinfection should be utilized between treatments.

Hand disinfection is divided into hygienic and surgical hand disinfection. For hygienic hand disinfection, the dried palms are completely wetted with a suitable disinfectant and rubbed in such a way that the front and back surfaces, nail folds, thumbs, intermediate finger areas, and fingertips come into contact with the agent (Figs 2-16 to 2-23). As a rule, 3 ml of disinfectant solution is used for this purpose. Hygienic hand disinfection is performed before and after each patient contact. Hygienic hand disinfection should also take place before aseptic work and after contact with infectious material.

Surgical hand disinfection should be performed by all persons who are directly involved in an operation in the sterile area. In contrast to hygienic hand disinfection, the forearms and wrists are also included in surgical hand disinfection (Fig 2-24). Thus, surgical hand disinfection takes significantly longer than hygienic hand disinfection but is performed with the same disinfectants. Washing the hands with soap is no longer part of surgical hand disinfection. If there is any contamination of the skin, it is recommended to take a 10-minute break after hand washing until surgical hand disinfection. Particular attention should be paid to ensuring that hands are sufficiently dried prior to disinfection and that complete wetting of all skin areas and nail folds is maintained, taking into account the specific exposure times specified in the manufacturer's instructions.

The sterile apron (over the surgical clothing) and sterile gloves must not be put on until the hand disinfectant has completely evaporated on the hands and forearms[2,3].

The sterile zone includes the patient's sterilely draped torso, the instrument table, and the assisting surgical staff. Sterile surfaces include the front of sterile aprons, the tops of sterile drapes, and the sterile covers of lamp handles. Within the sterile area, hands remain above the belly button at all times. Practice or clinic personnel who are not sterilely dressed must maintain a distance of at least 50 cm from the sterile area.

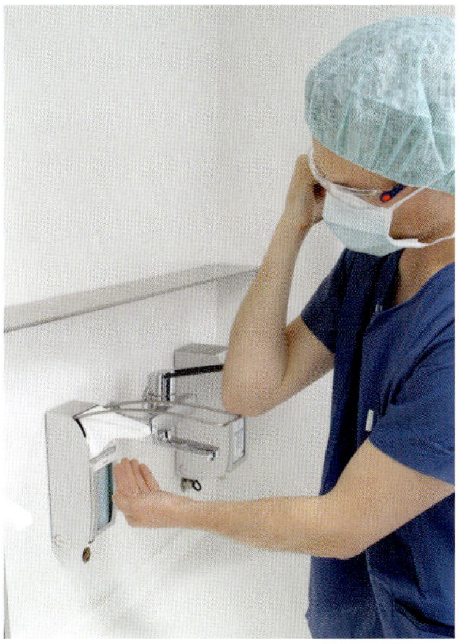

Fig 2-1 First, 5 ml of hand soap is placed in the palm of the left hand.

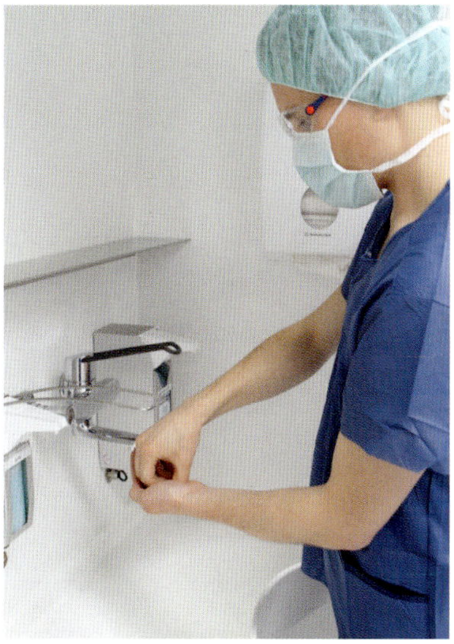

Fig 2-2 Then, the fingertips of the right hand are dipped into the palm of the left hand for 5 seconds and rubbed to decontaminate the fingernails.

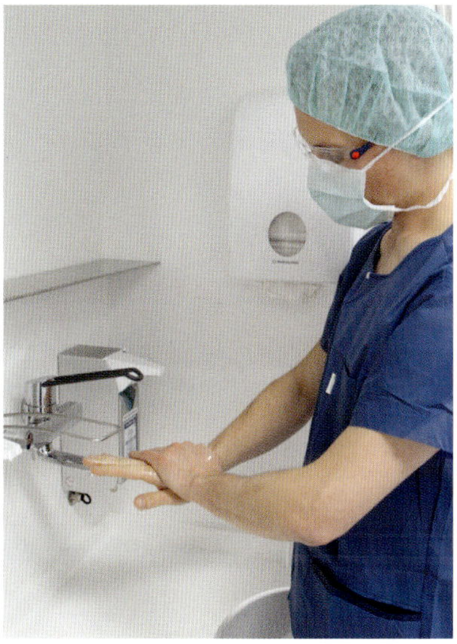

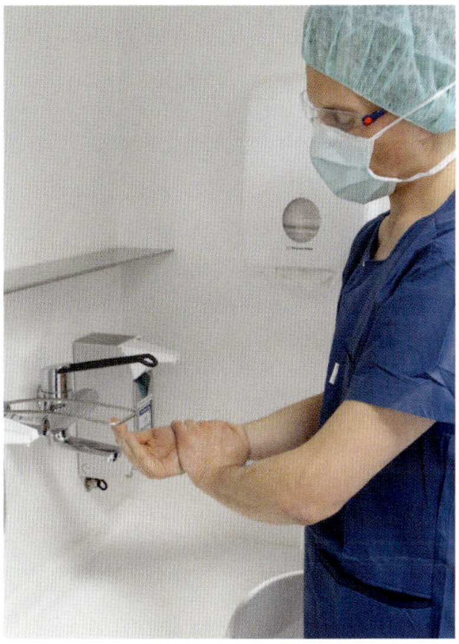

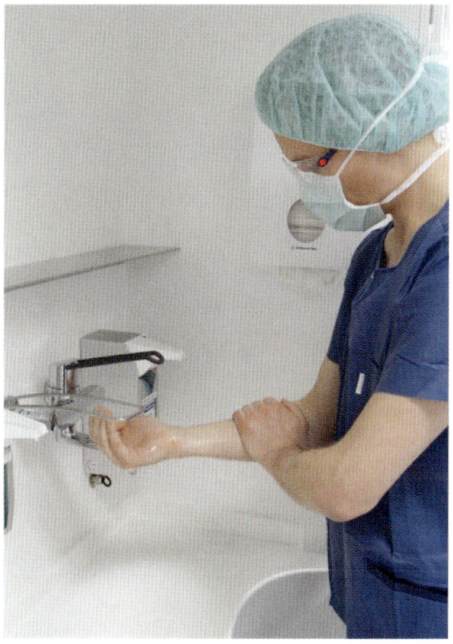

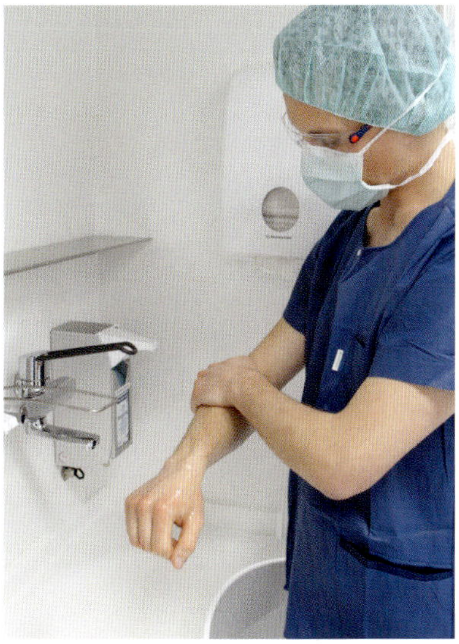

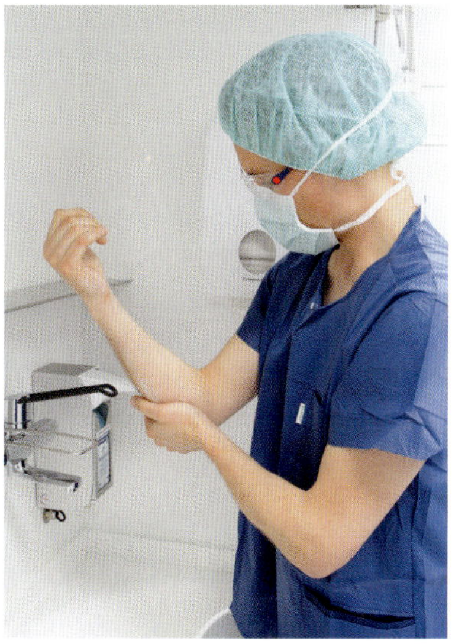

Figs 2-3 to 2-7 The hand soap should be spread on the right forearm for 10 to 15 seconds from the hand to the elbow using circular movements. This ensures that the entire skin surface is wetted with the hand soap.

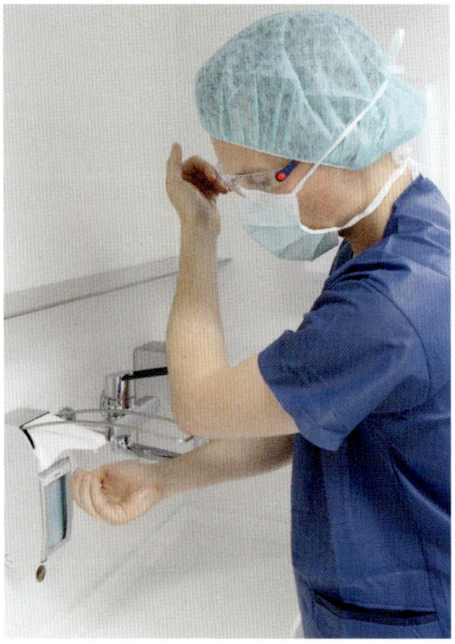
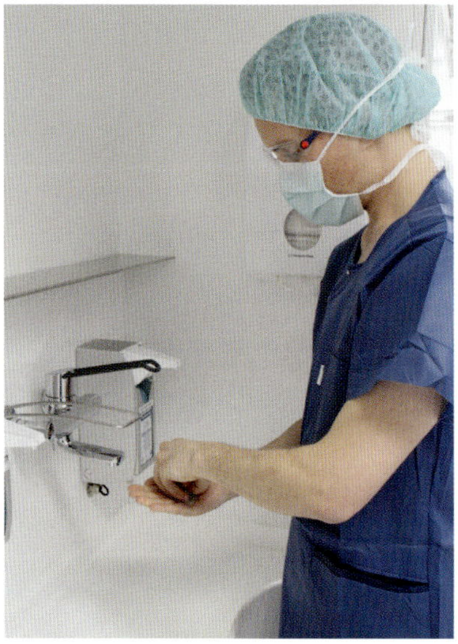
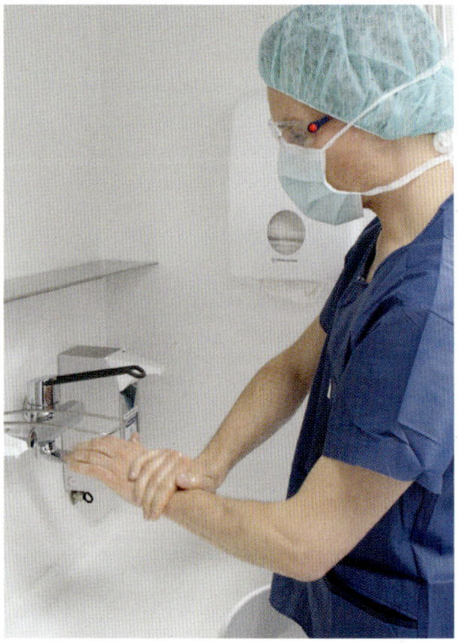
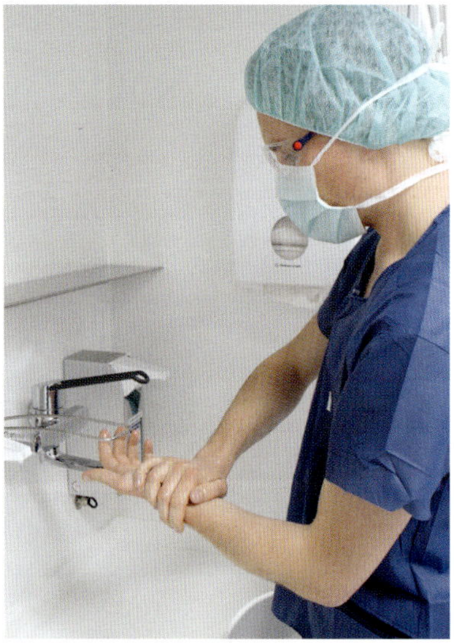
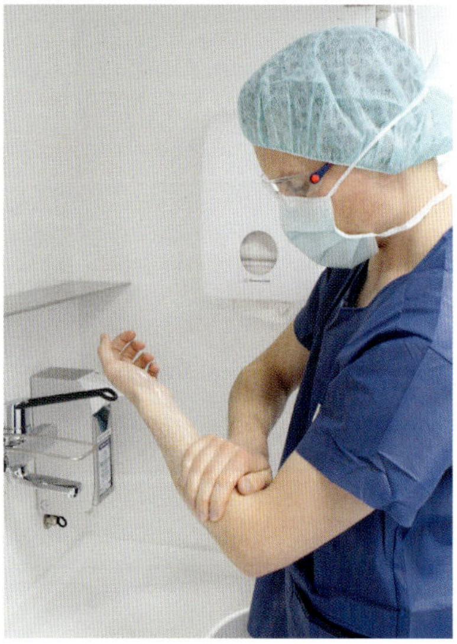
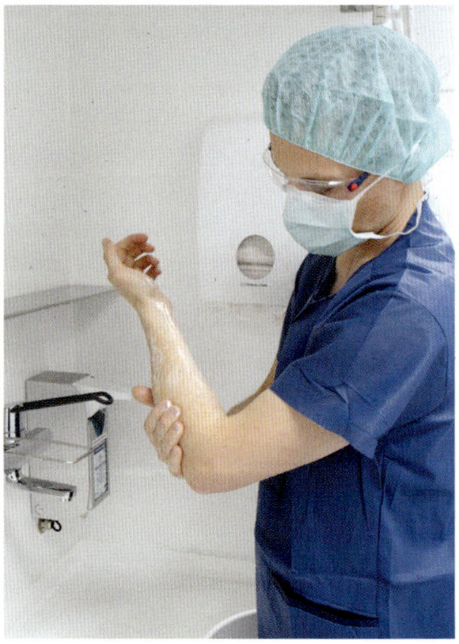
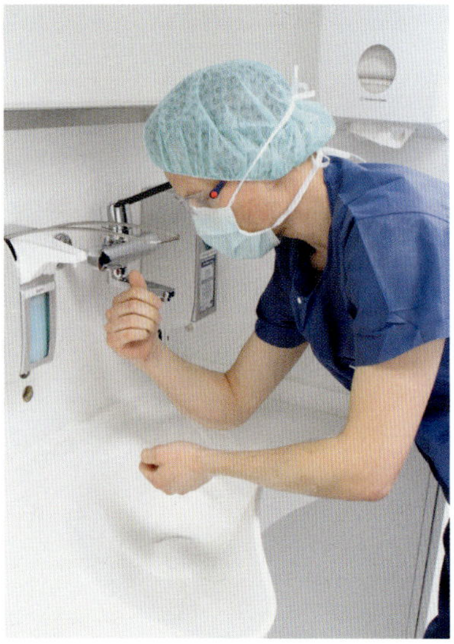
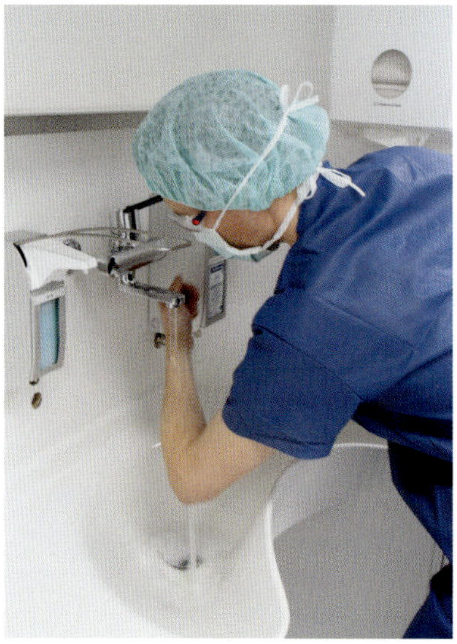

Figs 2-8 to 2-15 These steps are now repeated for the left hand and left forearm. The hand soap is then rinsed off the hands in the direction of the forearms and, after dripping off, carefully dabbed dry with a cloth in the same direction.

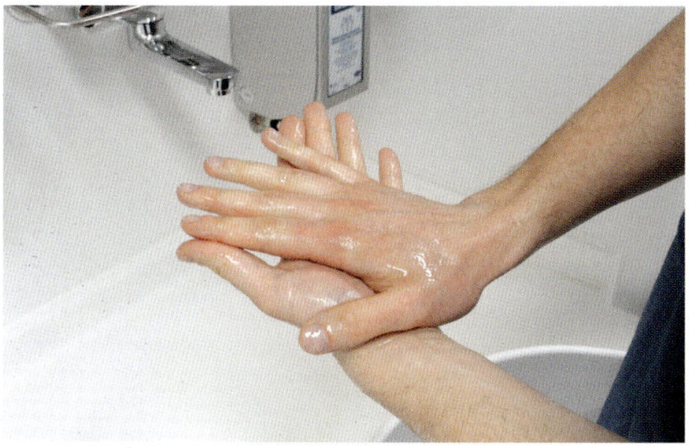

Fig 2-16 Hygienic and surgical hand disinfection begin by wetting the palms with a disinfectant.

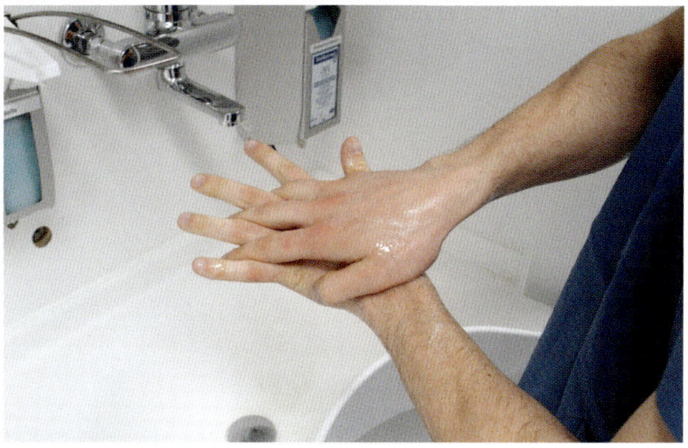

Fig 2-17 The back of the left hand, including the wrist, should be rubbed with the right palm using back and forth movements.

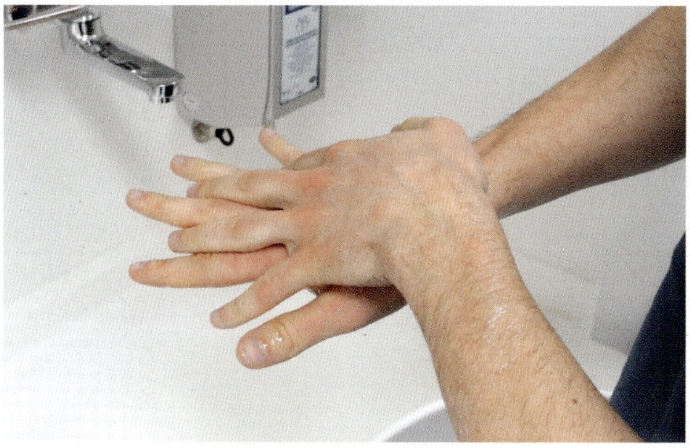

Fig 2-18 This is followed by the same for the other hand.

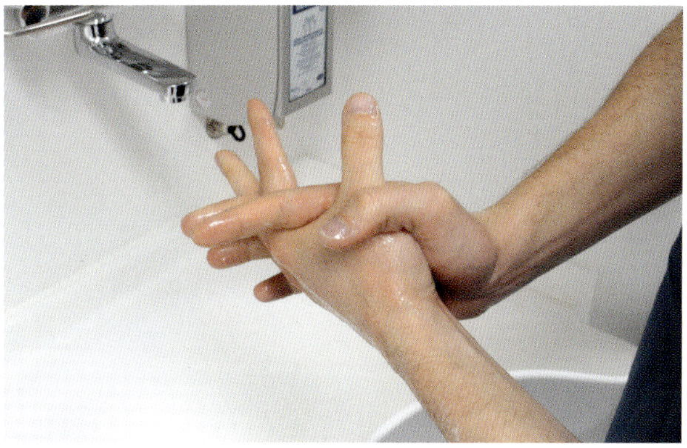

Fig 2-19 The palms of the hands should be rubbed together, with the fingers interlocking.

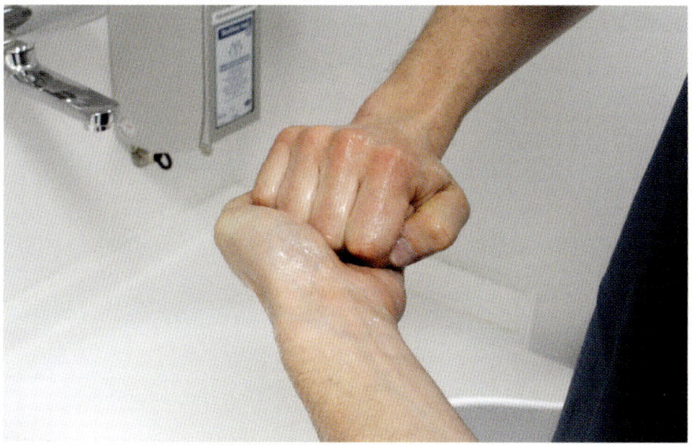

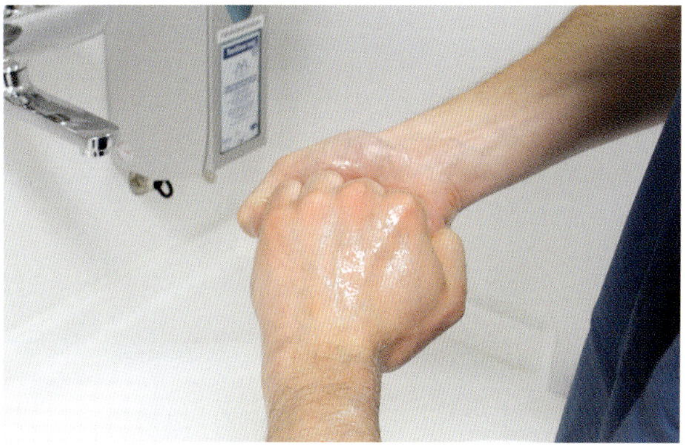

Figs 2-20 and 2-21 The backs of the fingers should each be disinfected in the palm of the other hand by moving them back and forth laterally.

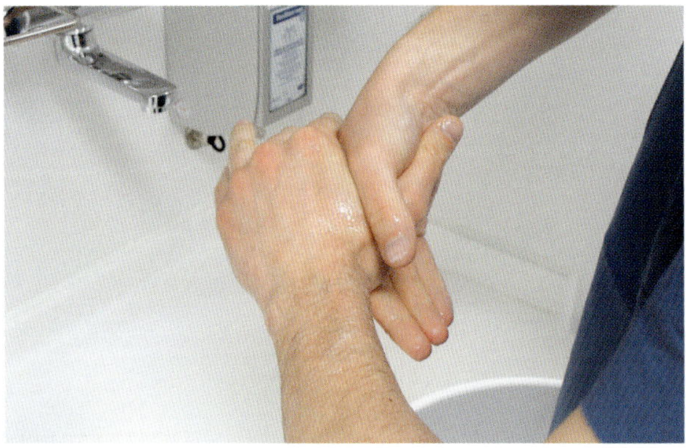

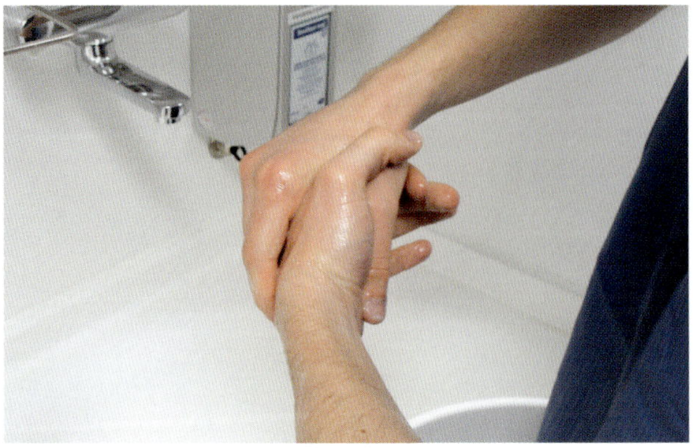

Figs 2-22 and 2-23 The thumb of the left hand should be rotated in the enclosed palm of the right hand, and vice versa.

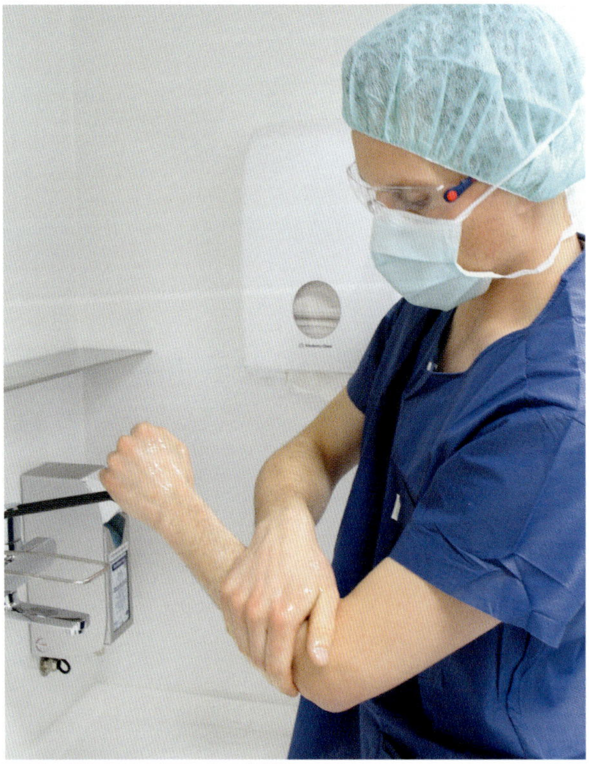

Fig 2-24 For surgical hand disinfection, the forearms and wrists should also be wetted with disinfectant solution beforehand, in addition to the palms.

Surgical instruments

Surgical instruments for oral surgery can be divided according to their functions. A rough distinction is made between holding instruments, grasping instruments, cutting instruments, preparation instruments, palpation instruments, rotating instruments, and suture instruments (including suture materials). The instruments can be combined in a basic tray or surgical tray for specific surgical procedures (for dentoalveolar, periodontal, and apical surgery, soft tissue surgery, etc), but can also be available sterilely packaged as individual instruments. The individual design of the surgical trays is in accordance with the preference of the specific surgeon.

Holding instruments

Holding instruments provide a better overview during the surgical procedure. For holding the adjacent soft tissue or mucoperiosteal flap, blunt retractors are preferred to sharp retractors (single, double, and multiple prongs) because the latter cause additional trauma to the soft tissue. Blunt retractors such as Langenbeck retractors (Fig 2-25), Middeldorpf cheek retractors (Fig 2-26) or vestibular hooks (Fig 2-27) are used to hold the cheek and lip, mostly during incision or suture placement. For surgical procedures on the floor of the mouth, the Brünings fenestrated tongue spatula (Fig 2-28) can also be used to hold the tongue. Once the mucoperiosteal flap has been mobilized, it is held away on the buccal side with the help of the Langenbeck retractor, and in the case of mandibular wisdom tooth removals, also with the Wilde retractor (Fig 2-29, Video 2-1), and lingually with Davis brain spatulas (Fig 2-30). Bone contact with the holding instrument at the level of the flap base is essential, otherwise there

Video 2-1 Insertion of the Wilde retractor after flap mobilization during surgical wisdom tooth removal in region 38.

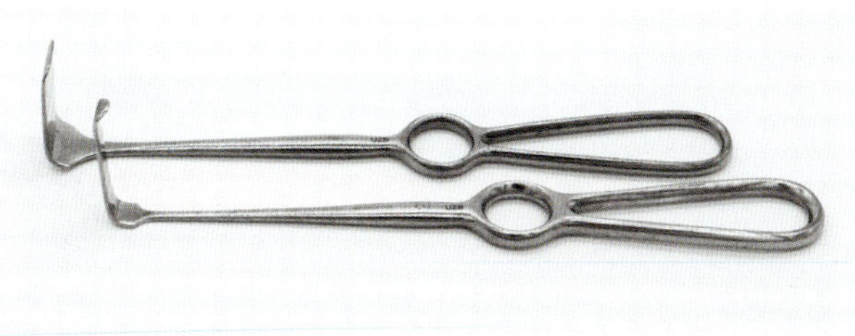

Fig 2-25 Langenbeck retractor (narrow and wide).

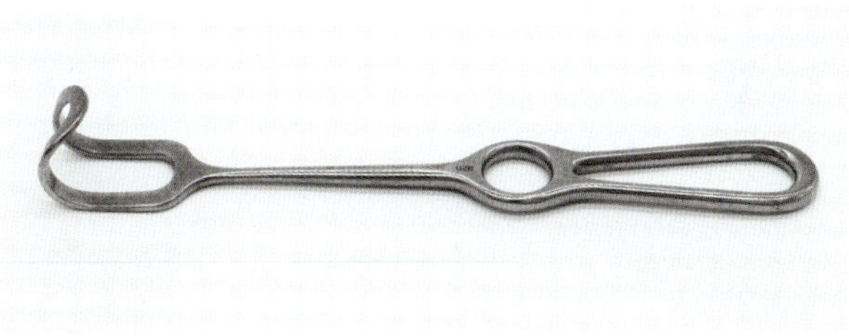

Fig 2-26 Middeldorpf cheek retractor.

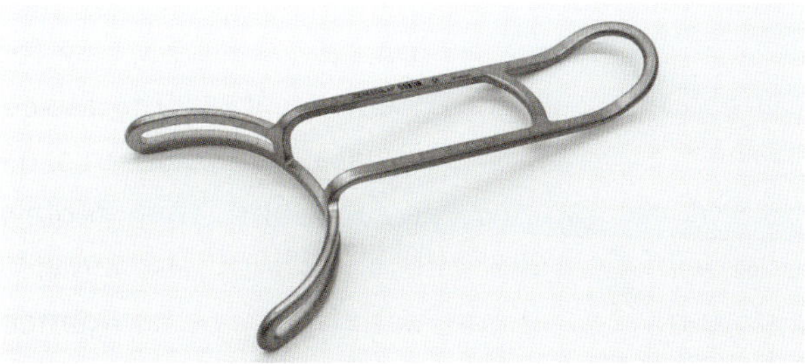

Fig 2-27 Vestibular hook.

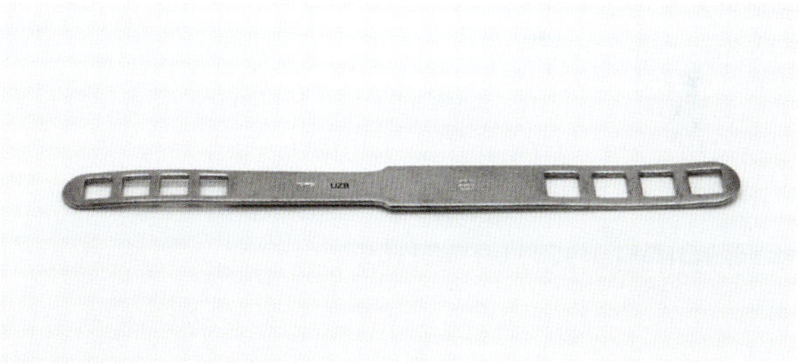

Fig 2-28 Brünings tongue spatula.

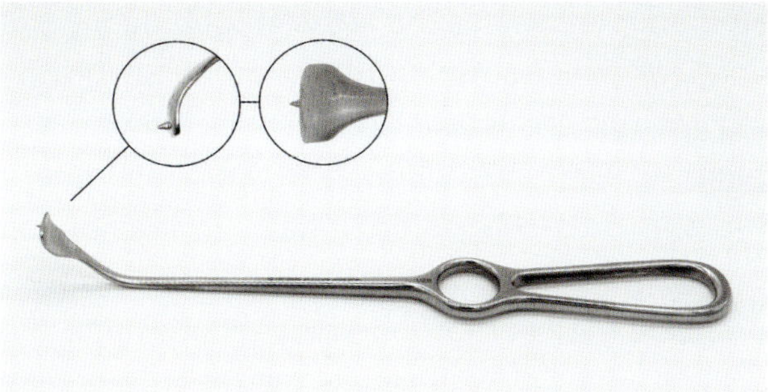

Fig 2-29 Wilde retractor.

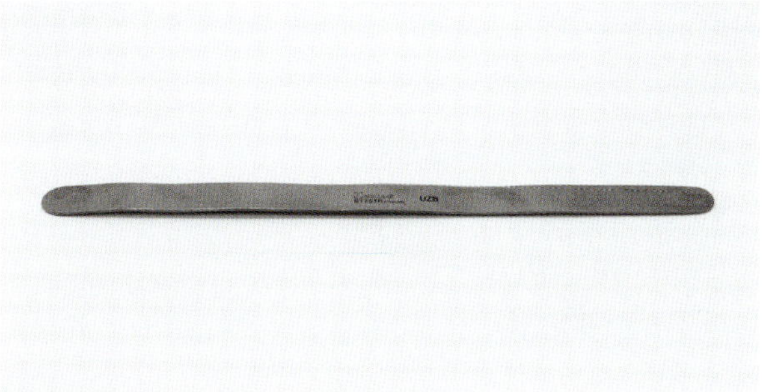

Fig 2-30 Davis brain spatula.

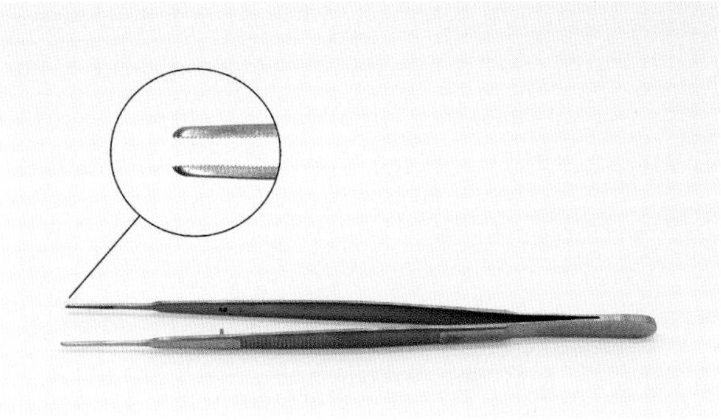

Fig 2-31 Anatomical forceps.

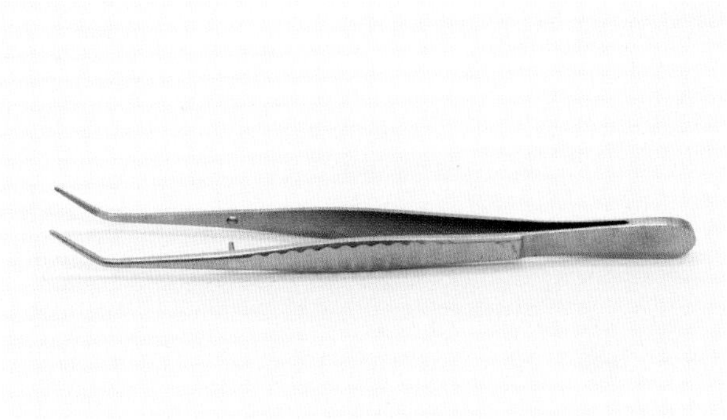

Fig 2-32 Dental forceps (not diamond coated).

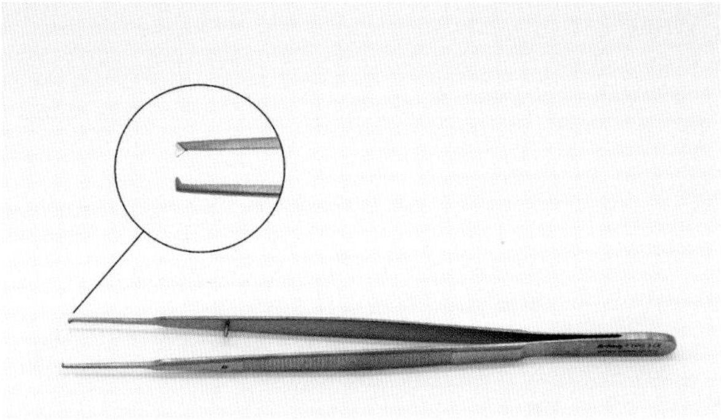

Fig 2-33 Surgical forceps.

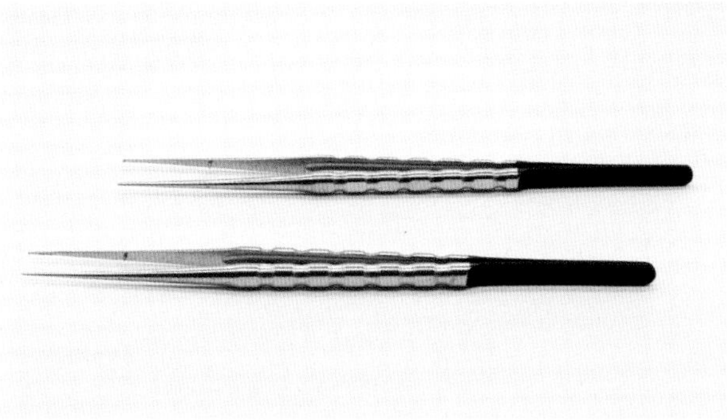

Fig 2-34 Microsurgical forceps.

is a risk of the flap tearing at the end of the incision if traction is applied.

Grasping instruments

The classic grasping instruments include forceps, which are available in different variants. The anatomical and dental forceps (Figs 2-31 and 2-32) have a transversely serrated working end and are used to grasp swabs, needles, drains or tamponades. However, in surgical forceps (Fig 2-33), the working end comprises interlocking serrations, which allows better grasping of the soft tissue. There are also microsurgical versions of both the anatomical and surgical forceps (Fig 2-34). Other grasping instruments such as vascular clamps, e.g. Halsted-Mosquito clamps (Fig 2-35), are used for grasping blood vessels during hemostasis as well as for fixation of holding sutures or swabs. They have a scissor-like handle with a locking device and a serrated working end, which may be straight or curved. The Backhaus towel clamp (Fig 2-36, Video 2-2) can be used for the fixation of sterile drapes as well as the suction tube during the surgical procedure. Another essential grasping instrument is the Luniatschek tamponade plugger (Fig 2-37, Video 2-3). This instrument has a V- or U-shaped tip at both its straight and curved working end, which can be used to insert drainage tubes or tamponades securely into the wound area. Other grasping instruments include forceps for tooth removal (Figs 2-38 and 2-39).

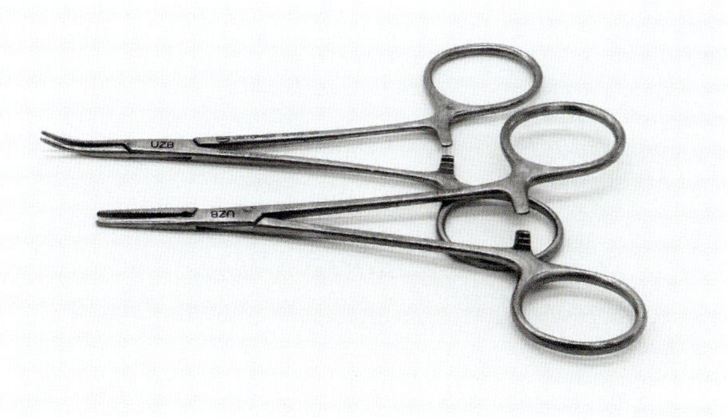

Fig 2-35 Halsted-Mosquito clamps.

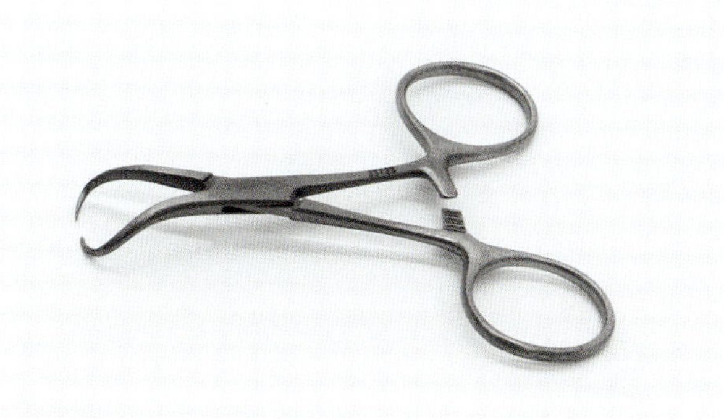

Fig 2-36 Backhaus towel clamp.

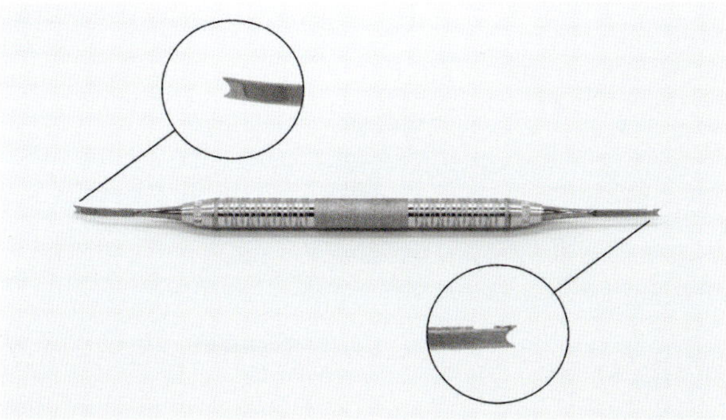

Fig 2-37 Luniatschek tamponade plugger.

Video 2-2 Fixation of sterile drapes and the suction tube with the Backhaus towel clamp.

Video 2-3 Insertion of an iodoform strip for drainage after wisdom tooth removal in region 48.

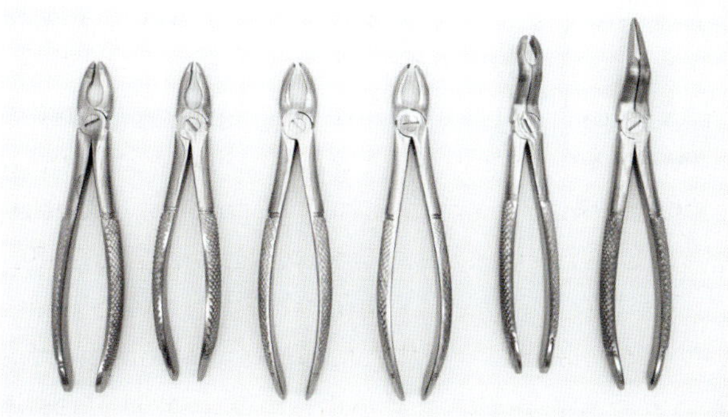

Fig 2-38 Maxillary forceps (from left to right): anterior forceps, premolar forceps, molar forceps for the first quadrant, molar forceps for the second quadrant, wisdom tooth forceps, and root remnant forceps.

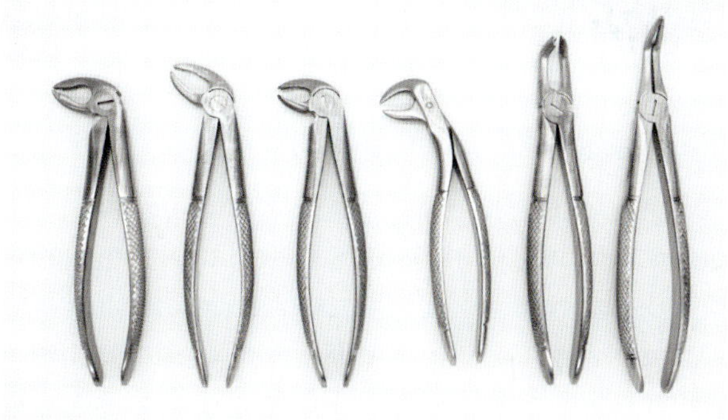

Fig 2-39 Mandibular forceps (from left to right): anterior forceps, premolar forceps, molar forceps, cow horn forceps, wisdom tooth forceps, and root remnant forceps.

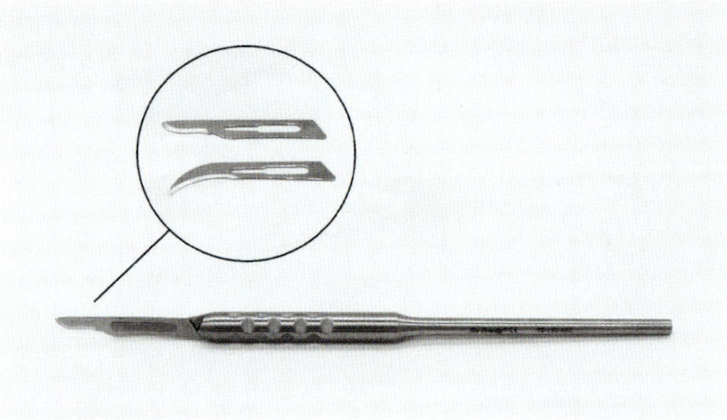

Fig 2-40 Scalpel blade holder with bulged (no. 15) and sickle-shaped (no. 12) blade.

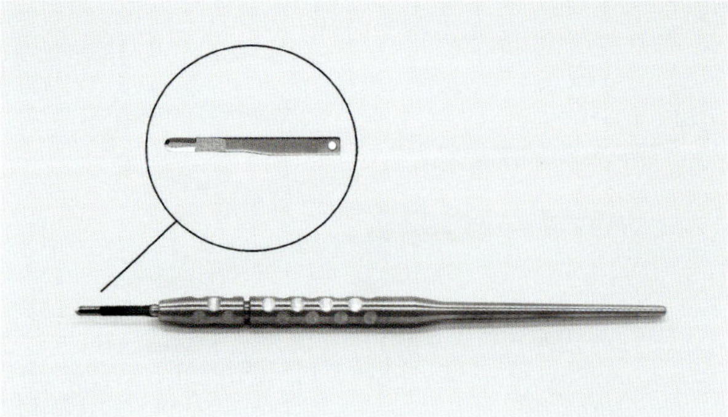

Fig 2-41 Scalpel blade holder with microsurgical blade.

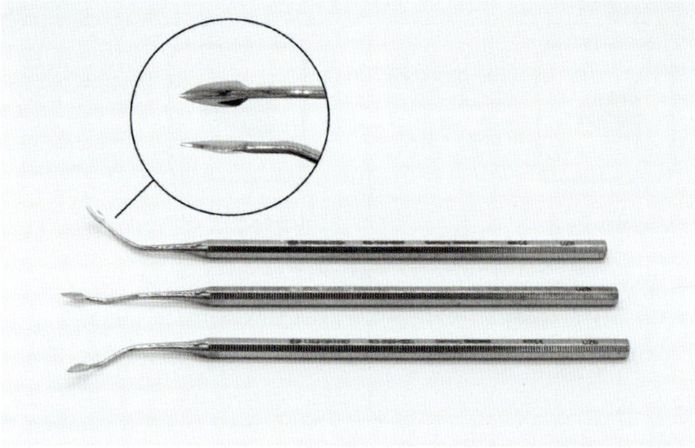

Fig 2-42 Desmotomes (straight and angled).

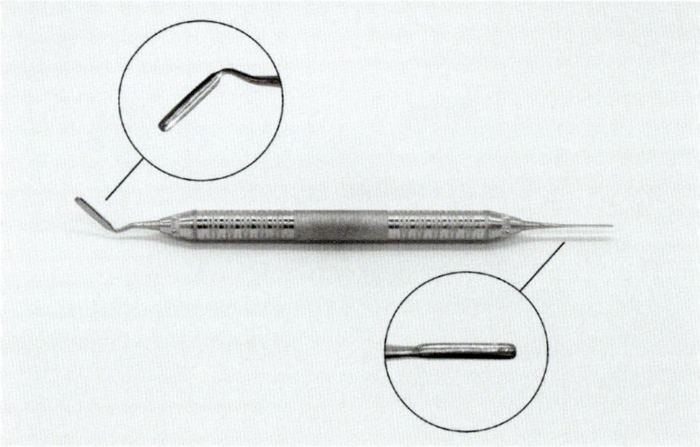

Fig 2-43 Periotome (with a straight and angled working end).

Cutting instruments

Cutting instruments include scalpels, which allow the sharp transection of soft tissue. Since scalpel blades blunt rapidly on contact with bone due to the usual incision pattern in oral surgery, disposable blades in various shapes (curved and sickle-shaped) with sterilizable blade holders are preferred (Fig 2-40). For microsurgical procedures such as gap flap formation or in extraoral tooth-preserving surgery, a narrow microsurgical blade that cuts on two sides is suitable (Fig 2-41, Video 2-4).

There are also blunter cutting instruments such as the desmotome (Fig 2-42) or periotome (Fig 2-43), which can be used to cut periodontal fibers in the area of the connective tissue attachment before tooth removals. However, cutting instruments also include scissors (Figs 2-44 to 2-46), which can be used in a variety of ways.

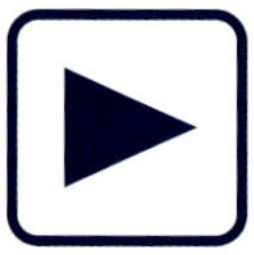

Video 2-4
Preparation of a palatal split flap.

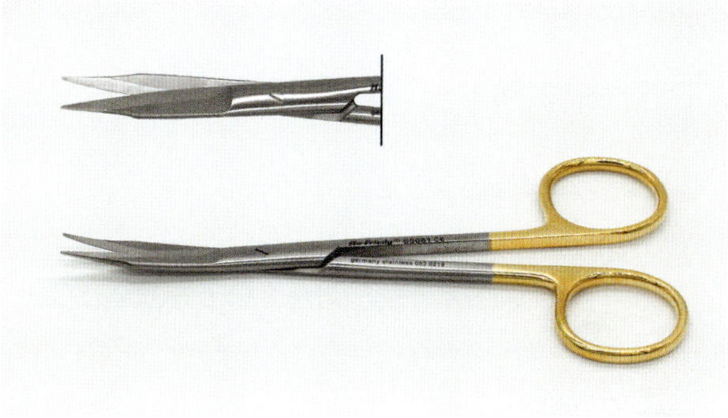

Fig 2-44 Goldman-Fox scissors (soft tissue scissors, dissecting scissors).

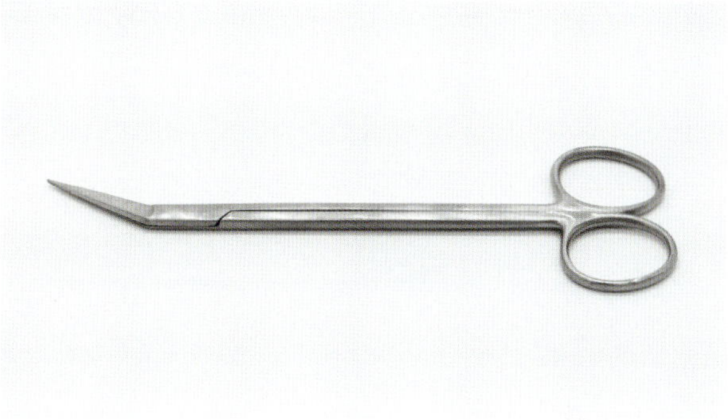

Fig 2-45 Thread scissors (angled, pointed/pointed).

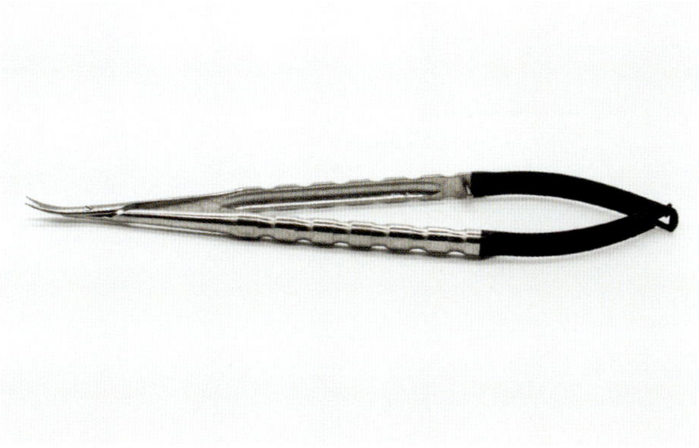

Fig 2-46 Microsurgical scissors.

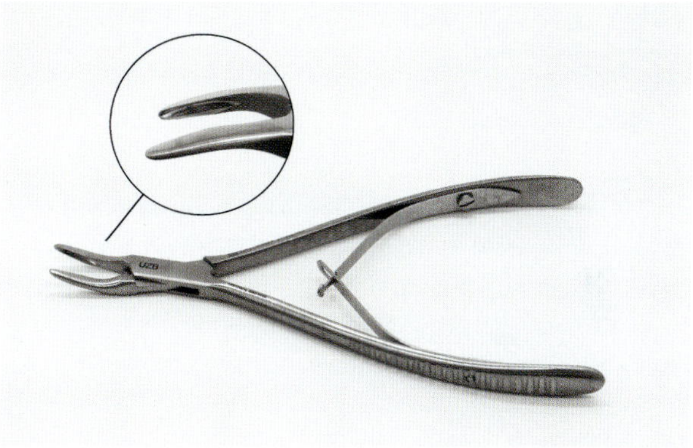

Fig 2-47 Luer bone rongeur.

They are used for soft tissue corrections as well as for dissections (loosening of the individual tissue layers by spreading the working ends) or for cutting off suture materials. The Luer bone rongeur (Fig 2-47) can be used to remove bone septa or to smooth sharp bone edges.

Preparation instruments

There are different variations of raspatories (Figs 2-48 to 2-54) that are primarily used to detach the mucoperiosteal flap from its bony base. In addition, they are also suitable for keeping soft tissue away during the use of rotating instruments. One raspatory favored by the authors is the Glickman raspatory (Fig 2-53, Video 2-5), which has two working ends: The triangular working end is suitable for mobilizing interdental papillae, while the oval working end is used primarily for detaching the mucoperiosteal flap in the marginal region. Other preparation instruments include bone curettes (Fig 2-55), which are used for the excochleation of granulation tissue and the extirpation of cyst epithelium. Elevators are another type of preparation instrument (Figs 2-56 to 2-60). The gouge-shaped working end is pushed into the periodontal gap, and the desmodont is expanded or widened by controlled rotational movements on the longitudinal axis of the instrument (supported on the *limbus alveolaris*), so that the tooth root can be dislocated by grasping it.

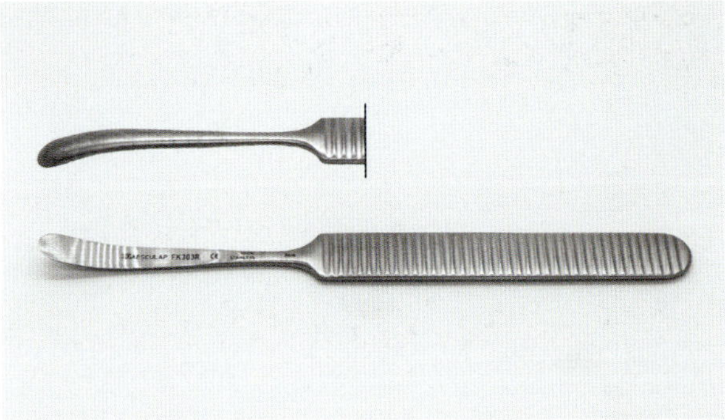

Fig 2-48 Williger raspatory.

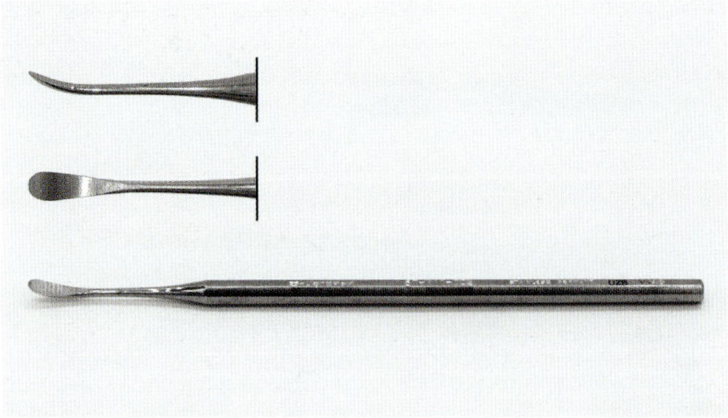

Fig 2-49 Partsch raspatory (short).

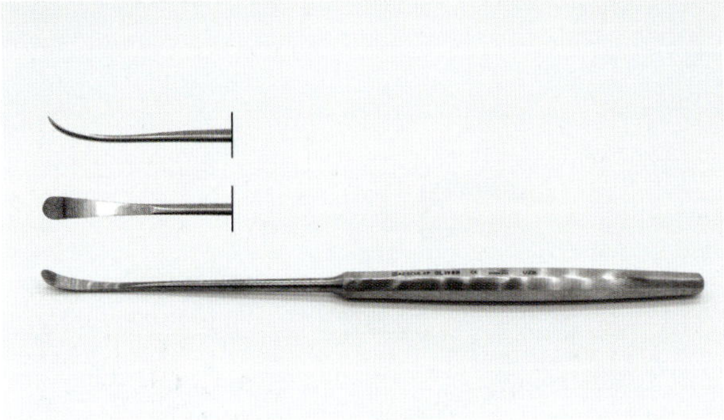

Fig 2-50 Partsch raspatory (long).

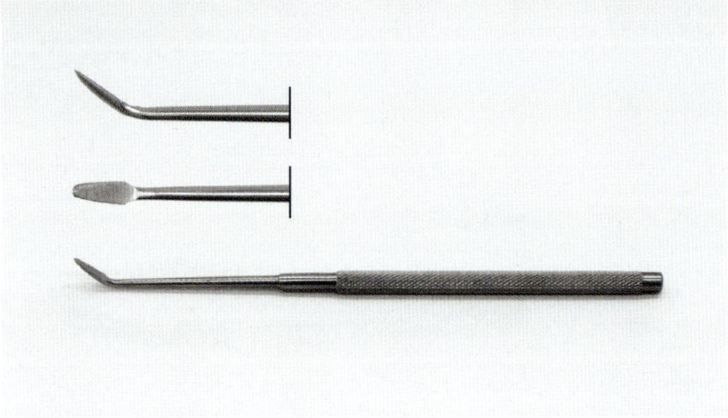

Fig 2-51 Papillary raspatory.

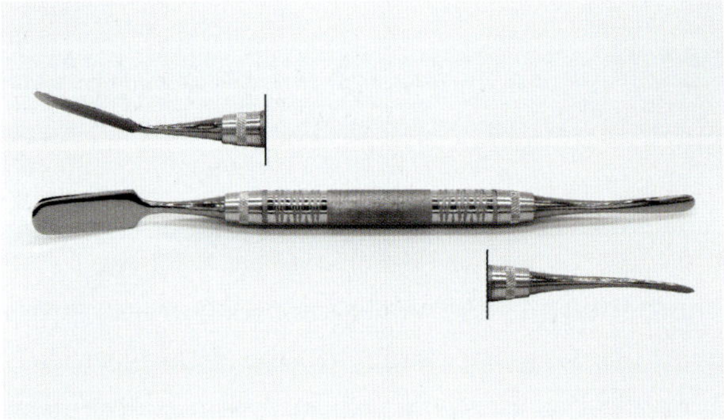

Fig 2-52 Prichard raspatory.

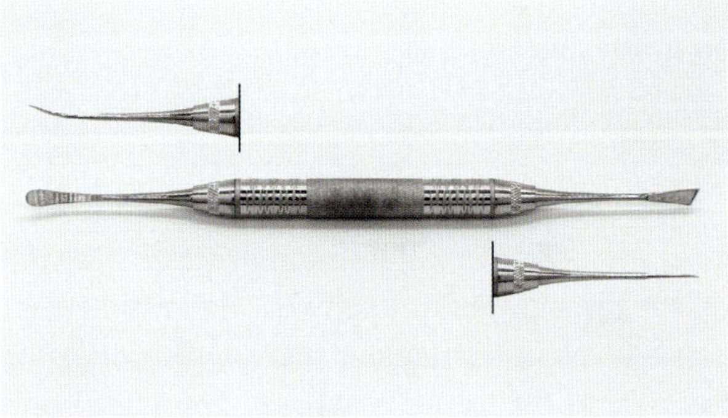

Fig 2-53 Glickman raspatory.

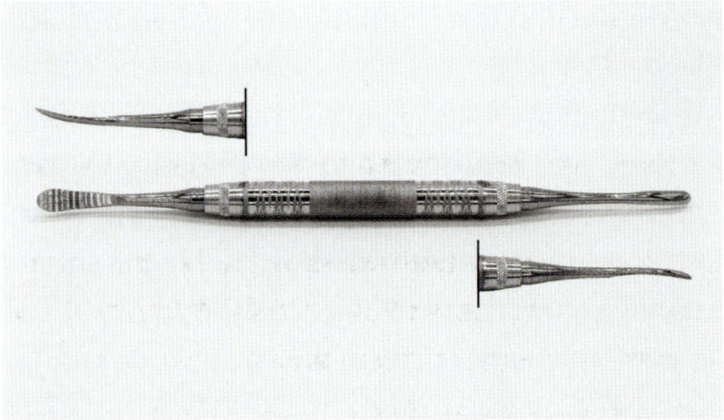

Fig 2-54 Freer elevator.

Video 2-5
Mobilization of the mucoperiosteal flap.

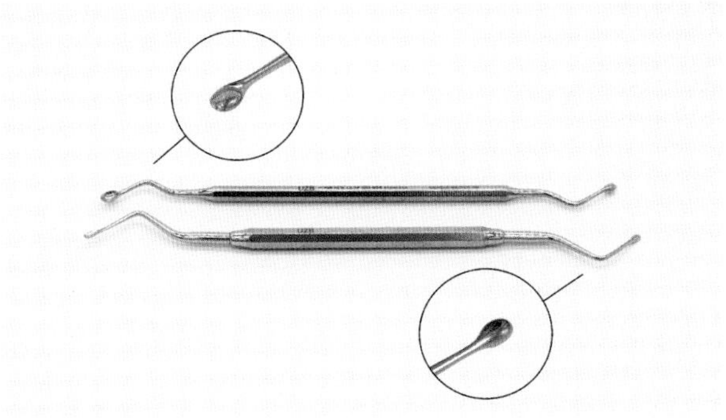

Fig 2-55 Hemingway bone curettes.

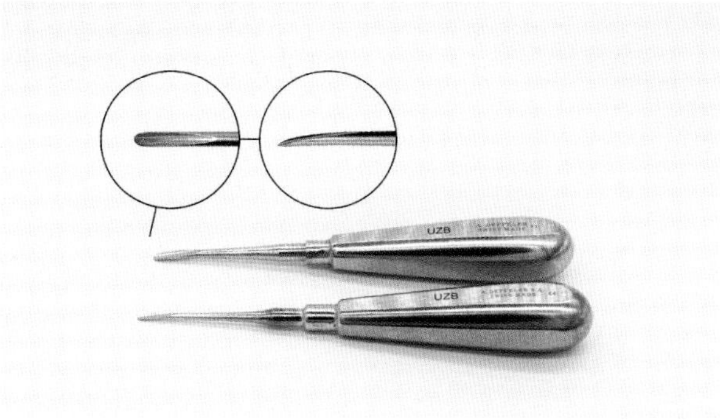

Fig 2-56 Deppler elevator (straight).

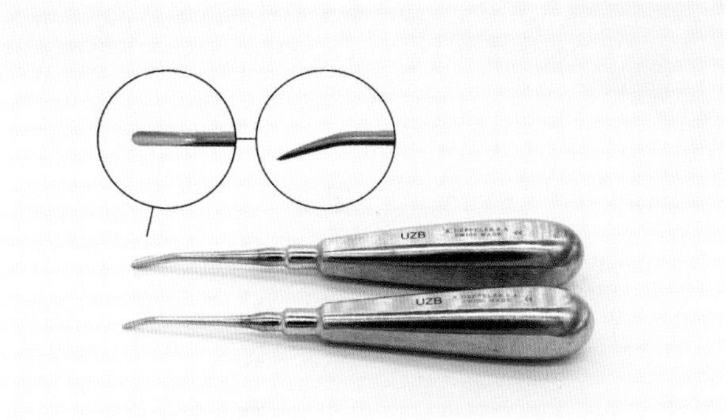

Fig 2-57 Deppler elevator (angled).

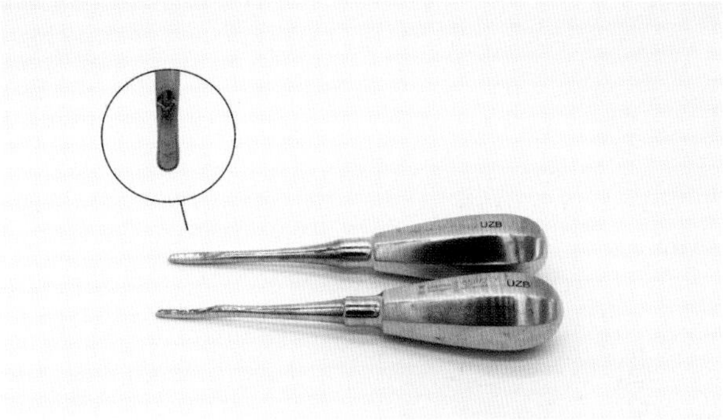

Fig 2-58 Bein elevator (straight).

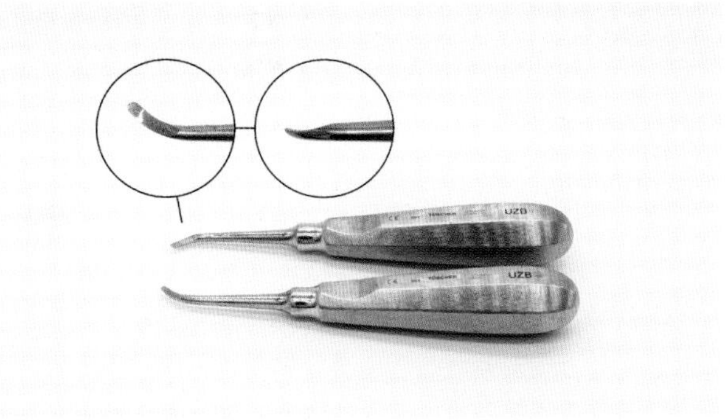

Fig 2-59 Miller root elevator.

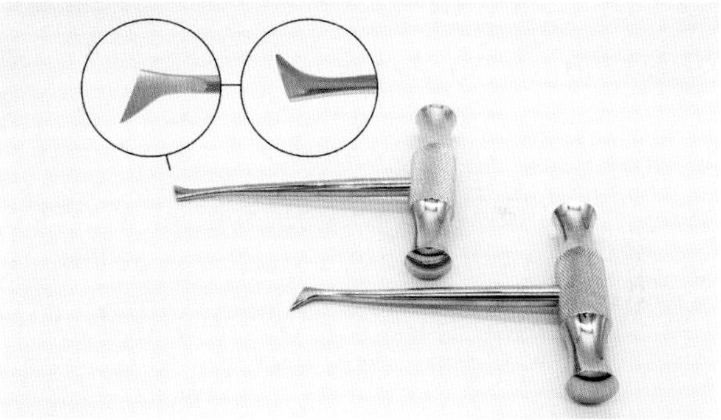

Fig 2-60 Winter elevator.

Palpation instruments

Classic dental palpation instruments such as the cow horn probe (Fig 2-61) are used in oral surgery, for example, to check the effect of local anesthesia. The periodontal probe (Fig 2-62) can also be used for this purpose. This probe is suitable for measuring distances or for probing fistula tracts. However, the most important probe is the Bowman lacrimal probe (Fig 2-63, Video 2-6), which can be used to visualize excretory ducts of the major salivary glands and also to verify or exclude an oroantral communication after tooth removal in the maxillary posterior region.

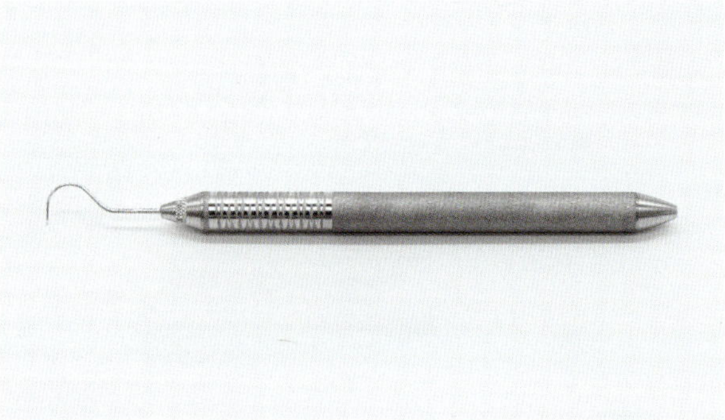

Fig 2-61 Cow horn probe.

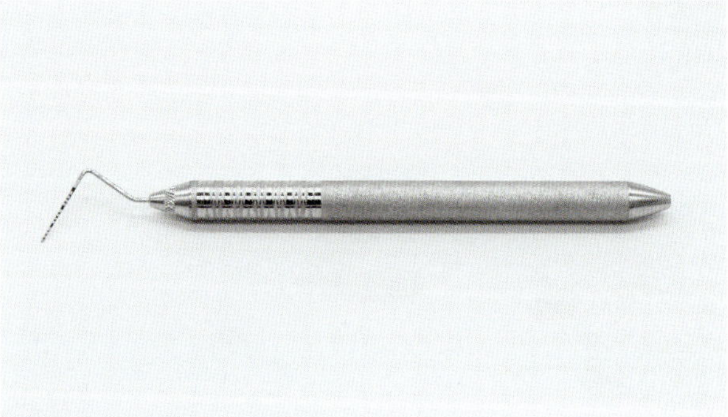

Fig 2-62 Periodontal probe.

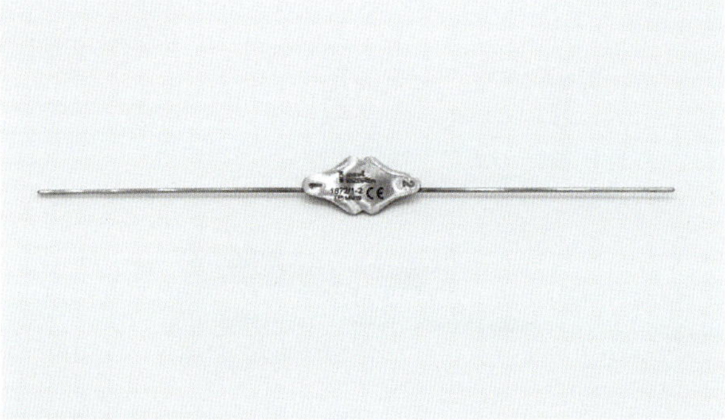

Fig 2-63 Bowman lacrimal probe.

Video 2-6 Probing the bony alveolar fundus to rule out an oroantral communication after the removal of tooth 16.

Rotating instruments

For the purpose of removing bone (osteotomy) or to smooth bone (osteoplasty), spherical rose drills of various sizes are used, which are mechanically driven by a sterilizable handpiece (Fig 2-64). Overheating on the bone must be avoided by cooling with sterile isotonic saline solution. Furthermore, Lindemann burs are used to decapitate teeth or to separate their roots (Video 2-7).

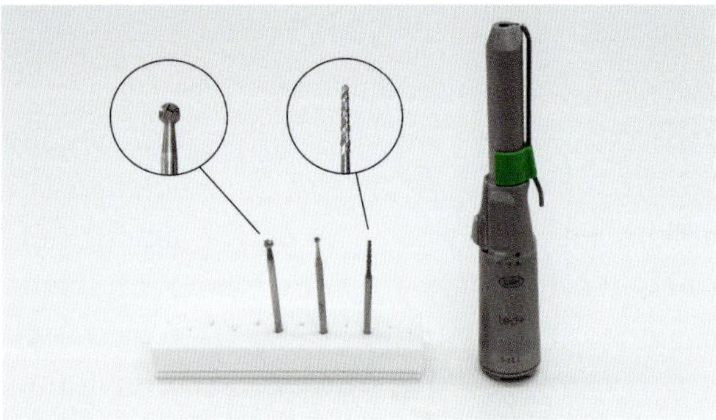

Fig 2-64 Handpiece with external cooling (from left to right): rose bur (descending sizes) and Lindemann bur.

Video 2-7 Osteotomy and decapitation during surgical removal of wisdom tooth 48.

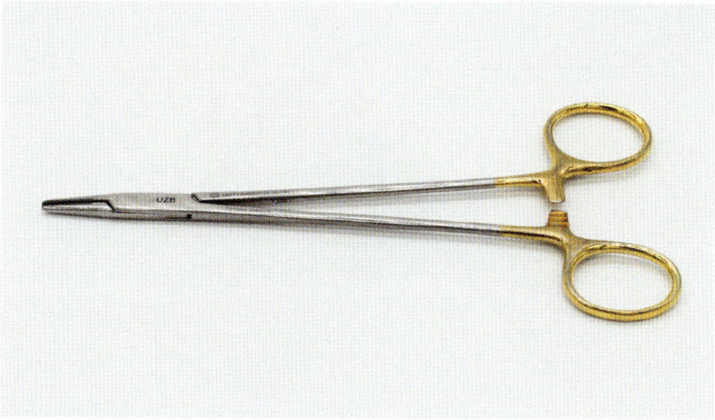

Fig 2-65 Mayo-Hegar needle holder.

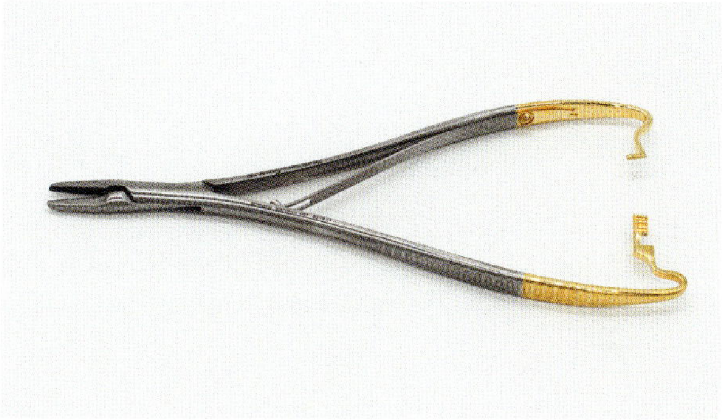

Fig 2-66 Mathieu needle holder.

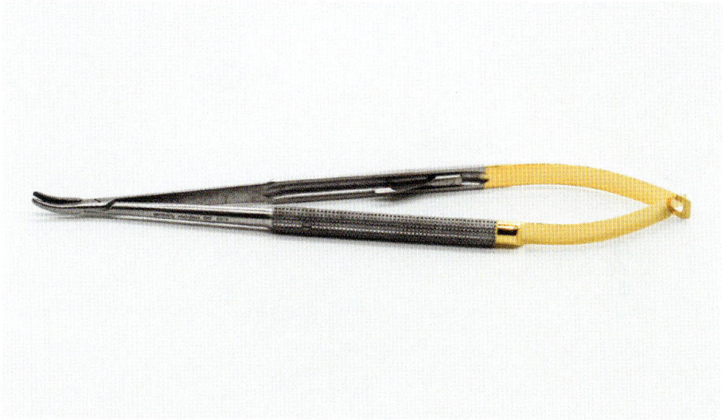

Fig 2-67 Microsurgical needle holder.

Suture instruments and suture materials

In oral surgery, closed needle holders or needle holders with a locking mechanism (Figs 2-65 and 2-66) are preferred to open needle holders, since the needle can be better fixed in the closed position during suture placement. This provides more comfort and safety, especially in an unclear surgical area. It must be noted that the size of the needle holder should correspond to the size of the needle and the thickness of the suture material. Specifically, this means that 6-0 sutures cannot be placed with macrosurgical needle holders and, conversely, 3-0 sutures cannot be placed with microsurgical needle holders (Fig 2-67). The size and shape of the needle holder determine their handling: some are held like scissors, some like pliers, and others like a pen (Figs 2-68 to 2-70). During suture placement, the needle should never be grasped with the needle holder in the area of the internally hollow needle shaft (reinforcement zone) because the needle will snap off and have to be discarded in the event of tooth or bone contact (Fig 2-71).

The selection of suture materials available on the market is large and very confusing, especially for beginners. In oral surgery, only so-called atraumatic sutures are used, i.e. sutures without a needle eye and without the thread having to be threaded in, but directly locked in the needle. The surgical needle basically consists of three elements (Fig 2-72): the needle tip; the needle body (with grooves) so that the needle cannot rotate in the needle holder; and the needle shaft (also called the reinforcement zone), which is hollow on the inside for securing the thread. The designation of a needle, which appears on the packaging (such as

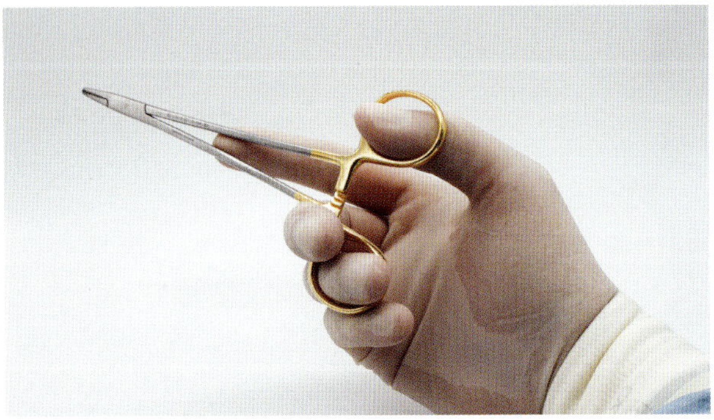

Fig 2-68 The needle holder is held in a scissor grip with the thumb and ring finger, and additionally stabilized with the index finger.

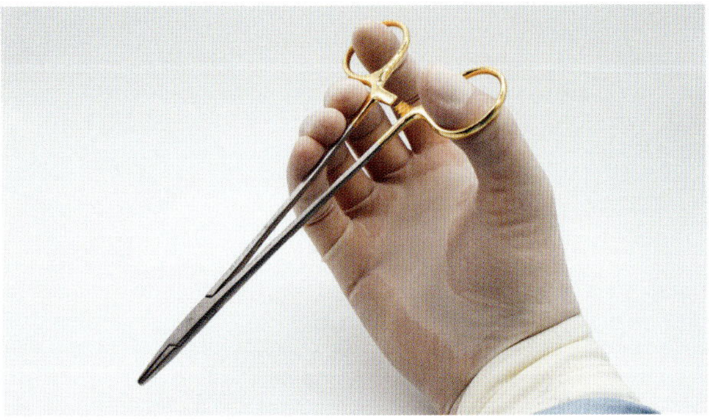

Fig 2-69 In some situations, however, it is more comfortable to hold the needle holder with the palm technique.

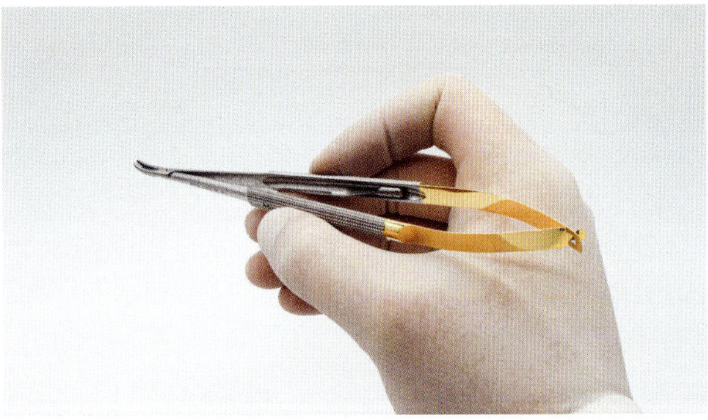

Fig 2-70 The microsurgical needle holder is held like a pen, which allows fine handling.

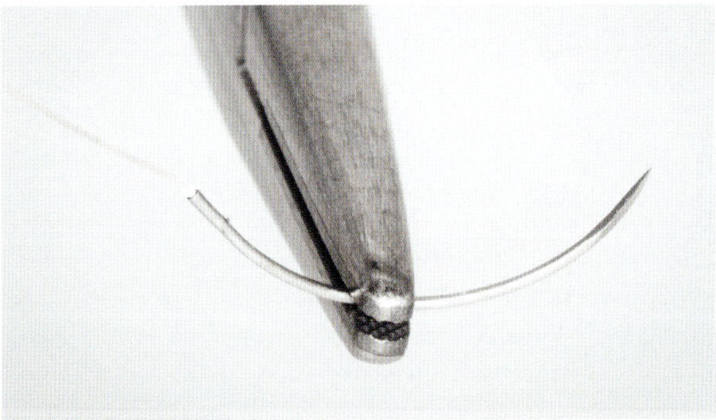

Fig 2-71 Correct locking of the surgical needle in the needle holder.

DS16), is made up of two letters and a number. This designation provides information about the shape, profile, point, and length of the needle. The first letter refers to the shape of the needle. Most surgical needles describe the part of a circular path (Fig 2-73): The best-known needle shapes are the H needle (1/2 circle), the D needle (3/8 circle), and the V needle (1/4 circle), with the D needle being the most suitable for oral surgery. Everyday life is made unnecessarily difficult with all other needle shapes. The second letter stands for the profile of the needle body, and the third letter, if present, for the specific needle tip (or point) (Fig 2-74). The best-known profiles are the R needle (R = round-body needle) and the S needle (S = cutting needle), which is ground to be triangular. Only S needles should be used for oral surgery. Other special needle profiles are not usually required. There are two variants of cutting needles. Manufacturers use a triangle symbol on the packaging to indicate the variant: if the triangle tip points upward, the cutting edge is located on the inner contour of the needle (conventional cutting), and if it points downward, the cutting edge is located on the outer contour of the needle (reverse cutting). For oral surgery, the reverse cutting needle is to be preferred because otherwise there is a risk of the

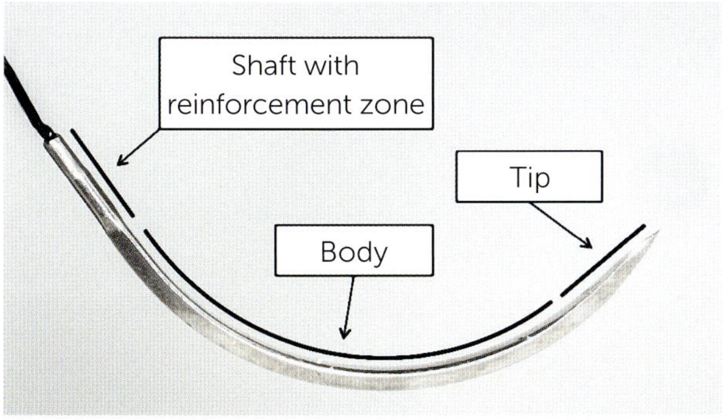

Fig 2-72 Structure of an atraumatic needle.

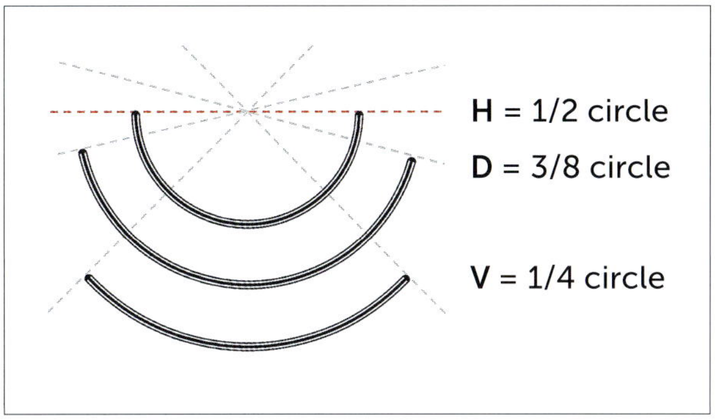

Fig 2-73 The most important needle shapes[1].

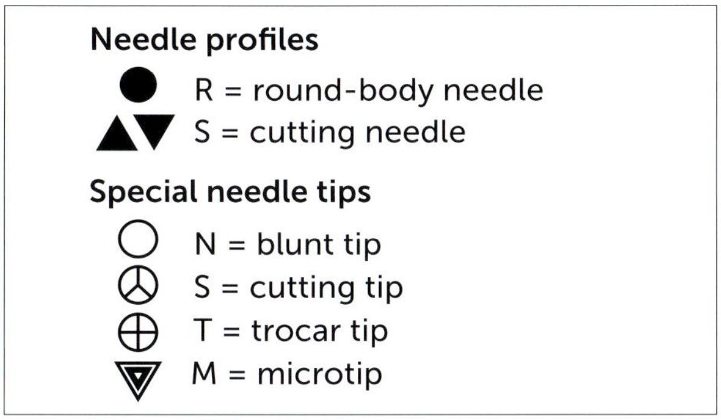

Fig 2-74 The most important needle profiles[1].

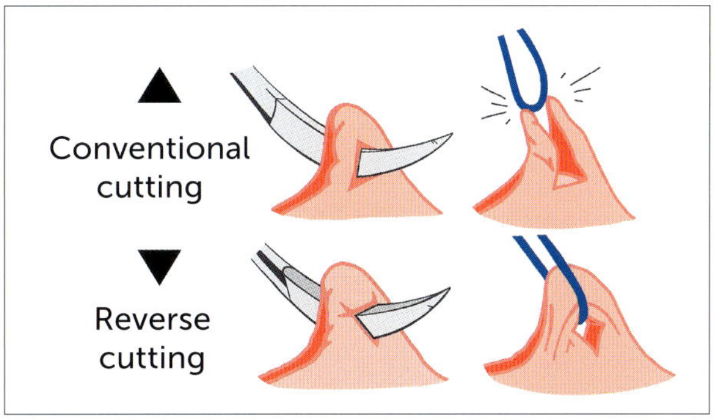

Fig 2-75 Conventional and reverse cutting needle bodies and their effect on soft tissue.

flap tearing (Fig 2-75). Finally, the number of the designation describes the length of the needle. It is difficult to suture releasing incisions with needles that are unnecessarily long; and with needles that are too short, the needle disappears completely buccally before it appears palatally or lingually (e.g. in papillae sutures). Therefore, the needle length for oral surgical procedures should ideally be between 16 and 19 mm.

The property of the surgical suture, and thus the choice of suture material, is influenced by various factors such as resorption behavior (Table 2-1), origin, texture, length, and thickness.

Table 2-1 Origin and resorption behavior of surgical sutures[1].

Resorption behavior	Origin	
	Synthetic	Natural
Non-resorbable	Polyester	Silk
	Cotton	Polypropylene
	Polyamide	Wire (steel)
Resorbable	Polyglycolic acid	
	Polyglactin	
	Polydioxanone	

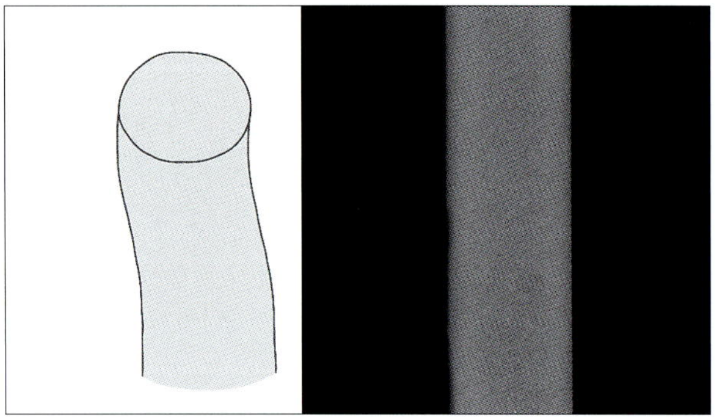

Fig 2-76 Monofilament thread.

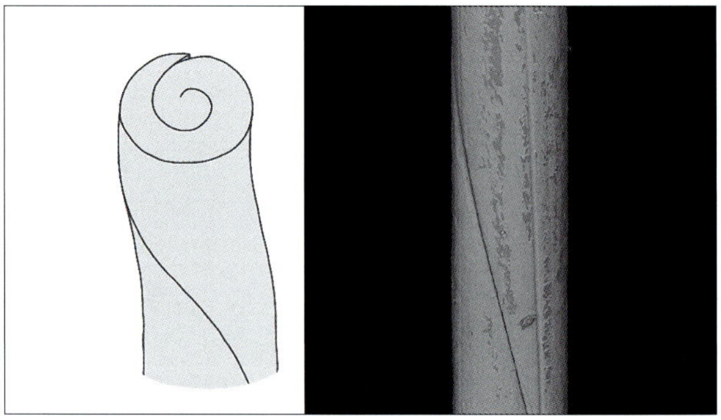

Fig 2-77 Twisted PTFE thread.

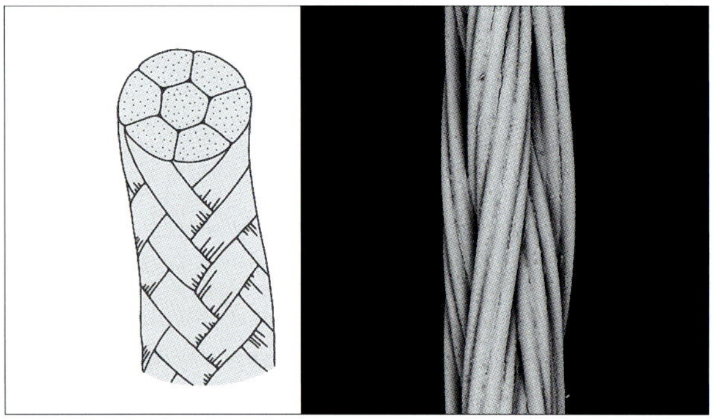

Fig 2-78 Multifilament thread.

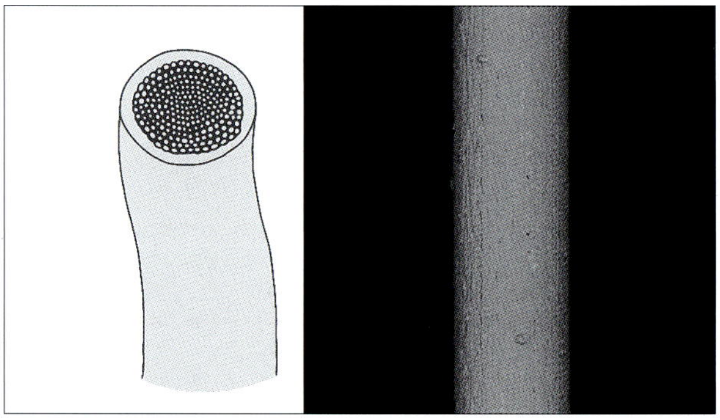

Fig 2-79 Pseudomonofilament thread.

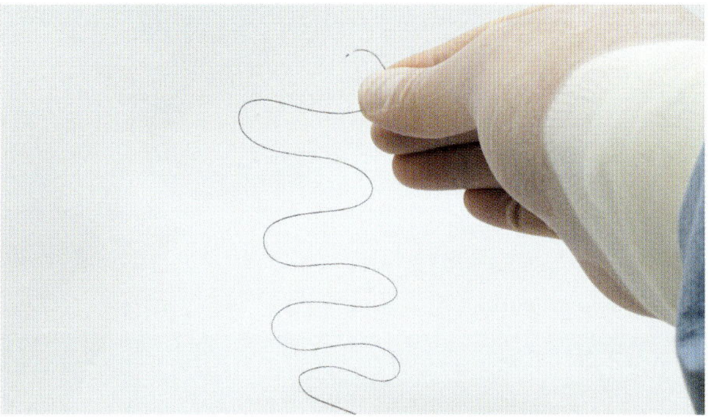

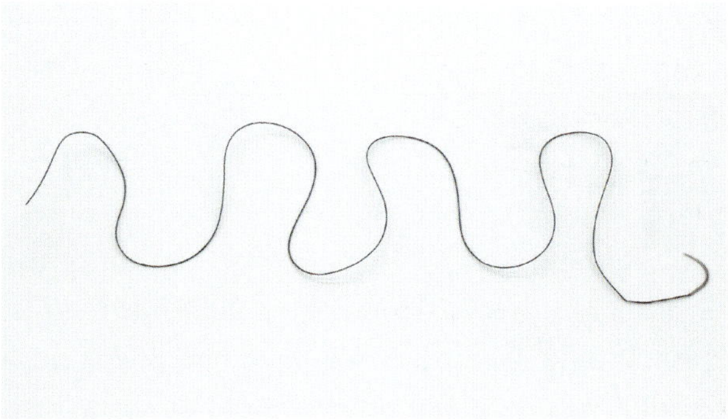

Figs 2-80 and 2-81 After removing the thread from the packaging.

Resorbable suture material is rarely used in oral surgery because its service life of up to several weeks is far too high and there is also a very high corresponding plaque accumulation. However, its use is justified in procedures in which several tissue layers have to be adapted (submucosal sutures) or in patients who can only be treated under intubation anesthesia due to their lack of cooperation (e.g. anxious and mentally ill patients or infants). The use of resorbable suture material eliminates the need for subsequent suture removal or further intubation anesthesia. In all other cases, however, non-resorbable suture material is to be preferred.

Furthermore, surgical sutures are characterized by their texture. A distinction is made between monofilament, pseudomonofilament, and multifilament threads. The monofilament thread (Fig 2-76) consists of a single plastic strand that has a hydrophobic surface. This ensures very smooth gliding through the tissue from the first to the last suture and results in low plaque accumulation during the healing phase. A special form of monofilament thread is the twisted polytetrafluoroethylene (PTFE) thread (Fig 2-77). This thread is characterized not only by its white color but also by its soft, tissue-friendly, and hydrophobic material, which makes it very pleasant to sew with. However, it is also characterized by a high purchase price. The multifilament thread consists of many fine filaments, which can be braided or twisted (Fig 2-78). As a result, the thread has a rather rough surface, which leads to additional trauma when it is pulled through as well as to higher plaque accumulation postoperatively. Furthermore, due to its hydrophilic property (capillarity), this type of thread absorbs more blood, saliva, and tissue fluid with each additional suture, which leads to poorer gliding properties. On the other hand, the multifilament thread is easier to knot, and the end of the thread is perceived by patients to be less irritating due to its greater suppleness. The pseudomonofilament thread is a multifilament thread that has been coated or impregnated on the surface (Fig 2-79). As a result, this is somewhat smoother and more hydrophobic than the multifilament thread, leading to less plaque accumulation. The pseudomonofilament thread thus represents a compromise between the properties of the monofilament and multifilament threads.

Threads can be ordered in various thicknesses. The range for oral surgical procedures is between 3-0 and 6-0 (USP designation). The higher the number, the thinner the thread, and vice versa. The use of a 6-0 thread is rather the exception in oral surgery. It requires microsurgical instruments and an optical magnification aid. As a general rule, thinner threads should be used in the esthetically visible region, and thicker ones in the posterior region.

All suture materials are supplied by the manufacturers in sterile packaging. The thread is wound on a spool made of cardboard or plastic. Monofilament suture material, in particular, tends to retain the shape of the spool after removal from the packaging (Figs 2-80 and 2-81). This does not exactly make suturing easier, especially for the first sutures, where the thread is usually still 40 cm long. In such cases, it is recommended to use sterile gloves to hold the needle between the thumb and index finger of one hand, and to pull the thread through the thumb and index finger of the other hand once (Video 2-8). By stretching the thread, the shape of the coil almost disappears and suturing becomes much easier.

Video 2-8
Stretching the surgical thread after removing it from the package.

References

1. Reichart PA et al. Curriculum Zahnärztliche Chirurgie. Band 1. Berlin: Quintessenz, 2001.
2. Schweizerische Zahnärztegesellschaft SSO. Qualitätsleitlinien: Praxishygiene, 2015. https://www.sso.ch/zahnaerzte/qualitaetsleitlinien.html (letzter Zugriff 04.06.2020).
3. World Health Organization (WHO). Surgical Handrubbing Technique, NewSurgicalA3, 2009.

Suturing techniques in oral surgery

3

Andreas Filippi

Many oral surgical procedures end with suture treatment – primarily to fix a mobilized and repositioned mucoperiosteal flap in its original position as far as possible; secondarily, however, to reduce the wound area of alveoli or to stabilize an alveolar or defect filling by means of sutures, if necessary; and last but not least, to enable stable soft tissue closure of alveoli or opened maxillary sinuses, if necessary[6,7].

Guiding and inserting the needle

The needle is grasped with the needle holder in the area of the needle body (not at the needle tip and not in the area of the reinforcement zone; see Section 2) and passed through or rotated through one side of the wound margin with a twisting motion. Depending on the situation and gingival biotype, the puncture should be made about 2 mm from the wound margin. If the needle cannot be passed through both wound margins in one stroke at this point, it is first pulled out of the soft tissue again with a twisting/rotating movement and then passed through the second part of the wound margin. Pure pulling movements on the needle should be avoided, as they can lead to both tearing of the wound edges and tearing of the suture directly at the needle.

Before starting to tie the knot, the suture should be pulled through far enough to ensure that about 4 cm still protrudes in order to save material when cutting it off.

The surgical knot

Each suture ends with a surgical knot. This prevents the suture from opening on its own during the wearing period, which could turn an intended primary wound healing into a secondary wound healing. Since wounds in the oral cavity are subject to constant mechanical pressure and traction (chewing, drinking, speaking, swallowing), and (unlike wounds in the dermis) cannot be immobilized, a surgical knot in oral surgery must remain stable for about a week until the suture is removed.

Various knotting techniques have been described for oral surgical procedures. However, across all levels of dental professional experience only one has proven successful, which consists of three consecutive knots.

The first knot is a double knot for rather thick (3-0 or 4-0) and multifilament suture material (Fig 3-1), and a triple knot for rather thin (5-0 or 6-0) and monofilament suture material (Fig 3-2). When tightening this first knot, the wound edges are adapted and brought into contact with each other. For the next knot, the suture must then be slackened slightly. During this process, the wound edges that have just been adapted must not move away from each other again. With thick multifilament suture material, due to the rough thread surface, the friction of a double knot is sufficiently great to prevent this from happening. With thin monofilament suture material, however, a triple knot is required to achieve the same friction of the smooth thread and thus prevent spontaneous dehiscence of the wound edges.

The second knot, regardless of the suture material used, is a single knot looped in the opposite direction of the first knot. Its function is to (re)adapt wound edges that may be somewhat distant from each other without having to start the suture from the beginning.

The third and last knot, also independent of the suture material used, is again a single knot that is looped once again in the opposite direction (or in the direction of the first knot). Its function is to prevent the first two knots from unraveling during the wearing period.

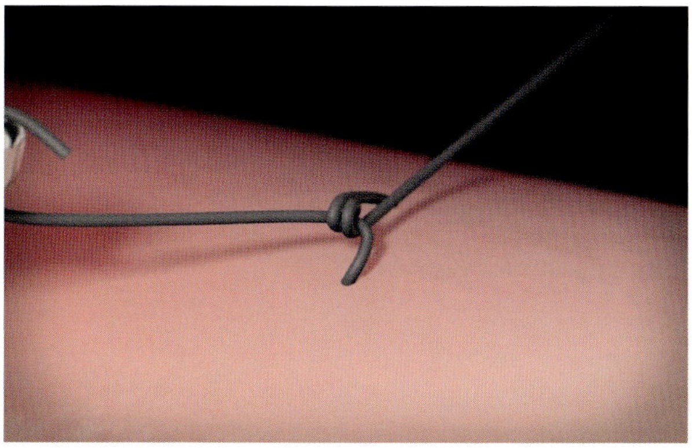

Fig 3-1 In multifilament sutures, the first knot is a double knot (from: Rasperini[5]).

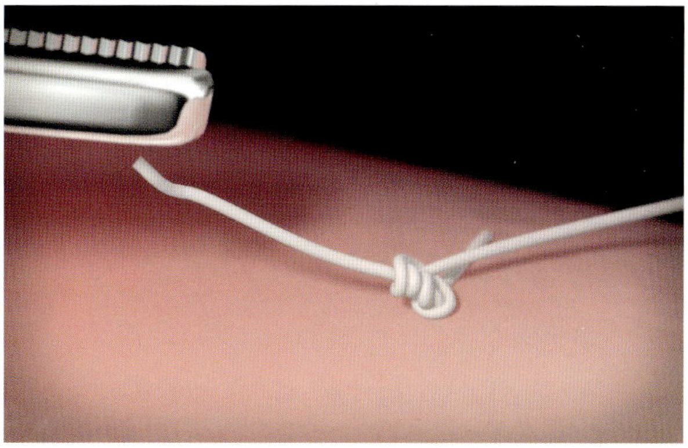

Fig 3-2 With monofilament suture material, the first knot is a triple knot (from: Rasperini[5]).

Cutting the suture after knotting

After the knot has been completed, the surgical assistant must cut the suture. The remaining amount of the protruding suture material should be an exact length so that the knot does not open on its own within the wearing period but also so that the ends of the suture do not disturb the patient. For multifilament suture material, this overhang should be 3 to 4 mm, and for monofilament suture material it should be 7 to 8 mm. Monofilament suture material that is cut too short pricks the surrounding mucosa, in a similar way to stubble. Multifilament suture material that has been cut too long is invasive and annoying, like a wool thread hanging into the oral cavity; often the patient will worry it with the tongue.

To ensure that the surgical assistant can always and reliably cut the suture with only one scissor cut, the surgeon should rotate the two ends of the suture once around its own axis by crossing the hands after tightening the last knot (Video 3-1). Then the cutting of the two suture ends with a scissor cut is always successful, which saves time and sometimes also nerves.

Video 3-1 Crossing the ends of the suture for easier cutting.

Suture techniques

A total of nearly 20 suture techniques have been described for oral surgical procedures, each with its own indication. Some, such as the single-button suture, are well known and widely used; other excellent suture techniques, less so. Some of these suture techniques are described in a little more detail below.

Single-button suture

The single-button suture (Videos 3-2 and 3-3) consists of two punctures through both wound edges (Fig 3-3). The thinner the gingival biotype and the further into the visible area the suture is, the more important it is that the knot does not lie directly on the incision at the end (Fig 3-4); the reasons for this are not to irritate the wound

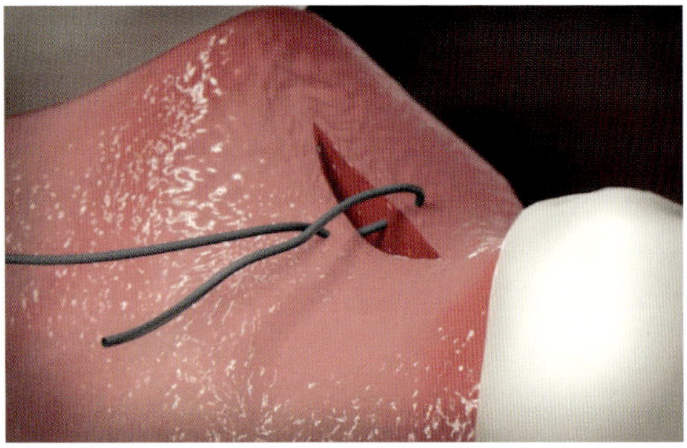

Fig 3-3 Single-button suture: two punctures (from: Rasperini[5]).

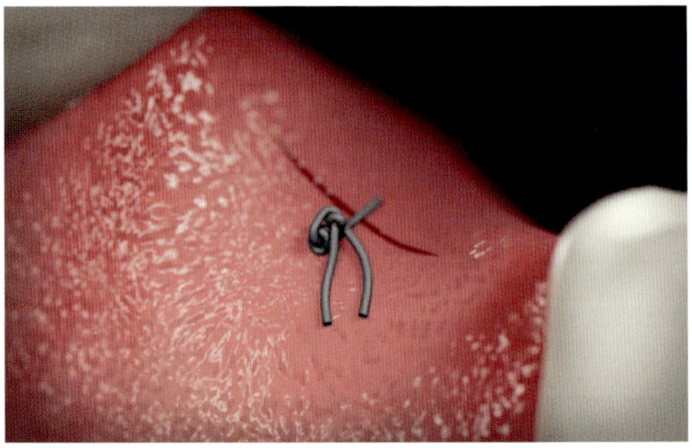

Fig 3-4 The knot should not lie on the incision but be moved away from it at the end by pulling the ends of the thread, if necessary (from: Rasperini[5]).

Video 3-2
Single-button suture (from: Rasperini[5]).

Video 3-3
Single-button suture.

unnecessarily in the healing phase and not to create a scar that is needlessly wide. To move the knot away from the incision, after cutting the ends of the sutures, one of the ends is grasped with a forceps. In the case of crestally located incisions, this pulling should always be performed in a buccal direction so that the suture is not unnecessarily irritating for the tongue (Fig 3-4).

Horizontal mattress suture

In contrast to the single-button suture, mattress sutures can absorb considerably more force and also hold considerably more force. Therefore, they should be favored whenever sutures are strategically important. Mattress sutures must not open or loosen during the healing phase. This is particularly important with soft tissue coverings of all kinds, e.g. after soft tissue maxillary sinus closure, soft tissue coverage of alveoli in antiresorptive treated patients, and after soft tissue coverage of extensive augmentations in the course of implantations.

All mattress sutures basically consist of four punctures, and they should all start buccally so that the suture ends do not unnecessarily disturb the tongue during the healing phase.

The horizontal mattress suture (Video 3-4) is so named because the four punctures are arranged in a horizontal plane (side by side) (Fig 3-5). The distance between the second and third as well as the first and fourth punctures must not be too small, otherwise the potential of this suture cannot develop sufficiently.

Today, a distinction is made between conventional and modified horizontal mattress suturing. The conventional horizontal mattress suture no longer plays a role in modern oral surgery because its geometry leaves unnecessarily wide connective tissue scars. When the suture

Video 3-4 Horizontal mattress suture (from: Rasperini[5]).

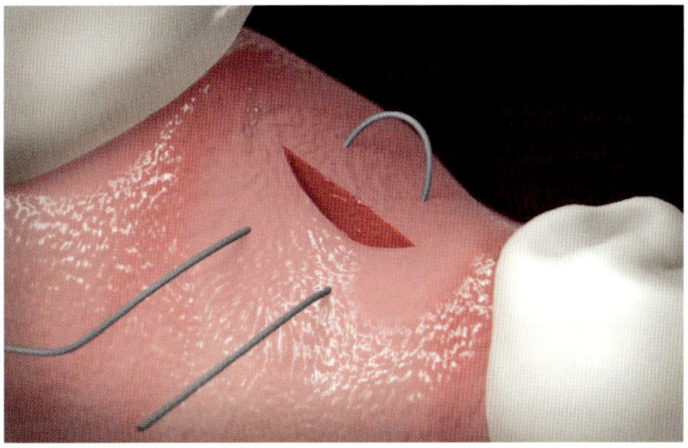

Fig 3-5 Horizontal mattress suture: four punctures (from: Rasperini[5]).

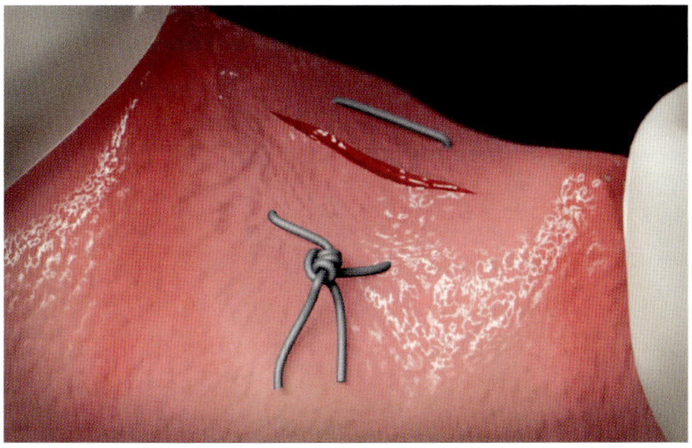

Fig 3-6 Horizontal mattress sutures often result in an unnecessarily wide scar (from: Rasperini[5]).

Video 3-5 Modified horizontal mattress suture (from: Rasperini[5]).

Video 3-6 Modified horizontal mattress suture.

is tightened during knot placement, the wound edges are not only adapted but are also somewhat raised, which leads to these undesirable results (Fig 3-6).

In the more recent modification of this suture (also called the Laurell-Gottlow suture) (Videos 3-5 and 3-6), after the fourth puncture and before the first knot, the needle is passed through the loop between the second and third puncture (Fig 3-7). It does not matter from which direction the needle is passed through the loop. Only then are the knots placed. The result

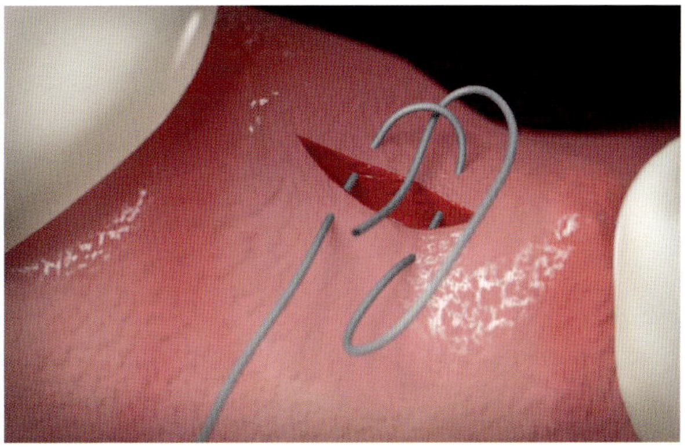

Fig 3-7 Modified horizontal mattress suture: The needle is passed through the loop before knotting (from: Rasperini[5]).

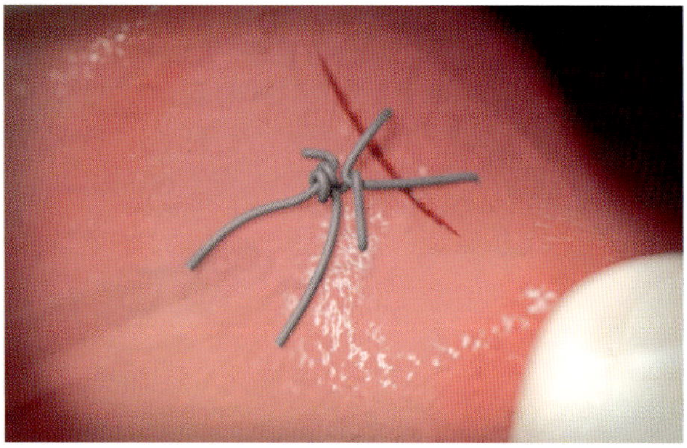

Fig 3-8 Modified horizontal mattress suture: The wound edges are perfectly adapted by the V-shaped suture guide (from: Rasperini[5]).

Video 3-7 Vertical mattress suture (from: Rasperini[5]).

Video 3-8 Vertical mattress suture.

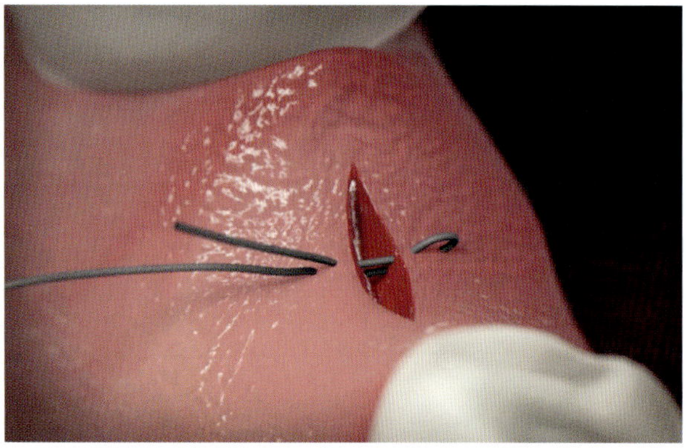

Fig 3-9 Vertical mattress suture: four punctures (from: Rasperini[5]).

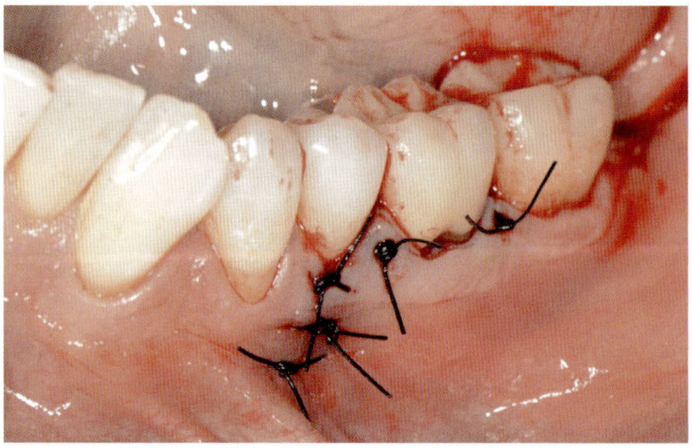

Fig 3-10 Situation after vertical mattress suture after apicectomy in region 36.

is correct when the loop comes to rest exactly at the knot, like the tip of a "V" (Fig 3-8). This can only be achieved if the knots are tightened from the buccal and not from the crestal side. The whole must not look like a "U" (when the suture is not tightened sufficiently) nor like an "X" (when the knots are not tightened from the buccal but from the crestal side). The two legs of the "V" then lie above the incision and press the two wound edges downward (Fig 3-8). This ensures a truly narrow and line-shaped scar.

Vertical mattress suture

The vertical mattress suture (Videos 3-7 and 3-8) also consists of four punctures and always starts buccally. The vertical mattress suture is so called because the four punctures are arranged in a vertical plane (one above the other) (Fig 3-9). It is particularly preferable to a single-button suture if the interdental papillae have been mobilized in the visible area in the course of incision guides and flaps, and it

Video 3-9 Double-loop suture (from: Rasperini[5]).

Video 3-10 Double-loop suture.

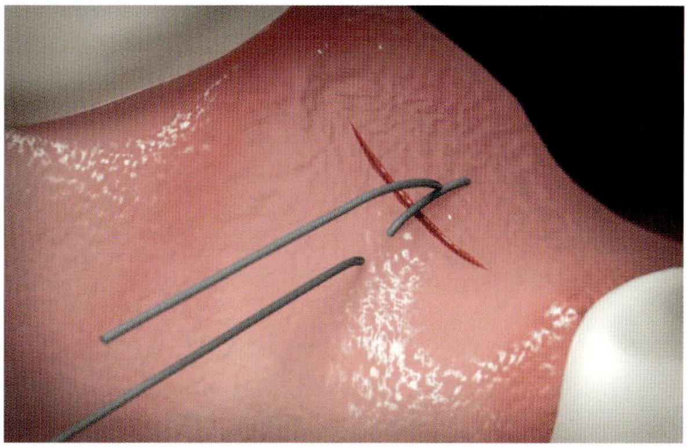

Fig 3-11 Double-loop suture: four punctures (from: Rasperini[5]).

must be ensured that they grow back in exactly the same place at the end of wound healing (Fig 3-10). A single-knot suture cannot guarantee this because part of the suture runs over the tip of the papilla and pushes it down slightly when the suture is closed[4].

Double-loop suture

The double-loop suture (Videos 3-9 and 3-10) also consists of four punctures and – for the same reasons – also starts buccally (Fig 3-11). A double-loop suture is always preferable to a single-button suture for the perfect functioning of the dentogingival closure after marginal incision or peri-implant soft tissue adaptation in implantation with transgingival healing. It is also excellent after surgical wisdom tooth removal[1]: The suture immediately distal to the second molar must guarantee a truly tight dentogingival closure to prevent lifelong increased probing depths in this area, which is difficult to control for plaque so far dorsally. The double-loop suture adapts the mobilized soft tissue in three superimposed planes and guarantees significantly better results than the single-button suture (Fig 3-12).

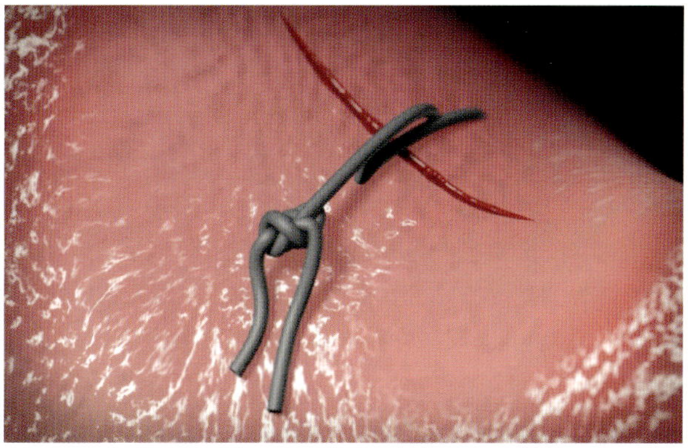

Fig 3-12 Finished double-loop suture (from: Rasperini[5]).

Cross suture

The cross suture (Video 3-11) also consists of four punctures and also starts buccally (Fig 3-13). It is indicated for the suture treatment of alveoli after conventional tooth removal (without opening). The cross suture has two functions: reduction of the wound area as well as stabilization of an inserted foreign material to protect it from spontaneous loss (depending on the indication, medical history, and case:

Video 3-11 Cross suture (from: Rasperini[5]).

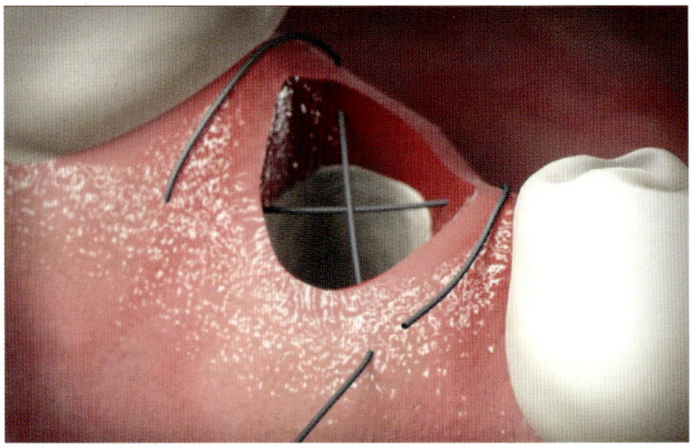

Fig 3-13 Cross suture (from: Rasperini[5]).

collagen, oxygenated cellulose [Tabotamp®; Ethicon, Norderstedt, Germany], non-absorbable tamponade or bone substitute material)[2,3]. In contrast to the horizontal mattress suture, this suture is passed obliquely through the alveolus from the buccal to the palatal side after the first puncture, and obliquely through the alveolus to the palatal side again after another puncture from the buccal side. The suture then runs supracrestally over the alveolus like a cross. A cross suture can also be achieved by first passing from the buccal side obliquely through the alveolus to the palatal side, and then horizontally offset from the palatal side again obliquely through the alveolus back to the buccal side. The geometry and thus the effect of the suture are practically identical at the end.

References

1. AWMF. S2k-Leitlinie Operative Entfernung von Weisheitszähnen. www.awmf.org (Stand August 2019).
2. AWMF. S3-Leitlinie Zahnärztliche Chirurgie unter oraler Antikoagulation/Thrombozytenaggregationshemmung. www.awmf.org (Stand August 2017).
3. Kämmerer PW, Stein JM (Hrsg.). Blutgerinnung – mit Blutungen richtig umgehen. Wissen kompakt 2019;13:171–219.
4. Kumar K, Sharma RK, Tewari S, Narula SC. Use of modified vertical internal mattress suture versus simple loop interrupted suture in modified Widman flap surgery: a randomized clinical study. Quint Int 2019;50:732–740.
5. Rasperini G. The Oral Surgery Suture Trainer. Berlin: Quintessenz, 2012. Verfügbar im Apple App Store.
6. Rueppell C, Meier R, Filippi A. Normale und gestörte Wundheilung nach Zahnentfernung. Quintessenz 2016;67:1225–1232.
7. Siervo S. Nahttechniken in der Oralchirurgie. Berlin: Quintessenz, 2007.

4

Incision guides and flap techniques

Fabio Saccardin

In order to gain adequate access to the surgical site, different incision guides and flap techniques are practiced. Standard operating procedures exist for most oral surgical interventions and are discussed in detail in this book. However, it is not always possible to implement such a standard procedure, so the dentist should have some basic knowledge of common incision and flap techniques, which is the subject of this chapter.

During the incision, the scalpel is held like a pen. Very little pressure is required to cut through the mucosa, including the periosteum. The incision is made perpendicular to the mucosal surface to allow precise adaptation of the wound edges later. Without exception, the incision should be made on a bony base. Incisions that pass over an expected bony defect (e.g. in cysts) should be avoided, as these frequently lead to wound dehiscence postoperatively. The length of an incision should be such that there is a sufficient overview of the surgical area without soft tissue tearing occurring at the end of the incision as a result of the hook traction, and also to ensure that structures that need to be anatomically protected, such as nerves or blood vessels, are not endangered by a wide extension. Furthermore, it should be possible to extend an incision intraoperatively. Oroantral communications after tooth removal in the maxillary posterior region are especially common and soft tissue coverage should be performed in the course of treatment. The incision chosen should also allow further surgical intervention at a later stage. Common errors in this regard include horizontal incisions at a future flap base, negatively affecting flap vascularization, loss of keratinized gingiva or displacement of the mucogingival boundary due to a soft tissue coverage where a future implant is surrounded by mobile mucosa.

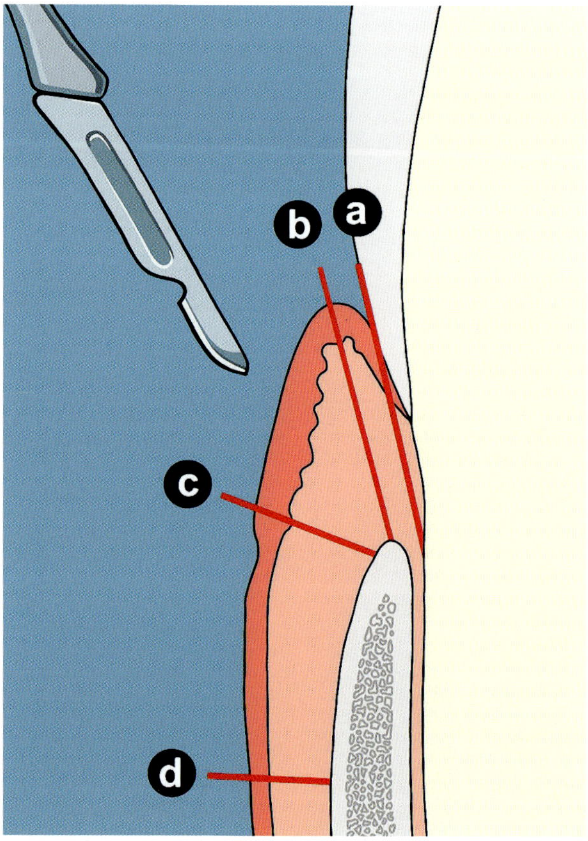

Fig 4-1 Primary incisions on the gingiva and mucosa: 'a' intrasulcular incision; 'b' marginal incision; 'c' paramarginal incision; 'd' mucosal incision.

Primary incisions

Primary incisions are usually performed in the gingival area. The incision can be intrasulcular, marginal or paramarginal (Fig 4-1). Only in exceptional cases are primary incisions required in the region of the mobile mucosa.

The intrasulcular incision (Figs 4-2 and 4-3), also called the sulcular or intracrevicular incision, is the gold standard in oral surgery and allows complete preservation of the marginal gingiva. The scalpel is aligned with the respective tooth axis and the blade is guided through the sulcus to the *limbus alveolaris* while maintaining constant contact with the tooth or root surface. The marginal and sulcular epithelium is preserved at the flap margin.

In the marginal incision (Figs 4-4 and 4-5), the incision is perpendicular to the mar-

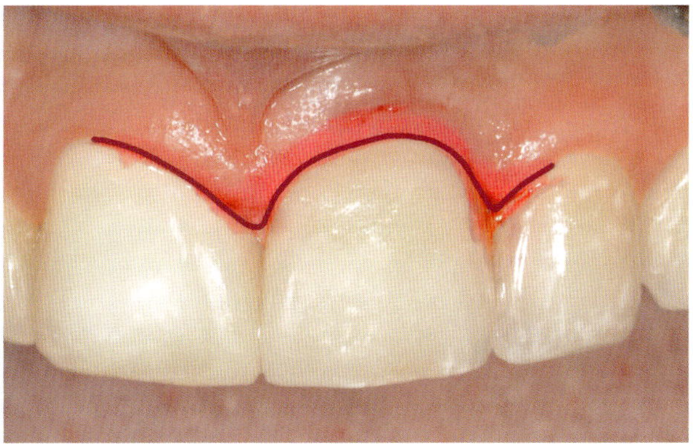

Fig 4-2 Intrasulcular incision in region 11 to 22 in the case of imminent sequestrectomy (condition after anterior tooth trauma).

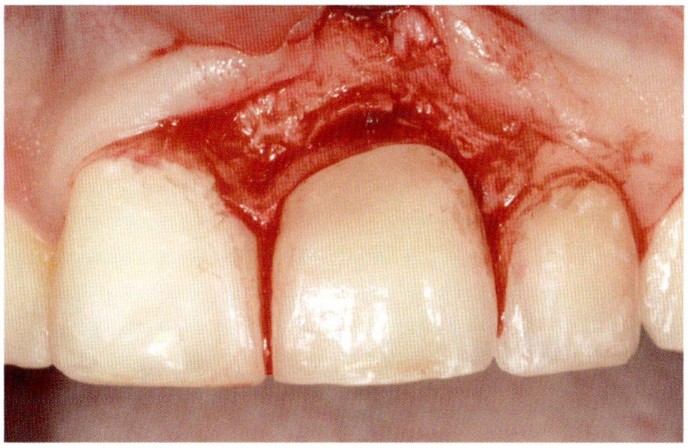

Fig 4-3 Labial bone sequestrum after incision and mobilization of the mucoperiosteal flap (same patient as in Fig 4-2).

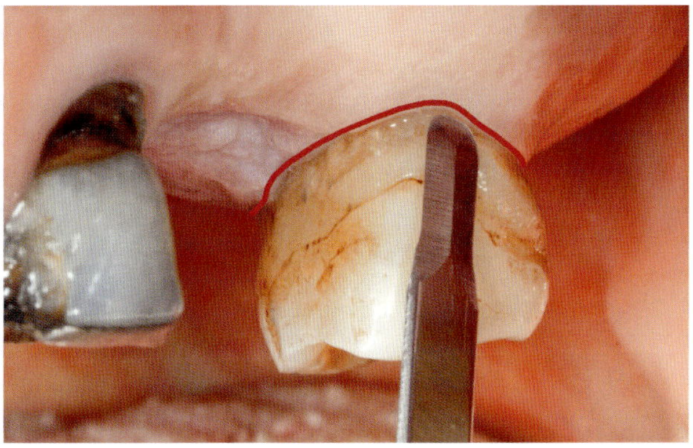

Fig 4-4 Circular marginal incision around tooth 27 that is planned for removal, followed by soft tissue coverage (condition after radiotherapy).

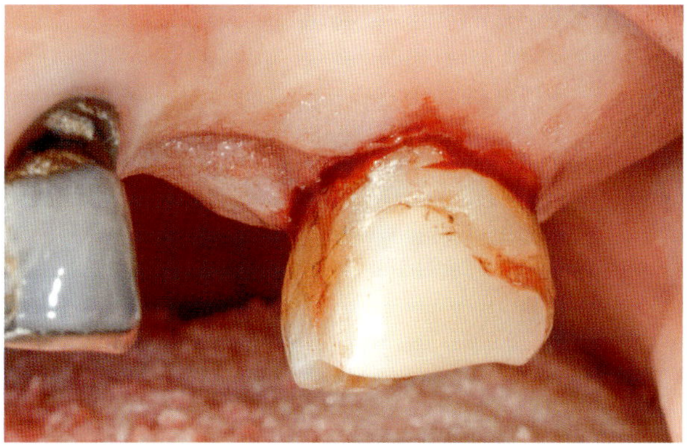

Fig 4-5 Marginal incision followed by removal of tooth 27 and formation of a trapezoidal flap for soft tissue coverage (same patient as in Fig 4-4).

ginal gingiva, so that after flap mobilization, the marginal and sulcular epithelium remain on the tooth surface. The flap margins are deepithelialized, which is particularly relevant in the case of soft tissue coverage, as otherwise a meeting of epithelialized wound margins does not lead to primary wound healing and carries the risk of wound dehiscence. If adjacent teeth are included in the incision, it is continued in a garland shape. It should be noted that the incision in the interdental area is guided to the neighboring tooth, and the blade is repositioned from there.

The paramarginal incision (Figs 4-6 and 4-7, Video 4-1), also called the submarginal incision, also runs in a garland shape approximately in the middle of the keratinized (attached) gingiva. The basic prerequisite is, of course, a sufficiently wide keratinized gingiva of at least 5 mm. In addition, the incision should not be made through a periodontal pocket. A preoperative survey of the probing values is therefore necessary.

The crestal incision is usually located in the center of an edentulous area on the alveolar ridge (Figs 4-8 and 4-9, Video 4-2). This inci-

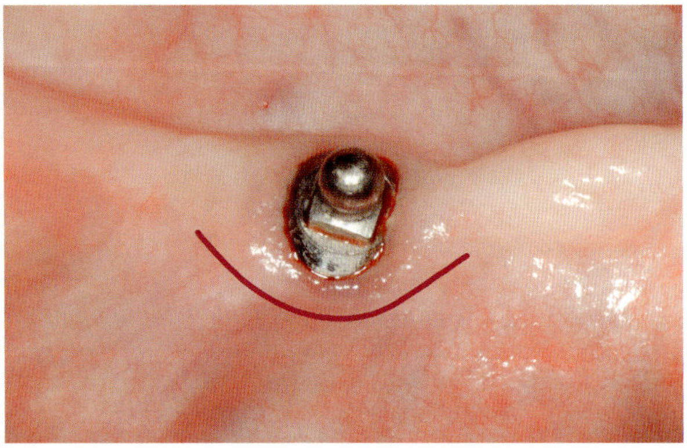

Fig 4-6 Paramarginal incision labial to the implant in region 43.

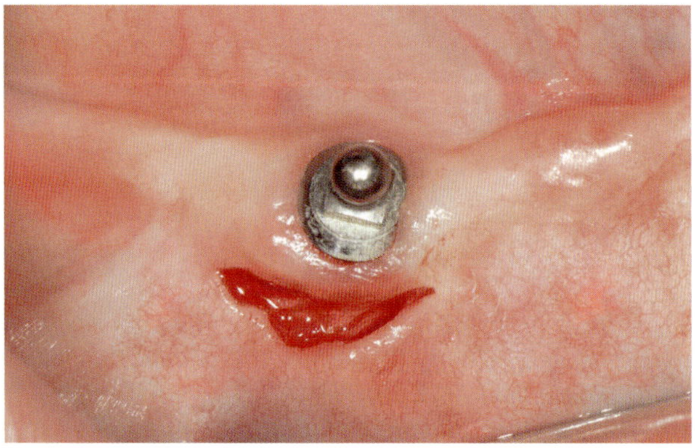

Fig 4-7 After incision and preparation of the recipient bed for free mucosal graft (same patient as in Fig 4-6).

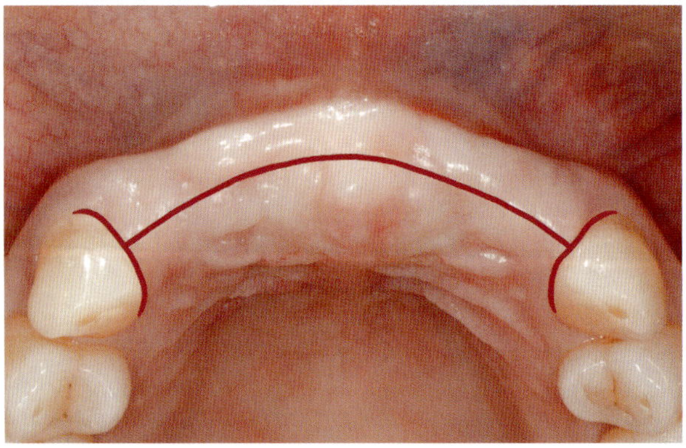

Fig 4-8 Crestal incision in region 12 to 22.

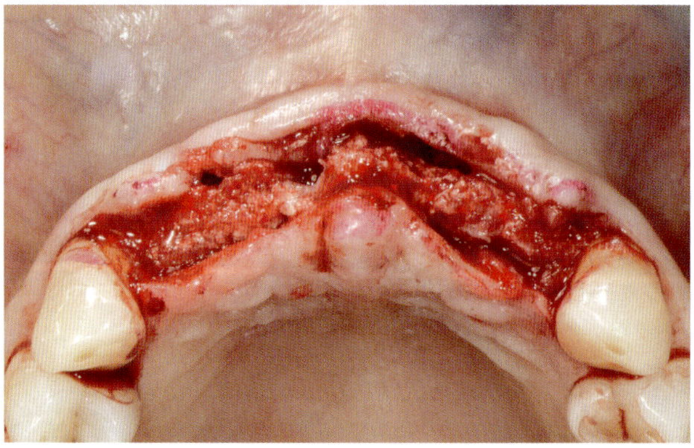

Fig 4-9 After mobilization of the mucoperiosteal flap labially and palatally (same patient as in Fig 4-8).

Video 4-1
Paramarginal incision in combination with a split flap.

Video 4-2
Crestal incision with intrasulcular relief on adjacent teeth.

sion is particularly useful in implantology. If two additional vertical releasing incisions are made after the crestal incision to form a trapezoidal flap, the primary incision must not be located too far orally, otherwise there is an increased risk of wound dehiscence due to the low flap vascularization.

The (intra-)mucosal incision is apical to the mucogingival border in the area of the mobile mucosa (Figs 4-10 and 4-11, Video 4-3). This

Video 4-3 Mucosal incision on right retromolar area for removal of a bone block.

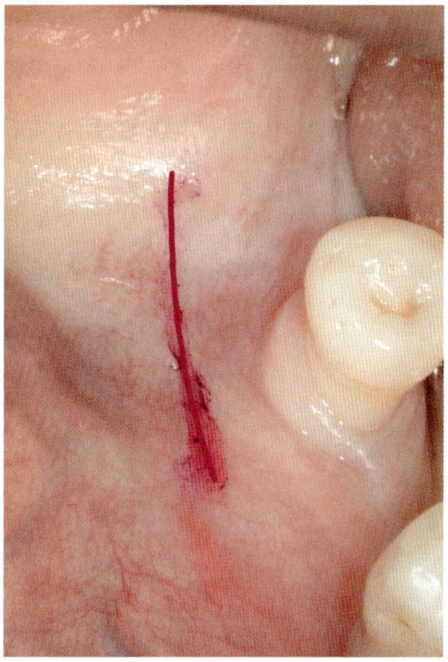

Fig 4-10 Mucosal incision.

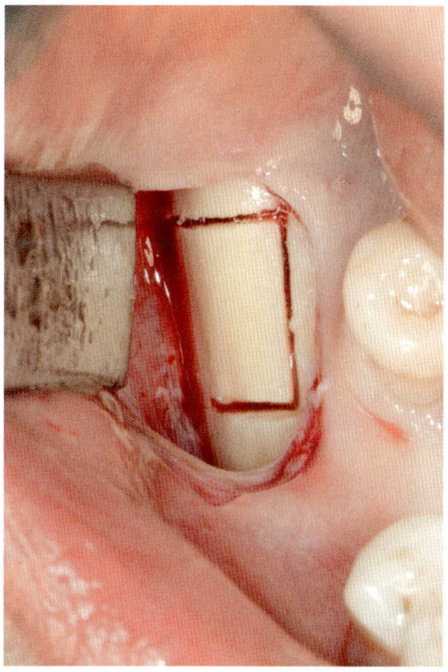

Fig 4-11 After mobilization of the mucoperiosteal flap and formation of predetermined breaking points for bone block harvesting (same patient as in Fig 4-10).

type of incision was used in the past, particularly in tooth-preserving surgery for apicoectomy or for open exposure and alignment of impacted teeth: Angle section according to Reinmöller, trapezoidal section modified according to Hauberisser, and arch section modified according to Partsch or Pichler were common here. Today, the (intra-)mucosal incision has hardly any indications, since it often lies over the bony defect in the case of extensive apical pathologies, and also shows wound dehiscence more frequently due to higher flap mobility. In addition, unsightly scar lines are produced.

Releasing incisions

After the primary incision, releasing incisions are often necessary to obtain an adequate view of the surgical area, but also to mobilize and hold the flap without tension. These incisions can be made in a horizontal or vertical direction.

The horizontal releasing incision (Figs 4-12 and 4-13) is simply a continuation of the primary incision already made at the gingival margin in the mesial and/or distal direction. A lateral extension by more than two adjacent teeth is usually not necessary. The advantage of this releasing incision is that vertical relief can be dispensed with and apically located anatomical structures, such as nerves and blood vessels, are thus spared.

In the vertical releasing incision (Figs 4-14 and 4-15), the incision is made from apical, usually in the region of the adjacent tooth, to mesial and/or distal of the primary incision (triangular flap and trapezoidal flap). Within the attached gingiva, however, the incision is angled so that it is perpendicular to the marginal gingiva. If this is not taken into account, pointed flap margins and possibly unsightly retractions at the gingival margin will result postoperatively. To minimize the risk of postoperative recession, the releasing incision should end in the mesial or distal third of the gingival margin of a tooth, and never median or at the lowest point of the gingival margin or even interdentally through the papilla. If an apically or coronally advanced flap is planned as part of a periodontal surgical procedure, the vertical releasing incision can also be designed in a C-shape, with the advantage that the flap can be more easily adapted later, and, above all, without tension. In general, the

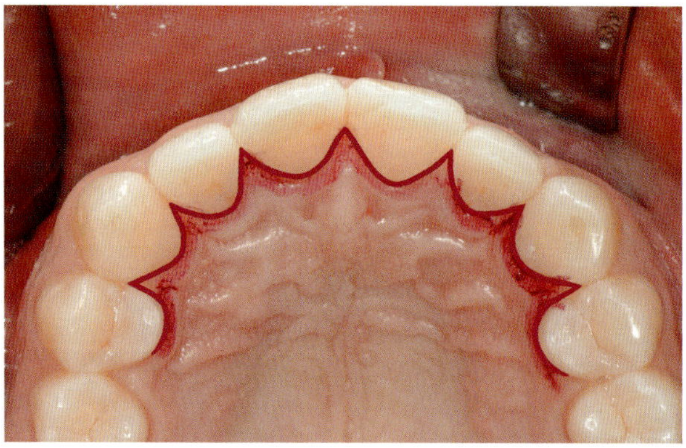

Fig 4-12 After intrasulcular horizontal releasing incision in the palatal region 14 to 24 during a cystectomy.

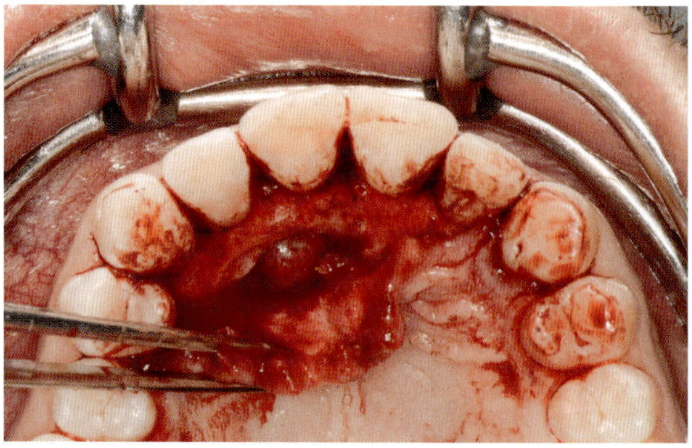

Fig 4-13 After preparation of the mucoperiosteal flap and visualization of the cyst bellows (same patient as in Fig 4-12).

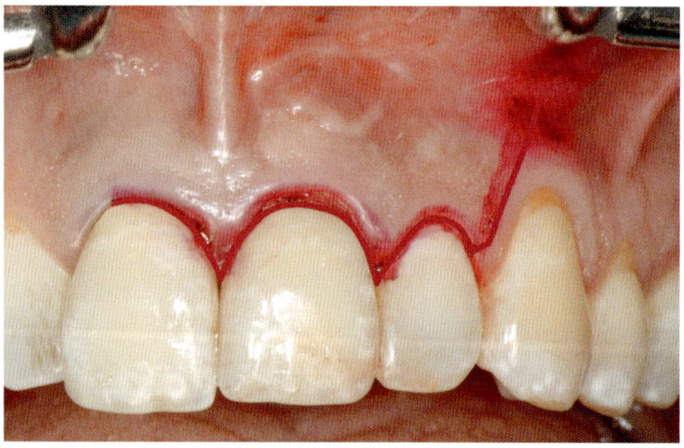

Fig 4-14 Intrasulcular incision starting from the distal third of tooth 11 to the distal third of tooth 22 with a vertical releasing incision (apical region 21 shows scar lines from a past mucosal incision; condition after apicectomy).

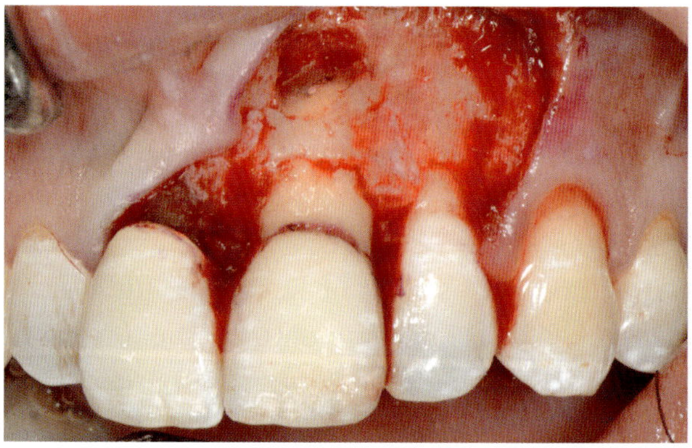

Fig 4-15 After mobilization of the mucoperiosteal flap and defect visualization for the upcoming revision of the retrograde root canal filling, including post resection of root apex 21 (same patient as in Fig 4-14).

major advantage of a vertical releasing incision over a horizontal one is that the widening of the surgical approach is localized.

Incisions in the esthetic region

Especially in the esthetic region in patients with a high smile line, recessions and unsightly scarring of the gingiva resulting from incorrect incision guides are unforgivable. Today, however, there is some predictability as to which incision pattern carries which postoperative recession risk. The intrasulcular incision (Fig 4-16) shows an average recession of 0.42 mm after 1 year, while the paramarginal incision (Fig 4-17) shows only 0.05 mm. No recessions were observed in the papilla base incision (Fig 4-18) within 1 year[4]. In general, changes in the periodontium due to incisions are expected mainly in the first year, after which the periodontal situation stabilizes over

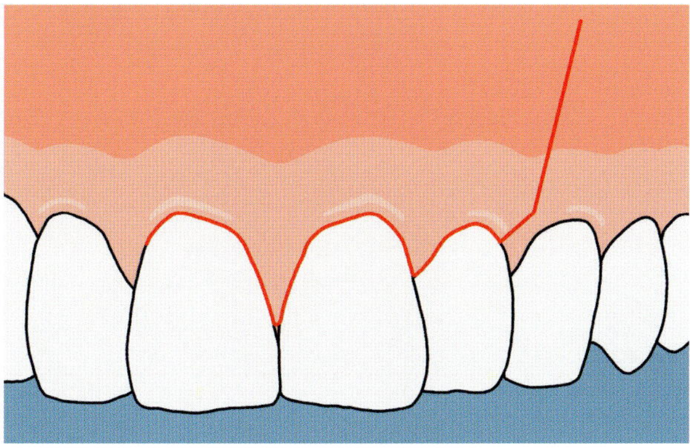

Fig 4-16 Intrasulcular primary incision with vertical relief in a triangular flap.

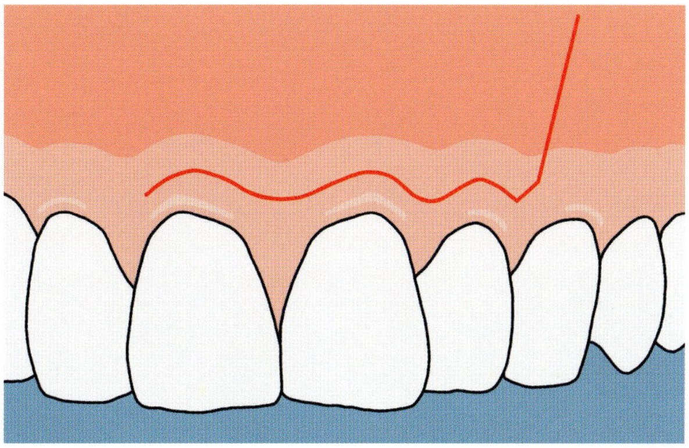

Fig 4-17 Paramarginal primary incision with vertical relief in a triangular flap.

an observation period of 5 years[3]. Even though recessions are less frequent and more discrete after a paramarginal incision, this incision often leaves unsightly scars that are exposed during laughter. Therefore, the papilla base incision is to be preferred in the esthetic region.

However, in addition to the incision route, the pressure during flap mobilization through the raspatory on the marginal bone, the exposure time of the bone (45 to 90 minutes), and the dehydration of the flap also play a decisive role[1,2].

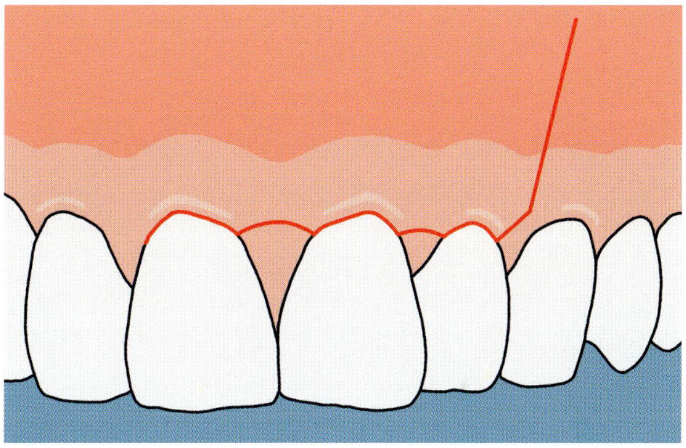

Fig 4-18 Papillary base incision as the primary incision with vertical relief in a triangular flap.

Abscess incisions

Submucosal abscesses due to acute exacerbation of infection must be incised and drained as part of emergency treatment. The location and direction of the incision must be carefully considered so that further oral surgery with flap formation is possible after the acute infection at the incision site has subsided. Therefore, horizontal incisions at the future base of the flap should be avoided because they negatively affect flap vascularization.

Primarily, vestibular submucosal abscesses in the maxilla should rather be opened via a vertical incision in the area of the future incision of a flap and palatally via an intrasulcular incision (Figs 4-19 and 4-20). If the incision site is not directly at the abscess, a blunt preparation with a raspatory must be prepared with constant bone contact up to the abscess, and the abscess spread. However, palatal abscesses are more frequently located medially and are poorly accessible for blunt preparation due to the curvature of the *palatum durum*, so that in these cases (para-)marginal incisions or those at the

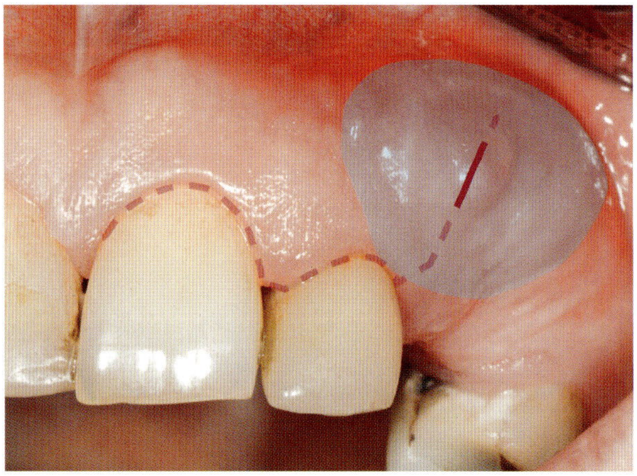

Fig 4-19 Submucosal abscess (marked here in red) starting from tooth 22, with the vertical incision in the area of the future incision guide in the case of flap formation.

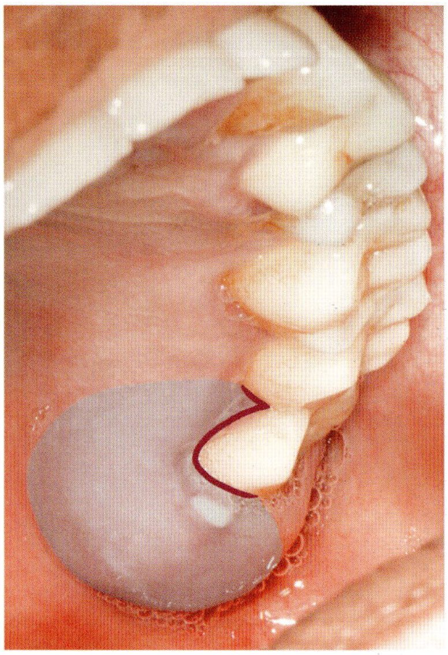

Fig 4-20 Intrasulcular abscess incision in the case of a palatally located submucosal abscess (marked here in red) starting from tooth 28.

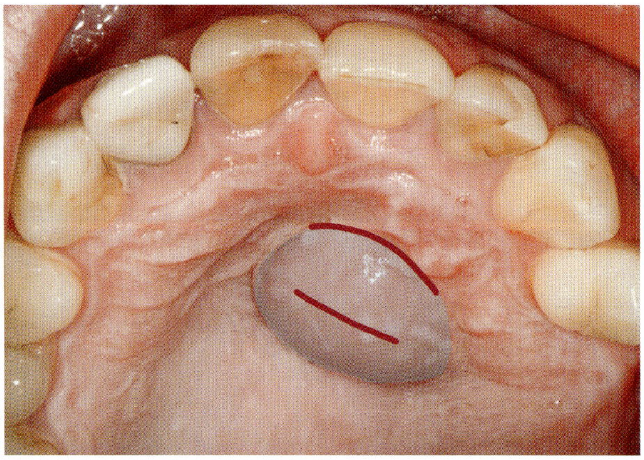

Fig 4-21 In exceptional cases, a poorly accessible abscess in the palatal region (marked here in red) can be opened by a marginal incision or at the *punctum maximum*, taking the palatal artery into consideration.

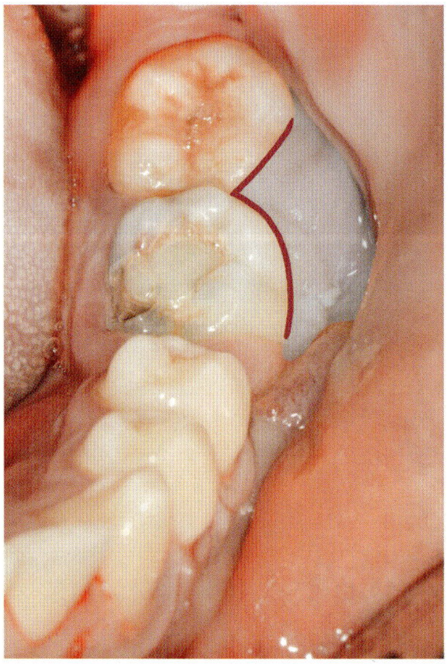

Fig 4-22 Paramandibular abscess (marked here in red) starting from tooth 36, showing the intrasulcular incision.

punctum maximum are permissible (Fig 4-21). The course of the palatal artery must be taken into account. If necessary, the future incision site can be punctured with a cannula to exclude a possible crossing of the incision with the palatine artery.

In the mandible, intrasulcular incisions are generally preferred in order to avoid blood vessels and nerves in the area of the mental foramen and the floor of the mouth, as well as the mimic musculature at the mentum (Fig 4-22). Again, the abscess is ultimately opened by blunt preparation with a raspatory via an intrasulcular incision (Fig 4-22).

After opening and spreading the abscess, the interior is irrigated with antiseptic until clear

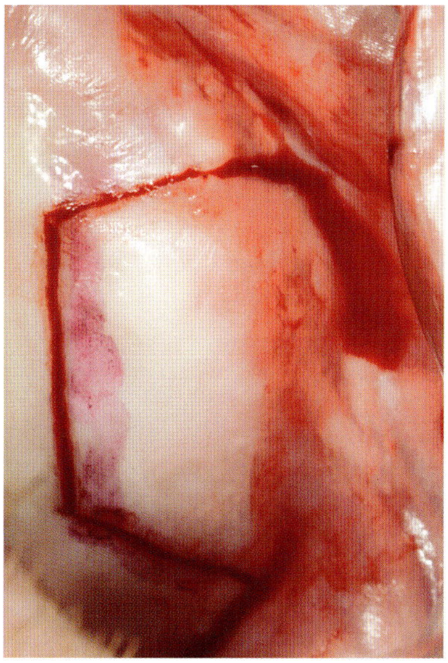

Fig 4-23 Trapezoidal mucoperiosteal flap after incision.

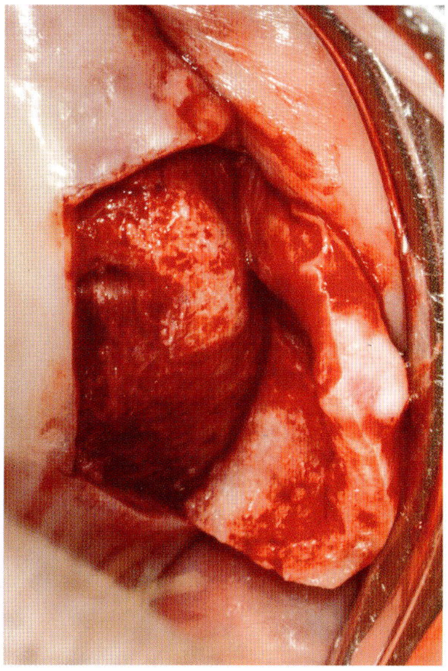

Fig 4-24 After detaching the mucoperiosteal flap from its bony base.

reflux is visible. This is followed by the insertion of a drain. Here, silicone tubes can be fixed with a suture, or iodoform/vaselinated cotton strips can be inserted to ensure postoperative pus drainage. After incision, an odontogenic focus must be treated promptly. In the case of submucosal abscesses with a tendency to spread (pronounced extraoral swelling, reduced jaw opening, pressure pain at the angle of the jaw or eye, reduced general condition, difficulty swallowing or fever) or with a general medical indication, adjuvant systemic antibiotic administration is recommended (usually amoxicillin with clavulanic acid, or clindamycin in the case of penicillin allergy). The first control should take place on the following day. The procedure of the local antiseptic measure, including drainage change if a cotton strip has been inserted, is repeated daily until there is no more leakage of pus.

Soft tissue flaps and mobilization techniques

In most oral surgical procedures, the surgical approach is via a soft tissue flap. Flaps are named according to their tissue composition (mucoperiosteal flap, mucosal flap), their future location (apically, coronally or laterally advanced flap), and their shape (trapezoidal flap, triangular flap).

In the mucoperiosteal flap, also called the full flap, the entire soft tissue, which consists of epithelium, subepithelial connective tissue, and periosteum, is detached from the bony support with a raspatory (Figs 4-23 and 4-24). This is facilitated if the incisions defining the flap overlap slightly so that the flap can be detached cleanly. If there is only one vertical releasing incision laterally of the primary incision, the flap is a triangular flap; if there are two vertical releasing incisions, the flap is a trapezoidal flap. In the case of a trapezoidal flap, care should be taken to ensure a sufficiently wide flap base so that sufficient flap vascularization is guaranteed postoperatively. With regard to the blood supply, the following applies: In the maxilla, vascularization takes place from cranial to caudal and in the mandible from distal to mesial. If scars are already present at the future flap base, a more generous extension of the flap is indicated.

After incision, the mucoperiosteal flap is carefully lifted from the bony base with only a lit-

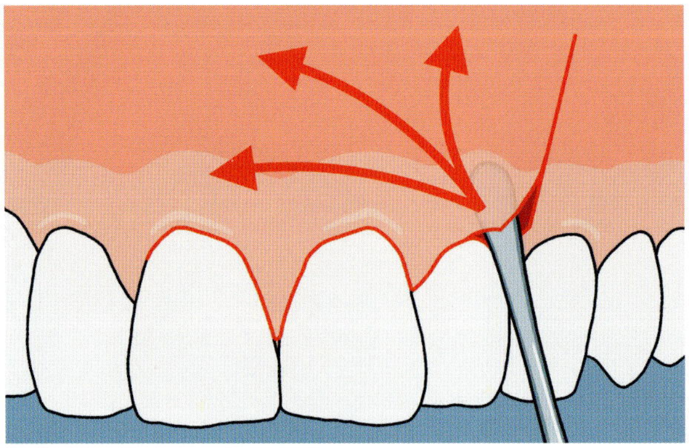

Fig 4-25 Instrument pressure that is directly applied on the marginal attachment damages the bone and the periodontium.

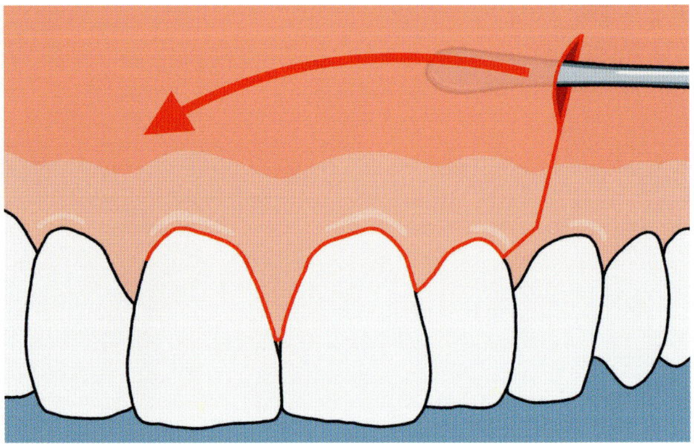

Fig 4-26 Mobilization is initially performed by tunneling preparation apical to the mucogingival margin.

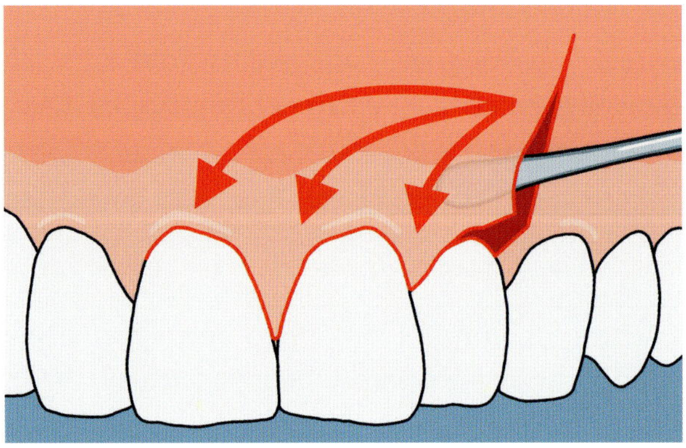

Fig 4-27 Only secondarily is the attached gingiva mobilized from the mucogingival border toward the sulcus.

tle pressure at the corners using a fine raspatory, then mobilized apically (Fig 4-25). The sharp working end of the raspatory should always be directed toward the bone. Tearing or bruising of the soft tissue should be avoided because it leads to more pronounced swelling and pain postoperatively. In addition, too much pressure from the instrument on the marginal bone causes recessions. Therefore, especially in the esthetic region, it is recommended to mobilize the flap by a tunneling technique, from lateroapical to the mucogingival border to coronal to the sulcus (Figs 4-26 and 4-27)[1].

The advantage of the mucoperiosteal flap is that the flap is very well vascularized due to the periosteum. However, detachment of the periosteum from its bony support results in some resorption of the alveolar bone.

The mucosal flap, also called the partial flap or the split flap, consists only of epithelium and subepithelial connective tissue of the mucosa. Residual portions of the subepithelial

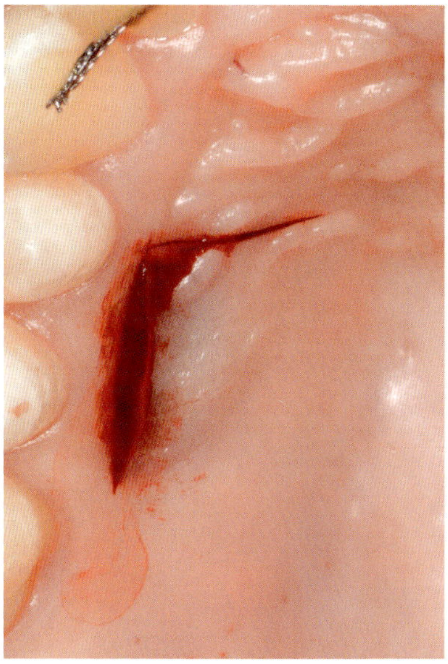

Fig 4-28 Triangular mucosal flap after incision.

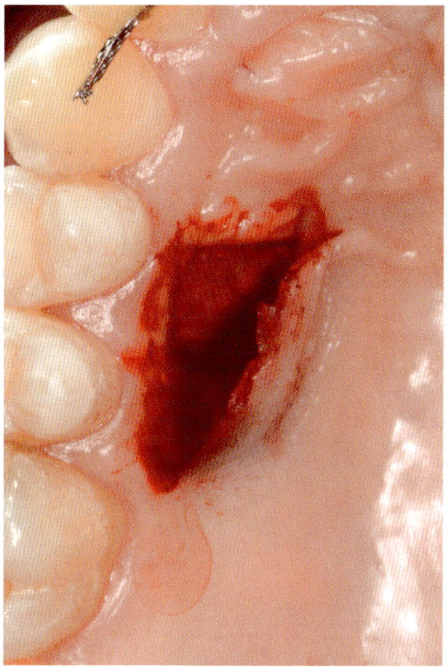

Fig 4-29 After sharp preparation of the mucosal flap.

connective tissue and the periosteum remain on the bone surface. Thus, the mucosal flap is thinner and somewhat less well vascularized than the mucoperiosteal flap. The preparation in this case is sharp, performed ideally with a microscalpel (Figs 4-28 and 4-29). Perforations must be avoided in the process. The greatest danger is in the region of the mucogingival border, where the mucosa is often very thin and frequently a bony prominence is present at the same time. The minimum flap thickness should not be less than 1 mm, otherwise the flap will no longer be sufficiently vascularized and there will be a risk of flap necrosis. This splitting technique is not easy, especially for beginners, and should therefore be learned at the beginning on a porcine jaw.

The great advantage of the mucosal flap is that the lack of periosteum ensures greater flap mobility. This enables tension-free wound closure, especially in the case of advanced flaps (apically, coronally or laterally). However, the mucosal flap can also be used to harvest a connective tissue graft.

References

1. Harrison JW, Jurosky KA. Wound healing in the tissues of the periodontium following periradicular surgery. J Endod 1991;17:425–435.
2. Levin MP, Grower MF, Cutright DE, Getter L. The effects of length of surgery on healing of full and partial thickness flaps. J Oral Pathol 1977;6:152–160.
3. Von Arx T, Alsaeed M, Salvi GE. Five-year changes in periodontal parameters after apical surgery. J Endod 2011;37:910–918.
4. Von Arx T, Vinzens-Majaniemi T, Bürgin W, Jensen SS. Changes of periodontal parameters following apical surgery: a prospective clinical study of three incision techniques. Int Endod J 2007;40:959–969.

Preoperative clarification

5

Jochen Jackowski, Hendrik Zeiß, Korbinian Benz

Medical law

All physicians come into contact with various areas of law during the course of their professional activity. In Germany, **medical professional law** regulates, among other things, access to the medical profession and the professional duties of physicians. It is part of **public law**.

Social law formulates the legal regulations governing the relationship between physicians and statutory health insurance funds, including the self-administration of physicians.

The **relationship** between the physician and the patient is assigned to civil law. Every medical treatment is based on an explicit or implicit treatment contract. The **German Civil Code (BGB)** contains regulations on the conclusion of such a contract and the resulting obligations. Particular attention must be paid to the physician's duty of care. This concerns both the actual treatment and the patient's information and documentation. Claims for damages by the patient may be based on a breach of the physician's duty of care.

In the course of professional practice, the physician also comes into contact with criminal law. As a rule, most physicians are not aware of this. **Criminal law** deals, in particular, with the potential realization of the criminal offences of bodily injury as a result of medical intervention and failure to render assistance on the basis of special medical skills.

All of the following statements are based on German legislation.

Duty of care

The physician's general duty of care is defined in **Section 630a (2) BGB**:

(2) Treatment shall be provided in accordance with generally accepted professional standards existing at the time of treatment, unless otherwise agreed.

The physician owes the patient appropriate treatment, i.e. medical activity, but not the desired result, i.e. the healing of the patient. A treatment is appropriate if it meets the **specialist standard**, which is a measure of medical care and provides information about the behavior that can be expected of a conscientious and attentive physician during therapy in the specific treatment situation from the professional point of view of that physician's specialty. It represents the respective state of scientific knowledge and medical experience that is necessary to achieve the medical treatment goal and has proven itself through testing (BGH NJW-RR 2014, 1053, 1054).

The state of knowledge of medical science is determined by:

- Guidelines of the medical societies and the German Medical Association,
- Guidelines of the professional societies,
- Recommendations,
- Experts in the respective fields.

Self-determination and information

In the context of information in the medical field, a distinction is made between intervention information (also self-determination information), therapeutic information (also security information), and economic information.

Intervention information

Self-determination information is linked to the patient's personal right to decide whether or not to consent to a medical intervention. Its high significance in daily practice results from the fact that, in principle, every medical intervention – even those carried out completely *lege artis* – violates the physical integrity of the patient. This is of relevance under criminal law and gives rise to civil liability on the part of the physician (BGH NJW 1989, 1538, 1540; BGH NJW 1987, 1481, 1481), which only ceases to apply if the patient effectively consented to the procedure before it was performed. In this regard, **Section 630d (1) Sentence 1 BGB** states:

> *(1) Before carrying out a medical measure, in particular an intervention in relation to the body or health of the patient, the person treating the patient is obliged to obtain the patient's consent.*

The essential element of self-determination information arises from the understanding of the relationship between the physician and the patient. Based on the patient's **right to self-determination**, patients have the right to know what they are suffering from and what therapeutic strategy the physician is pursuing to alleviate their suffering. Of great importance in this context is the **duty of physicians** to inform patients, because only patients who have been informed carefully and in detail can give their self-determined consent to a medical intervention. Consent given by a patient is invalid if the patient was not informed or if the information provided was inadequate. **Section 630d (2) BGB** establishes this connection between consent and information:

> *(2) The validity of consent requires that the patient or, in the case of Paragraph 1 Sentence 2, the person entitled to consent, has been informed prior to consent in accordance with Section 630e Paragraphs 1 to 4.*

Following this understanding, **Section 630e (1) BGB** stipulates:

> *(1) The person providing treatment is obliged to inform the patient of all circumstances essential to consent. This includes, in particular, the nature, scope, implementation, expected consequences, and risks of the measure as well as its necessity, urgency, suitability, and prospects of success with regard to the diagnosis or therapy. The information must also refer to alternatives to the measure if several medically equally indicated and customary methods can lead to substantially different burdens, risks or chances of recovery.*

The types of self-determination information developed by case law were taken up by the legislator even before the introduction of the Patients' Rights Act as part of the German Civil Code, namely diagnostic information, progress information, and risk information. Despite the legal regulation, this categorization is not obsolete, because it shows the physician the necessary steps of the clarification. However, the three types of information mentioned here cannot be clearly distinguished from one another, and there may be overlaps with therapy/security information.

Diagnostic information

The patient must be informed of the medical findings by the physician as part of the diagnostic clarification. Patients must be told that they are ill and what disease they are suffering from. The diagnostic information includes the probable consequences of the disease and the urgency of therapy. In individual cases, it may be necessary to provide only limited information or none at all to a patient suffering from an incurable, fatal disease. The physician must not burden a patient with uncertain suspected diagnoses.

Progress information

In the progress clarification, the type, scope, and execution of the planned intervention are explained to the patient in detail. According to the established case law of the **Federal Court of Justice (BGH)**, patients must know, on the whole, what they are consenting to. Patients must be informed of the risks of the intervention that are not entirely outside the realm of probability, insofar as these are not apparent to a medical layperson anyway from the nature of the intervention and may be of significance to their decision making. The task of the informing physician is to give the patient a general idea of the severity of the intervention with its specific risks. These must neither be glossed over nor aggravated (BGH NJW 2019, 1283, 1284).

The particular known consequences of an intervention must be mentioned. Both temporary (e.g. hematoma formation, pain) and permanent (e.g. the creation of a gap after tooth removal, scarring, functional impairment) consequences must be presented.

In the area of intersection between information on the course of the procedure and information on the risks, the patient is provided with information on the **prospects of success** of the planned therapy and on possible **treatment alternatives**, which also include a possible decision not to undergo the procedure. This part of the clarification is particularly emphasized in **Section 630e (1) Sentence 2 BGB**. In particular, in the case of a relative indication for surgery, the patient must be informed that surgery may be avoidable by conservative treatment (OLG Hamm VersR 2011, 625) or that several options for care are available with significantly different physical and psychologic demands on the patient or different risks and prospects of success (OLG Hamm, MedR 2018, 409, 411).

Risk information

The degree of risk disclosure depends on the urgency of the surgical intervention. Stricter standards apply to interventions for diagnostic purposes than to urgent procedures that may be necessary to save lives. In any case, however, risk disclosure requires informing the patient about the complications and side effects of the intervention that can be expected according to medical knowledge, as well as the risk of failure. The greater the risk of failure, significant complications or deterioration of the patient's state of health, the more detailed the information must be for the patient about the planned intervention and possible alternatives (BGH NJW 1988, 1514, 1515; BGH NJW 1981, 633, 633).

The patient must be informed about the essential risks of an intervention even if there is no therapeutic alternative to the planned intervention. Even in the case of a vital indication for an intervention, the patient's right to self-determination requires that the physician leave the patient the option of deciding independently about the intervention and refusing an intervention, if necessary, even if such a decision is medically unreasonable (BGH NJW 1994, 799, 800; BGH judgment of 28.11.1957, 4 StR 525/57).

Information must be provided about the specific risks of an intervention. This also includes rarely occurring complications if these are associated with significant consequences for the patient. For example, the risk of osteomyelitis must be explained prior to wisdom tooth removal (BGH NJW-RR 2003, 1606, 1606).

Execution of the information

Section 630e (2) to (5) BGB deals with the question of how information must be provided:

(2) The information must

1. be given verbally by the person providing treatment or by a person who has the necessary training to carry out the measure; in addition, reference may also be made to documents that the patient receives in text form,

2. be given in sufficient time to enable the patient to make a considered decision on consent,

3. be understandable to the patient. Copies of documents signed by the patient in connection with the information or consent must be given to the patient.

(3) The patient does not need to be informed if this is exceptionally unnecessary due to special circumstances, in particular if the measure cannot be postponed or the patient has expressly waived the right to information.

(4) If the consent of an authorized person is to be obtained in accordance with Section 630d (1) Sentence 2, this person must be informed in accordance with Paragraphs 1 to 3.

(5) In the case of Section 630d (1) Sentence 2, the essential circumstances in accordance with (1) must also be explained to patients in accordance with their understanding, insofar as they are capable of receiving the explanation due to their level of development and ability to understand, and insofar as this is not contrary to their best interests. Paragraph 3 applies accordingly.

This gives rise to the following points for the physician to consider in the context of patient clarification:

1. Who must provide the information?

As a matter of principle, the patient must be informed by the person providing treatment as defined by the law, i.e. by the patient's contractual partner. The provider of a medical facility must ensure that the physician providing the information is sufficiently professionally qualified and that proper information is thus provided. Even a physician who is still in training but who has appropriate theoretical knowledge is considered professionally qualified. The physician responsible for the planned therapy must be satisfied that the patient has been properly informed before the procedure is performed.

2. Who must be informed?

An informed consent always refers to the person who has to consent to the intervention. If patients have reached the age of majority, they are informed themselves, whereas in the case of minors, both parents must always be involved in this process. The use of an interpreter may be necessary in the case of foreigners. In the case of a patient who is incapable of giving consent, **Section 630d (1) Sentence 2 BGB** determines the addressee of the information:

(1) (...) If the patient is incapable of giving consent, the consent of a person authorized to do so must be obtained, unless a living will pursuant to Section 1901a (1) Sentence 1 permits or prohibits the measure. Further requirements for consent under other regulations remain unaffected. If consent cannot be obtained in time for a measure that cannot be postponed, it may be performed without consent if it corresponds to the patient's presumed will.

Section 630e (4) and (5) BGB additionally stipulate that the beneficiary must be informed in the same way as a patient who is capable of giving consent. Patients who are incapable of giving consent must be informed themselves within the scope of their ability to understand.

3. When must information be provided?

To ensure that the patient's right to self-determination is protected, information must be provided in good time so that the patient has sufficient time to weigh up the pros and cons of the intervention (BGH NJW 1994, 3010, 3010). The more serious the intervention, the sooner the patient must be informed. In the case of elective surgery under inpatient conditions, an explanatory discussion should be held with the patient as soon as the date of the procedure is agreed. Otherwise, in the case of inpatient procedures, it is usually sufficient to provide information on the day before the procedure, whereby the term "day" must be taken literally and the information must be provided by around 5:00 pm. As a rule, information on the evening before the intervention or on the day of the intervention itself is not sufficient (BGH NJW 1998, 2734, 2734). In the case of outpatient and diagnostic procedures, information on the day of the procedure is generally sufficient. In this case, there should be at least one hour between the information and the intervention so that the patient can reach a decision in a self-determined manner. Clarification only on the operating table is not sufficient (BGH NJW 2000, 1784, 1787).

4. How must the patient be informed?

In a personal physician–patient consultation, the patient is informed verbally. The patient has the option of asking questions. According to the Patients' Rights Act, written (text) documentation is not required. However, the documentation requirements pertaining to the information have been considerably increased by the legislator. In the case of an exclusively verbal explanation, it was previously in the physician's own interest to document this in the medical record in case of requiring it as evidence at a later date. Now, **Section 630f (2) BGB** expressly stipulates that, among other things, **"explanations and consents" must be included in the patient's file**. If reference is made to documents to support the explanation (e.g. schematic diagrams of the planned operation), **Section 630e (2) Sentence 1 (1) BGB** stipulates that these must be provided to the patient in text form. The term "text form" refers to **Section 126b BGB**, which requires the use of a text document that clearly shows who the issuer is, and which is concluded by a signature (including facsimile) or in some other way. If such documents are used to accompany an explanation, they must be handed over to the patient. It is sufficient to hand over an identical duplicate. **If, however, the patient signs the document, then Section 630e P (2) Sentence 2 BGB stipulates that a copy of it has to be provided to the patient!**

The following therefore applies to the **routine use** of text information in daily practice: The use of text information is still recommended, even if the Federal Court of Justice is critical of it (see BGH NJW 1985, 1399). The Federal Court of Justice has always tried to ensure that information is provided in a personal discussion between the physician and the patient, and that it is not limited to the handing out of text information (BGH NJW 1994, 793). The requirement for verbal information is standardized by law. In difficult cases, the discussion should be conducted with witnesses and in any case documented in the patient's file. The patient should be given the text information before the discussion about informed consent, because it may result in a so-called **question burden** on the patient (cf. BGH, NJW 2000, 1784). However, this will only be the case if the patient has had the opportunity to read the text information carefully before the consultation. Afterwards, the physician should inform the patient in a clarification discussion with the help of graphic representations. It is advisable to individualize the text information with handwritten notes, underlining, providing additions, etc, during the consultation. After the patient and the physician have signed the Declaration of Consent (Fig 5-1) form, a complete and legible copy must be made and given to the patient.

Consequences of omitted or incorrect information

Failure to provide information or incorrect information does not in itself give rise to civil liability on the part of the treating physician. Treatment carried out without effective consent only gives rise to liability if it has resulted in damage to the patient's health (BGH NJW 2008, 2344, 2345). However, the performance of an indicated and *lege artis* surgical intervention is sufficient for this (BGH NJW 1987, 1481, 1481).

The accusation of omitted or faulty information and thus of ineffective consent thus becomes a 'lifeline' for a patient who does not succeed in proving a concrete treatment error on the part of the physician. In this way, the physician's liability is still to be justified because, from the patient's point of view, the desired healing success did not occur, or other complications occurred that are not accepted as inevitable. Therefore, all physicians should inform their patients as comprehensively as possible and document this in a provable manner in order to counteract the aforementioned argument. According to **Section 630h (2) BGB**, the burden of proof for a proper explanation of the procedure lies with the practitioner.

(2) The practitioner must prove that consent has been obtained in accordance with Section 630d and that information has been provided in accordance with the requirements of Section 630e. If the information provided does not meet the requirements of Section 630e, the practitioner may plead that the patient would have consented to the procedure even if the information had been provided properly.

If the practitioner is unable to prove this, the patient's **hypothetical consent** can still be invoked. To do this, the practitioner must explain why the patient would have consented to the procedure even if the patient had been properly informed (severity of the illness, prognosis of success). The patient may plead that, had proper information been provided by the practitioner, the patient would have had a genuine decision-making conflict, from which a refusal of the therapy appears understandable (BGH NJW 1991, 1543; BGH NJW 1991, 2344; BGH NJW 1982, 700). In court proceedings, the patient should be heard by the court in person on this point (BGH NJW 2005, 1364; BGH NJW 1990, 2928).

Withdrawal of consent

After a patient has effectively consented to a procedure on the basis of proper informed consent, the patient may revoke the consent that was given at any time. This is expressly regulated in **Section 630b (3) BGB**:

(3) Consent may be revoked informally at any time and without giving reasons.

Declaration of consent for dental surgical procedures

Patient: ________________________________ Patient no.: _______________

The following procedure is to be performed on me:
____
____
____
Special findings (e.g. hepatitis, HIV, etc): ______________________________
Medications: ______________________________

I have had the opportunity for a detailed discussion with: ____________________________
Name of surgeon

I was informed of the following risks:

- Success rate of root tip resection O
- Wound healing disturbance (swelling, pain, postoperative bleeding) O
- Opening of the maxillary sinus O
- Sensitivity disturbances in the area of treatment O
  - Inferior alveolar nerve O
  - Lingual nerve O
  - Mental nerve O
- Risk of jaw fracture O
- Damage to neighboring teeth and tooth germs O
- Other risks ______________________________ O

Furthermore, we would like to draw your attention to the fact that in very rare cases, injuries to the inferior alveolar nerve, lingual nerve, and mental nerve can occur during a conduction anesthesia.

After local anesthesia, the ability to react and thus the ability to drive is significantly reduced!

The tissue from the surgical area is usually submitted for histopathologic examination.

Pathology institution: ____

I have no further questions.

________________________ ____
Date Signature of patient or legal representative

Fig 5-1 Documentation of preoperative information and patient consent.

Of course, the patient's right only applies before the procedure is performed or, in the case of ongoing treatment measures, for the future. Subsequent revocation of consent cannot deprive the patient of the justifying basis for the intervention.

Therapeutic information

Therapeutic information must be distinguished from intervention information. While the latter serves as the basis for the patient's effective consent to treatment, the former is part of the physician's duty to treat. In the context of therapeutic information, the physician is obliged to inform the patient about all circumstances that are necessary to ensure the success of the treatment, and to ensure that the patient behaves appropriately (BGH VersR 2005, 227, 228) (recommendations for carrying out check-ups, advice on appropriate lifestyle, information on medication).

With the Patients' Rights Act, **Section 630c (2) BGB** established the obligation of the practitioner to provide therapeutic information:

> *(2) The treating party is obliged to explain to the patient in an understandable manner at the beginning of the treatment and, if necessary, in its course, all circumstances essential for the treatment, in particular the diagnosis, the probable health development, the therapy, and the measures to be taken at and after the therapy.*

A breach of this duty can lead directly to civil liability on the part of the physician if it can be proven that damage to the patient's health is causally attributable to the breach of duty. A breach of the duty to provide therapeutic information may also constitute a gross treatment error. This is particularly the case if the patient is threatened by considerable damage as a result of the failure to provide information (BGH NJW 2005, 427; BGH NJW 1989, 2318).

Economic information

The physician is also obliged to provide the patient with economic information. **Section 630c (3) and (4) BGB** regulate this:

> *(3) If the treating party knows that a complete assumption of the treatment costs by a third party is not ensured or if there are sufficient indications for this according to the circumstances, the treating physician must inform the patient in writing about the probable costs of the treatment before the beginning of the treatment. Further formal requirements from other regulations remain unaffected.*

> *(4) The patient does not need to be informed if this is exceptionally unnecessary due to special circumstances, in particular if the treatment cannot be postponed or the patient has expressly waived the right to information.*

This statutory provision is primarily due to the fact that, in Germany, the vast majority of the population has statutory health insurance and assumes that medical treatment is not associated with costs that must be borne directly by the patient. Patients entitled to benefits and privately insured patients also assume that they do not have to pay the costs of treatment 'from their own pocket' because they are fully reimbursed by their respective insurers. On the basis of **Section 630c (3) BGB**, it is urgently recommended that every patient be informed of the anticipated costs of therapy if it is not entirely certain that the costs will be covered by a third party. This applies without exception to private patients or self-paying patients because a possible obligation to pay the treatment costs by a third party is never certain.

Documentation

The **duty of documentation** is another component of the physician's duty of care. Even before the Patients' Rights Act, it was established case law that **detailed, careful, and complete documentation** of medical treatment/surgery is one of the physician's essential duties to the patient. The documentation is at the same time a professional obligation according to **Section 6 MBO-Z** (Musterberufsordnung-Zahnärzte) and partly even a legal obligation (e.g. in Section 43 StrlSchVO, Section 29 (2) RöntgVO, Section 19 ArbStoffVO, Section 37 (3) JarbSchG). **Section 630f BGB** now contains the following regulations:

(1) The treating party is obliged to keep a patient file in paper format or electronically for the purpose of documentation in direct temporal connection with the treatment. Corrections and changes to entries in the patient file are only permissible if, in addition to the original content, it remains recognizable when they were made. This must also be ensured for patient records kept electronically.

(2) The attending physician is obliged to record in the patient file all measures and their results which, from a professional point of view, are essential for the current and future treatment, in particular the medical history, diagnoses, examinations, examination results, findings, therapies and their effects, interventions and their effects, consents, and explanations. Physician's letters shall be included in the patient file.

(3) The treating physician shall keep the patient file for a period of ten years after completion of the treatment unless other retention periods exist according to other regulations.

The purpose of the documentation is to safeguard **therapy, accountability, and preservation of evidence**. In terms of content, the documentation must cover **anamnesis, diagnosis, and therapy**. In the context of preserving evidence, the **documentation of the clarification and the operation report** should be emphasized, in particular.

The question of whether a medical treatment error has occurred is primarily assessed on the basis of the documented course of treatment. For this reason, case law places high demands on the **format of medical documentation**, which must be clear to the specialist. It is not required that documentation be comprehensible to the layperson. Likewise, it is also inadvisable to use documentation that lacks punctuation, is difficult to read or is written by a dental assistant. However, the more careful the documentation, the greater its evidential value. However, the documentation must be submitted in direct chronological connection with the treatment or procedure. Subsequent corrections or additions are permissible, provided that the content and time of the change and the original documentation are recognizable.

A breach of the documentation obligation may give rise to a claim for damages by the patient for the costs of an unnecessarily performed duplicate examination. In addition, missing or incomplete documentation may result in a reduction of the burden of proof in favor of the patient pursuant to **Section 630h (3) BGB**.

Criminal law relevance of medical conduct

Bodily injury

Injury to the body of another is punishable by law. The **Criminal Code (StGB)** contains a number of provisions **(Sections 223 to 229 StGB)** for the various degrees of this criminal liability.

However, this does not mean that every physician has 'one foot in jail' when carrying out medical activities. In addition to the objective facts, punishment for bodily injury requires unlawful and culpable action. The bodily injury is not unlawful if there is **effective consent** of the patient to the medical intervention. Civil law principles apply to the question of whether the patient has given effective consent. Effective consent and thus **proper patient information** are thus doubly relevant, so to speak; on the one hand for civil liability and on the other for criminal liability.

If there is no effective consent due to lack of proper information, the intervention may possibly be justified by assuming **hypothetical consent**. The prerequisite for this is that the patient would have consented to the intervention even in the case of not having been properly informed.

If the patient is not in a position to consent to the medical intervention, for example, because the patient is suffering from dementia, **presumed consent** may be considered as a justification. For the assumption of presumed consent, the individual, hypothetical will of the patient must be determined.

If there is a lack of effective consent, it must still be determined in criminal law terms whether the physician also acted **culpably**. The Criminal Code distinguishes between intentional and negligent bodily injury. An **intentional bodily injury** may be present if the physician acts against the express will of the patient. This is the case, for example, if there is no effective consent and the physician knows full well that the patient does not want the intervention. Only in the case of intentional bodily injury do the so-called qualifications known to the Criminal Code come into consideration, for example, dangerous bodily injury or bodily injury resulting in death.

Negligent bodily injury requires that physicians disregard the care to which they are obligated according to the circumstances and their personal abilities. The accusation of negligence may relate to the intervention itself, but also to the consent.

Glossary

ArbStoffVO	Ordinance on Working Substances
BGB	German Civil Code
BGH	Federal Court of Justice
JarbSchG	Youth Employment Protection Act
MedR	Medical Law
NJW	New Legal Weekly
NJW-RR	Rechtssprechungs-Report Civil Law
OLG	Higher Regional Court
RöntgVO	Radiograph Ordinance
StGB	Criminal Code
StrlSchVO	Radiation Protection Ordinance
VersR	Insurance Law

Preoperative radiographic diagnostics

6

Dorothea Dagassan-Berndt

X-rays are ionizing rays that can potentially cause tissue damage. Due to this, the prior justification of every radiographic exposure is necessary. There are three stages in the indication process:

- Stage 1 involves the basic justification of radiographic exposure for medical purposes,
- Stage 2 involves justification with respect to general diagnostic or therapeutic procedures,
- Stage 3 involves individual application (Swiss Radiation Protection Ordinance Art. 27–29).

Overview

There are several radiology techniques utilized for the imaging of dental hard tissue, including:

- intraoral (periapical, bitewing or occlusal) radiographs,
- panoramic radiographs,
- skull radiographs, and
- cone beam computed tomography (CBCT).

Compared with general radiology, the radiation exposure of these procedures is relatively low and mainly qualifies as low dose. As it does for all radiographs, the principle of ALARA (As Low As Reasonably Achievable)[7] also applies to dental radiology. Accordingly, the procedure that results in the lowest radiation dose for the patient for the existing problem should always be selected. In addition, the existence of previous radiographic images should be ascertained in order to avoid the unnecessary duplication of radiographic images.

The basic principle for all oral surgery procedures is that correct and complete imaging should be carried out of all the tissue to be treated, including all the relevant neighboring structures. Distortion-free images are fundamental to provide an adequate view of patients' anatomy in order to meet the requirements of patient assessment, diagnostics, treatment planning, and the management of risks in oral surgery.

There is a risk of projection-related distortions with periapical, bitewing or occlusal intraoral radiographs, and they are usually too small for sufficient imaging of the entire surgical site and the relevant neighboring structures (Fig 6-1). In the case of a small surgical area, an orthogonal imaging technique should be implemented in order to capture the anatomical structures with as little distortion as possible.

In general, the panoramic radiograph provides a good "standardized" overview of all relevant structures and is the most common type of radiograph used prior to oral surgery. This two-dimensional (2D) image is low dose (approximately 4 to 75 mSv), has relatively good resolution (approximately 5 to 9 LP/mm), and is relatively inexpensive[6,8]. For the taking of a panoramic radiograph, the ideal position of the patient's head is predetermined and can be said to be standardized. In addition to providing a complete view of the anatomy of the dentoalveolar region, the panoramic radiograph provides insight into the neighboring anatomical structures and is able to show calcifications in the region of the soft tissue. Soft tissue calcifications can be visualized in approximately 4% to 6% of cases[2,3,14,18]. These usually correspond to findings such as calcifications of the styloid or stylomandibular ligament complex as well as arteriosclerotic calcifications, tonsilloliths or sialoliths[2,18]. The detection of cervical calcifications is understood to be an important contribution to prophylactic diagnostics[5]. For these reasons, all panoramic radiographs indicated for oral surgical procedures should be evaluated in this context.

Since its introduction about 20 years ago[1,15], CBCT has been an established procedure for visualizing special positional relationships of anatomical structures or pathologies in three dimensions. CBCT is used for surgical plan-

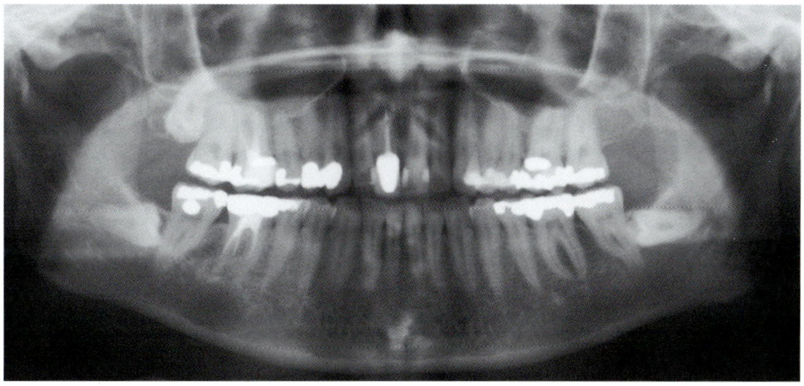

Fig 6-1 Radicular cyst apical to region 46: This would not be completely depicted, or even at all, on an intraoral radiograph.

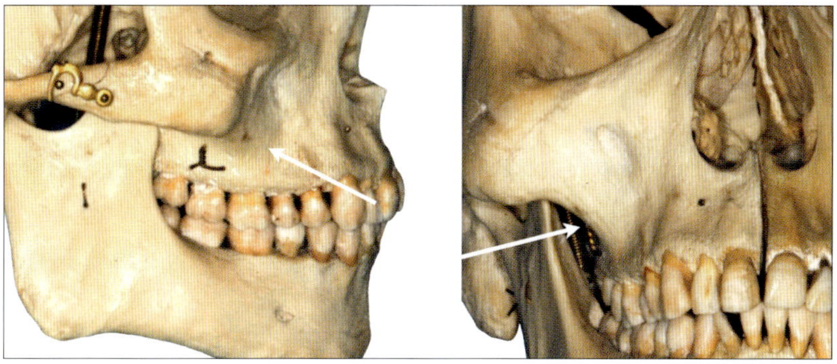

Fig 6-2 Anatomy of the inserting zygomatic arch in the maxillary posterior region.

ning in selected cases and helps significantly to inform about specific risk situations. A volume size that is adapted to the specific problem, the selection of appropriate setting parameters, and good availability make CBCT an important imaging technology for use in oral surgery.

Application

Preoperative radiographic diagnostics depends on the planned procedure. For simple tooth removals, the entire tooth with the adjacent anatomical structures should be completely imaged. In the maxillary posterior region, intraoral radiographs present the challenge of superimposition with portions of the zygomatic arch inset on the facial wall of the maxillary sinus (Fig 6-2). This often overlaps with the root tips of the maxillary first and (occasionally) second molars, making diagnosis difficult due to the strong summation effect. Alternatively, an eccentric image can be taken of this area; however, this could result in a detrimental distortion of the structures. For these reasons, a panoramic radiograph may be more suitable than a periapical, bitewing or occlusal intraoral radiograph.

Where the roots of a maxillary tooth are close to the maxillary sinus, it is important to be able to assess the condition of the maxillary sinus without any doubt before oral surgery takes place (Figs 6-3 and 6-4). The subsequent therapy in the event of a possible maxillary sinus opening (immediate closure vs maxillary sinus irrigation with secondary closure) must be clearly evident from the preoperative radiograph.

Surgical tooth removals require imaging of the entire surgical area in addition to imaging of the tooth. In the mandible, the course of the mandibular canal must be clearly shown on the radiograph. The caudal border of the mandibular canal is more frequently mineralized and is therefore easier to visualize than the cranial border[9] (Fig 6-5).

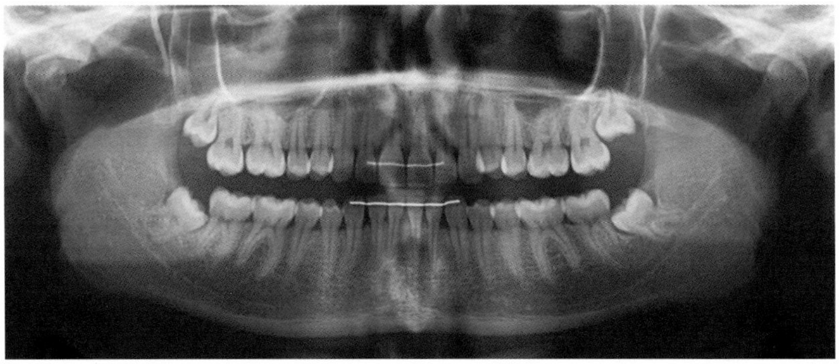

Fig 6-3 Condition of the maxillary sinus before surgical removal of the maxillary third molars: Shadowing of the maxillary right sinus in maxillary sinusitis.

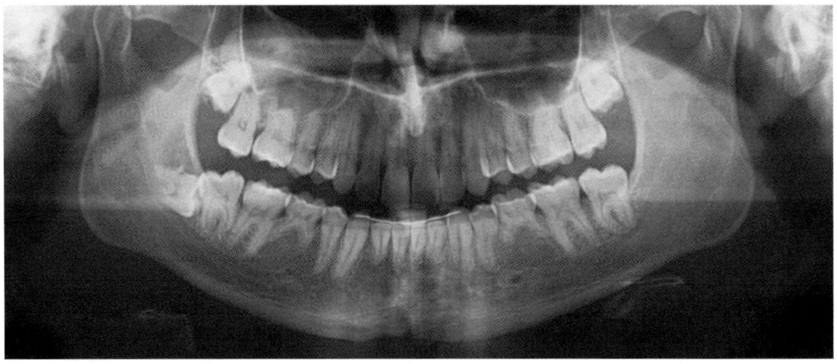

Fig 6-4 Shadowing of the maxillary right sinus in the presence of a pseudocyst.

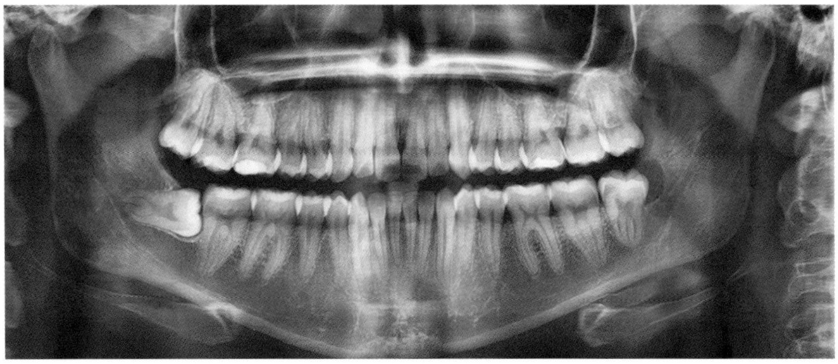

Fig 6-5 The caudal border of the mandibular canal is more visible than the cranial border.

Surgical wisdom tooth removal requires radiographic evaluation with complete visualization of the tooth as well as the relevant surrounding anatomical structures[10]. Further three-dimensional (3D) radiographic diagnostics is only indicated when conventional 2D radiographs shows evidence of a direct positional relationship to structures at risk, or where pathologic changes are present. In addition, it is indicated when the practitioner requires further spatial information in terms of risk assessment, intervention planning, or for intraoperative orientation[10].

Indications of such a risk situation are, in particular[4]:

- Overlapping of the wisdom tooth root tips with the mandibular canal (Figs 6-6 and 6-7),
- Deflection or interruption of the cortical line of the mandibular canal in the immediate vicinity of the root tip (Figs 6-8 and 6-9),
- Darkening of one or more roots,
- Pathologic changes (cysts, resorption phenomena on adjacent teeth).

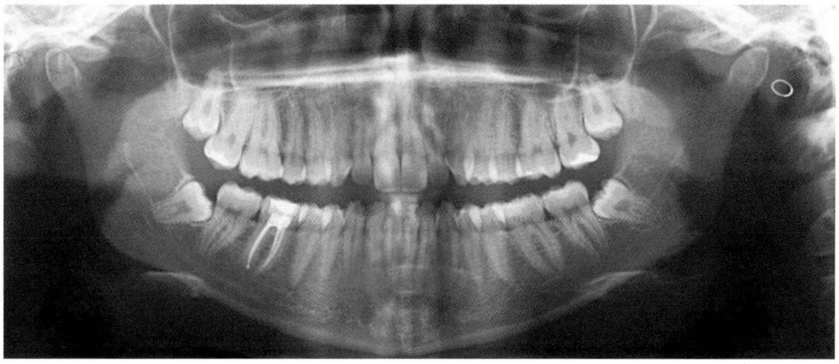

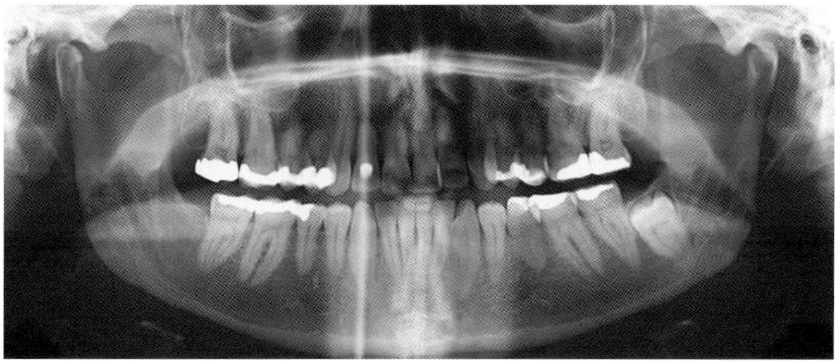

Figs 6-6 and 6-7 Overlay of root tips with the mandibular canal.

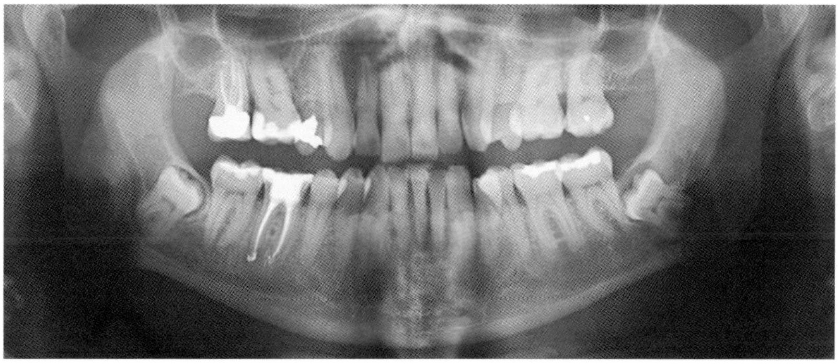

Fig 6-8 Deflection of the mandibular canal.

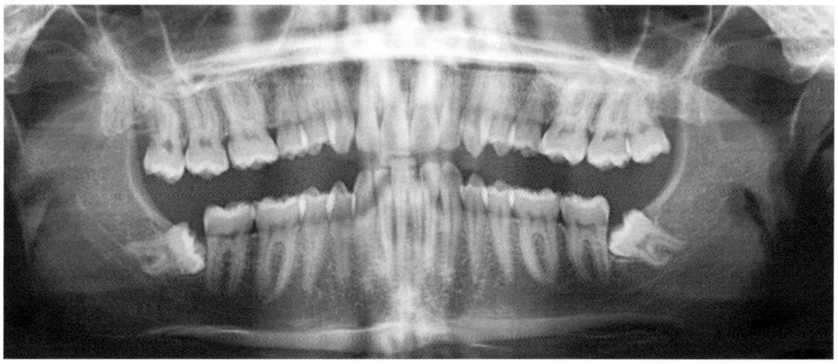

Fig 6-9 Interruption of the white line in the immediate vicinity of the root tip.

Resorptions by wisdom teeth on neighboring second molars are only insufficiently visualized on panoramic radiographs (Fig 6-10). Horizontally displaced wisdom teeth and marginal bone resorption at the distal root surface of the second molar are indications of possible resorptions[13], which according to the current literature have an approximate frequency of 20%[15-17]. In a

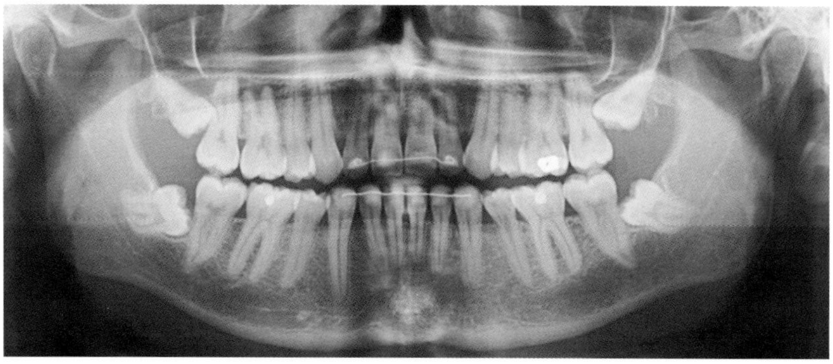

Fig 6-10 Panoramic radiograph: Mandibular wisdom teeth with suspected resorption on the neighboring teeth.

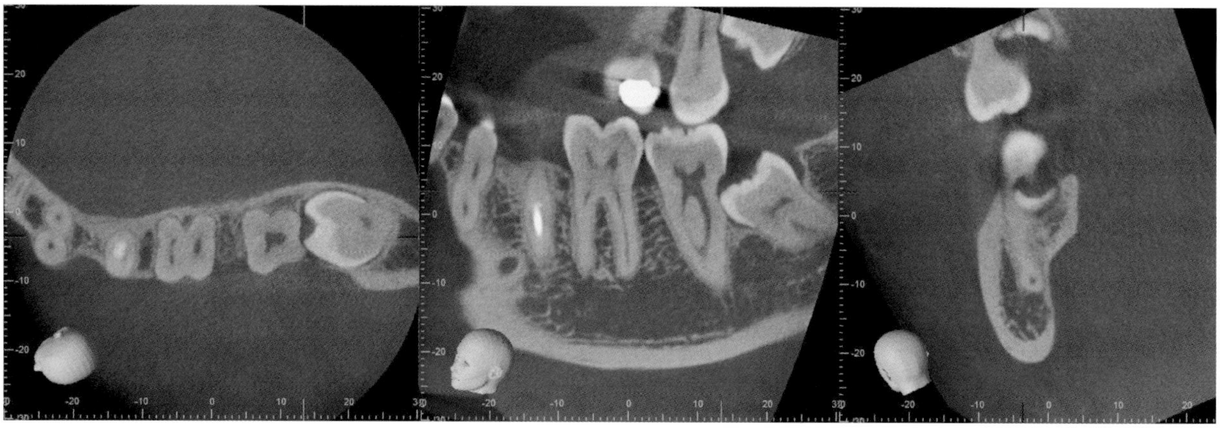

Fig 6-11 CBCT of the mandibular left region 38 with resorption at neighboring tooth 37.

panoramic radiograph, the basal portions of the maxillary sinus are visualized, which allows an assessment of these structures with regard to most pathologic findings[16,17,19].

In special cases, diagnosis by means of CBCT is necessary because an accurate assessment of some situations, such as the aeration situation over the *ostium naturale*, cannot be made on a 2D image (Fig 6-11).

In summary, panoramic radiography is the most frequently used radiographic technique in oral surgery. However, special anatomical or pathologic conditions may require the use of CBCT to aid preoperative diagnostics.

References

1. Arai Y, Tammisalo E, Iwai K, Hashimoto K, Shinoda K. Development of a compact computed tomograohic apparatus for dental use. Dentomaxillofac Radiol 1999;28:245–248.
2. Ariayi AS, Berndt D, Lambrecht JT. Weichgewebskalzifikationen auf der Panoramaschichtaufnahme. Schweiz Monatsschr Zahnmed 2009;119:1009–1013.
3. Baumann-Bhalla S, Meier RM, Burow A, et al. Erkennung von Kalzifikationen der Arteria carotis auf der Panoramaschichtaufnahme zur Prävention cerebrovaskulärer Insulte. Schweiz Monatsschr Zahnmed 2012;122:1023–1029.
4. Dula K, Bornstein MM, Buser D, et al. SADMFR Guidelines for the use of cone-beam computed tomography/digital volume tomography. Swiss Dent J 2014;124:1170–1183.
5. Friedlander AH, Garrett NR, Chin EE, Baker JD. Ultrasonographic confirmation of carotid artery artheromas diagnosed via panoramic radiography. J Am Dent Assoc 2005;136:635–640.

6. Granlund C, Thilander-Klang A, Ylhan B, Lofthag-Hansen S, Ekkestubbe A, Ylhan Lofthag-Hansen E. Absorbed organ and effective doses form digital intra-oral and panoramic radiography applying the ICRP 103 recommendations for effective dose estimations. Br J Radiol 2016;89:20151052.
7. ICRP. Recommendation of the International Commission on Radiological Protection. ICRP Publication 26, Oxford: Pergamon Press, 1977.
8. Kadesjö N, Lynds R, Nilsson M, Shi XQ. Radiation dose from X-ray examinations of impacted canines: Cone beam CT vs two-dimensional imaging. Dentomaxillofac Radiol 2018;47:20170305.
9. Kubilius M, Kubilius R, Vrinauskas V, Zalinkevicius R, Tözuüm T, Joudzbalys G. Descriptive study of manidbular canal visibility. morphometric and densitometric analysis for digital panoramic radiographs. Dentomaxillofac Radiol 2016;45:20160079.
10. Kunkel M, Fritz U, Pistner H, et al. S2k-Leitlinie Operative Entfernung von Weisheitszähnen. DGZMK 2019. https://www.dgzmk.de/documents/10165/1373255/007-003_S2k_Weisheitszaehne_Langversion_2019.pdf/9ae672cc-6d7d-411b-9ed1-90652a3dee6b (letzter Zugriff am 11.06.2020).
11. Malina-Altzinger J, Damerau G, Grätz KW, Stadlinger B. Evaluation of the maxillary sinus in panoramic radiography – a comparative study. Int J Implant Dent 2015;17:1–7.
12. Mathew AL, Pai KM, Sholarpurkar AA. Maxillary sinus findings in the elderly: a panoramic radiographic study. J Contemp Dent Pract 2009;10:E041–E048.
13. Matzen L, Schropp L, Spin-Neto R, Wenzel A. Radiographic signs of pathology determining removal of an impacted mandibular third molar assessed in panoramic image or CBCT. Dentomaxillofac Radiol 2016;28:20160330.
14. Monsour OA, Romaniuk K, Hutchings RD. Soft tissue calcifications in differential diagnosis of parities superimposed over the mandible by dental panoramic radiography. Aus Dent J 1991;36:94–101.
15. Mozzo P, Procacci C, Tacconi A, Martini PT, Andreis IA. A new volumetric CT machine for dental imaging based on the cone-beam technique: preliminary results. Eur Radiol 1998;8:1558–1564.
16. Oenning ACC, Melo SLS, Groppo FC, Haiter-Nero F. Mesial inclination of impacted third molars and its propensity to stimulate external root resorption in second molars – a cone-beam computed tomographic evaluation. J Oral Maxillofac Surg 2015;73:379–386.
17. Oenning ACC, Neves FS, Alencar PNB, Prado RF, Groppo FC, Haiter-Nero F. External root resorption of the second molar associated with third molar impaction: comparison of panoramic radiography and cone beam computed tomography. J Oral Maxillofac Surg 2014;72:1444–1455.
18. Ribeiro A, Keat R, Khalid S, et al. Prevalence of calcifications in soft tissue visible on a dental pantomogram. a retrospective analysis. J Stomatol Oral Maxillofac Surg 2018;119: 369–374.
19. Wang D, He X, Wang Y, et al. External root resorption of the second molar associated with mesially and horizontally impacted mandibular third molar: evidence from cone beam computed tomography. Clin Oral Invest 2017;21:1335–1342.

Tooth removal techniques

7

Andrea Zürcher

Indications

The indication for the removal of one or more teeth is made considering the medical history as well as the clinical and radiologic findings. This includes:

- Deeply decayed or severely destroyed teeth,
- Persistent complaints or pathologic processes in teeth with *lege artis* endodontic treatment,
- Failure after or contraindication to root tip resection,
- Advanced marginal periodontitis (e.g. teeth with a high degree of looseness or exposed furcation),
- Orthodontic indications (e.g. dental crowding),
- Hyperdontia,
- Non-preservable teeth after dental trauma (e.g. longitudinal fracture),
- Focal restoration prior to immunosuppression/radiotherapy/chemotherapy/antiresorptive drugs,
- Teeth that have caused extensive infection (e.g. lodge abscess),
- Teeth adjacent to tumors.

Contraindications

Absolute contraindications are:

- Acute phase of myocardial infarction,
- Severe heart failure,
- Acute leukemia or agranulocytosis.

Temporary contraindications are:

- Hemorrhagic diatheses (thrombocytopathies, thrombocytopenias, coagulopathies, vascular hemorrhagic diatheses),
- Acute infections (e.g. abscess),
- During radio- or chemotherapy.

Specific risks

- Injury to the surrounding soft tissue,
- Fracture of crowns and roots,
- Fracture of bone lamellae or tuberosity avulsion,
- Maxillary sinus opening,
- Damage to weakened adjacent teeth (e.g. teeth with partial crowns, crowns, fillings, or periodontally diseased teeth),
- Thermal injury caused by rotary instruments,
- Dislocation of teeth or root debris into adjacent structures (e.g. maxillary sinus, soft tissue, lodges),
- Ingestion or aspiration of a tooth or tooth fragments,
- Temporomandibular joint dislocation,
- Mandibular fracture,
- Nerve damage caused by local anesthesia (inferior alveolar nerve/lingual nerve).

Local anesthesia

Depending on the location (maxilla or mandible, anterior or posterior region) as well as the type of removal (simple removal with an elevator or forceps or surgical removal), appropriate conduction and/or infiltration anesthetics are performed (Table 7-1).

Step-by-step clinical procedure

The practitioner must first ensure that the correct tooth is removed. The removal of a tooth can be performed in a sitting or standing position. Generally, the practitioner is on the right side of the patient. For the removal of teeth in the right mandible, the 11 o'clock position has proven to be effective (for right-handed patients).

Table 7-1 Overview of local anesthesia.

Position/tooth	Anesthesia
Maxillary anterior and canine	Infiltration anesthesia labial (for serial extractions, conduction anesthesia – infraorbital nerve) and conduction anesthesia (nasopalatine nerve)
Maxillary premolar	Infiltration anesthesia (buccal and palatal)
Maxillary molar	Infiltration anesthesia (buccal) and conduction anesthesia (greater palatine nerve)
Mandibular anterior and canine	Infiltration anesthesia (labial and lingual)
Mandibular first premolar	Conduction anesthesia (mental nerve), infiltration anesthesia (lingual)
Mandibular second premolar	Conduction anesthesia (inferior alveolar, lingual, and buccal nerve)
Mandibular molar	Conduction anesthesia (inferior alveolar, lingual, and buccal nerve)

The mandible is held in place with the thumb, index finger, and middle finger of the left hand. Removing teeth in the maxilla is performed in the 9 o'clock position. The index finger and thumb stabilize the alveolar process during this procedure.

After checking the effect of the local anesthetic (Fig 7-1), the periodontal fibers are loosened with a periotome or desmotome (Fig 7-2). For a truly minimally invasive removal (e.g. in the course of tooth transplantation), the fibers are sharply cut with a scalpel. Elevators of ascending size are used to mobilize the tooth in the socket. The elevator is advanced in the longitudinal direction of the tooth as deep as possible into the periodontal gap, and protected from slipping with a finger of the other hand. After bone contact with the *limbus alveolaris*, the elevator is carefully rotated with controlled force. This stretches the elastic bony wall of the alveolus, and the tooth begins to loosen. Terminal teeth can often be mobilized and removed with the elevator. If extraction forceps are required to mobilize the tooth, forceps of an appropriate size for the tooth are selected (see Section 2) and applied in the longitudinal axis to the root. The branches of the forceps are advanced as far as possible apically and placed below the cementoenamel junction (Fig 7-3). Tilting and rotating movements are performed with a controlled amount of force. The tilting movements tear through the periodontal fibers and expand the alveolus. Primarily, teeth with a round root cross-section (maxillary anterior teeth and canines; mandibular premolars) are rotated at least initially; teeth with an oval root cross-section or multirooted teeth (maxillary premolars and molars; mandibular anterior teeth, canines, and molars) are tilted from oral to vestibular. Controlled combination movements depending on the bone resistance are advisable. In addition, a slight traction is applied in the direction of the longitudinal axis of the root (Fig 7-4).

Removal of primary teeth

A primary tooth is removed with special primary forceps. Due to the more elastic bone as well as the usually existing resorption of the roots, this is done with less force than in the permanent dentition. To protect the permanent tooth germ, the use of elevators or deep curettage of the alveolus should be avoided.

Removal of anterior teeth

- Maxillary anterior and posterior teeth are primarily removed with rotational movements (Figs 7-1 to 7-4).
- Mandibular anterior teeth are primarily tilted labially and lingually (no rotational movements are made due to the slender oval/dumbbell-shaped roots).

Removal of premolars

- Maxillary premolars are primarily tilted palatally and buccally (first premolars are often multirooted).
- Mandibular premolars are initially loosened using rotational movements, then primarily tilted lingually and buccally.

Removal of molars

- Maxillary molars are tilted palatally and buccally. If the roots are strongly divergent, they are separated with a rotating instrument under water cooling (Y-shaped) and removed individually (Figs 7-5 and 7-6, Video 7-1).
- Mandibular molars are tilted lingually and buccally; first molars are tilted more buccally. If the roots diverge strongly, they are separated (from buccal to lingual) and removed individually (Figs 7-7 and 7-8).

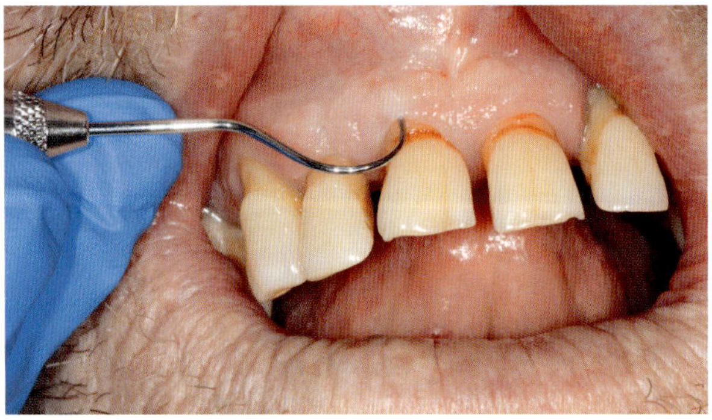

Fig 7-1 Checking the effect of the local anesthetic with a cow horn probe.

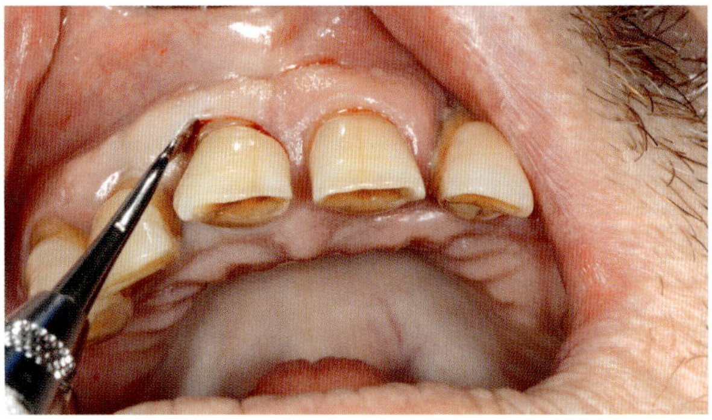

Fig 7-2 Loosening the periodontal fibers with a periotome.

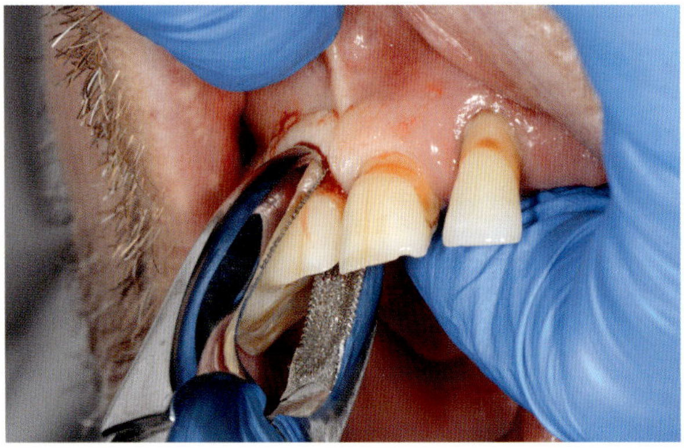

Fig 7-3 Attaching the anterior forceps: The branches of the forceps are placed below the cementoenamel junction.

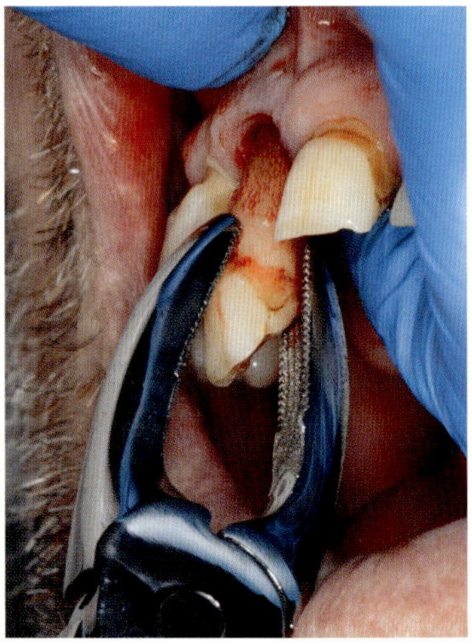

Fig 7-4 Removal of tooth 11 by a rotational movement and traction in the direction of the longitudinal axis.

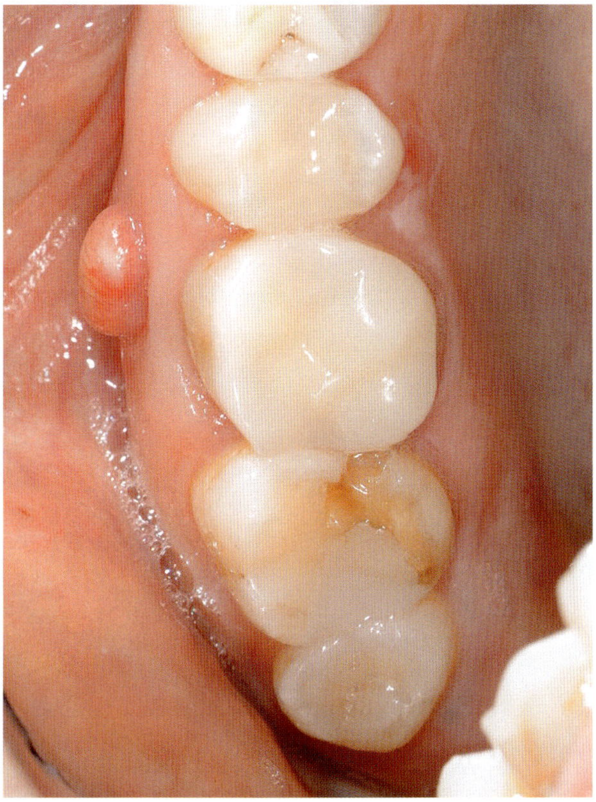

Fig 7-5 Initial situation at region 16.

Video 7-1 Removal of tooth 16 with decapitation and separation.

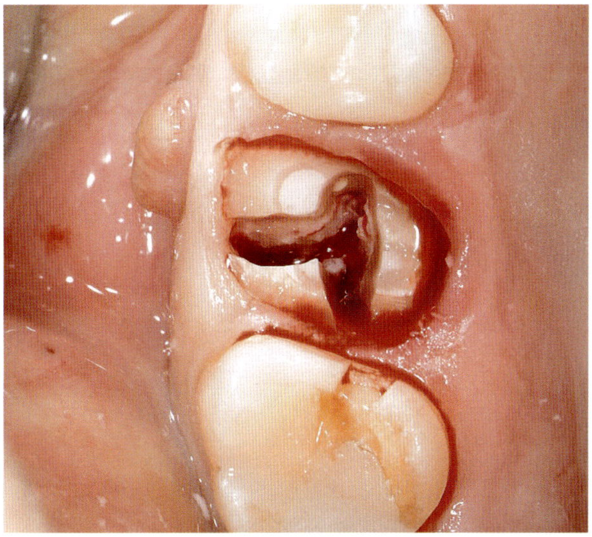

Fig 7-6 After decapitation and Y-shaped separation of the roots.

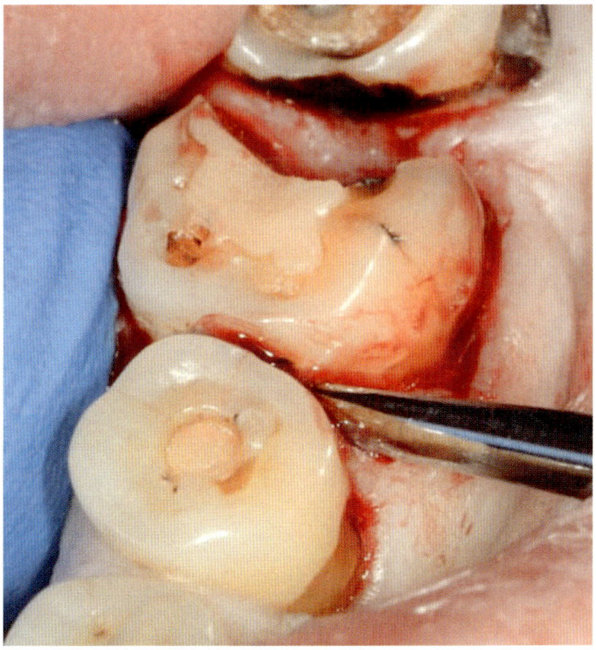

Fig 7-7 Loosening of the tooth with an elevator (under lingual protection with the left index finger).

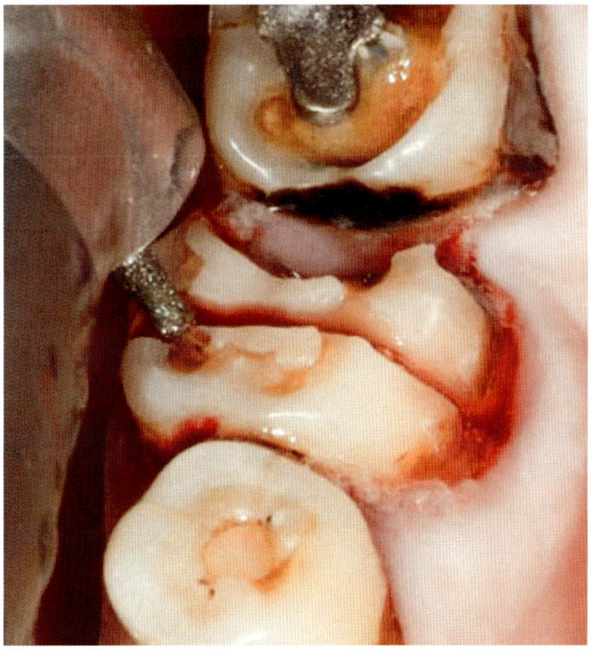

Fig 7-8 Separation of the tooth in a buccolingual direction under cooling with sterile isotonic saline.

Serial extractions

In serial extractions (Figs 7-9 to 7-12), the alveolar walls must be carefully smoothed after tooth removal to avoid sharp bone edges that could later perforate the mucosa during mechanical loading by the prosthesis. Irregular mucosal edges are corrected, and the wound edges are adapted with single-button sutures or the wound area is closed with staggered papilla sutures (Fig 7-12).

Minimally invasive tooth removal

In principle, each tooth should be removed with as little tissue damage as possible. This is not always possible with fractured teeth or root remnants. With the aid of the Benex extraction system (Helmut Zepf Medizintechnik, Tuttlingen, and Hager & Meisinger, Neuss, Germany) (Figs 7-13 to 7-17, Video 7-2), the root remnant can be removed in a vertical direction by applying an axial traction force along its longitu-

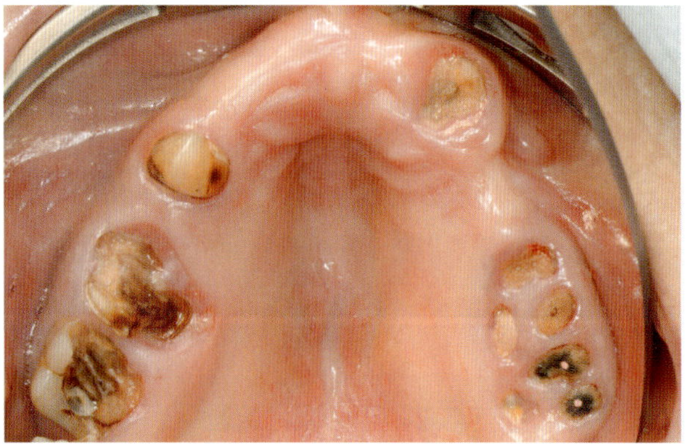

Fig 7-9 Initial clinical situation: Residual teeth in the maxilla that are not worth preserving.

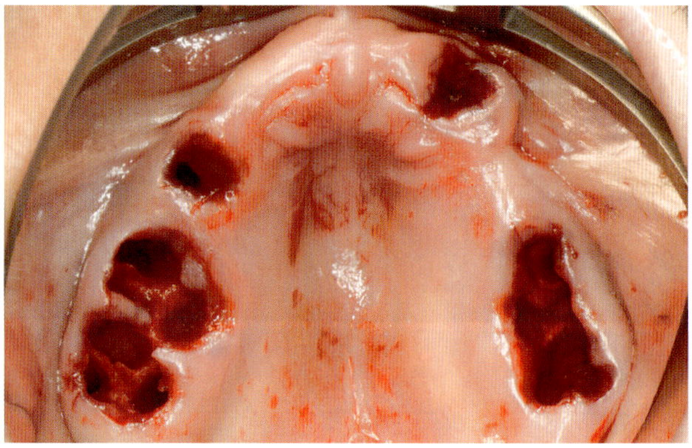

Fig 7-10 After removal of the remaining teeth, the alveoli are inspected.

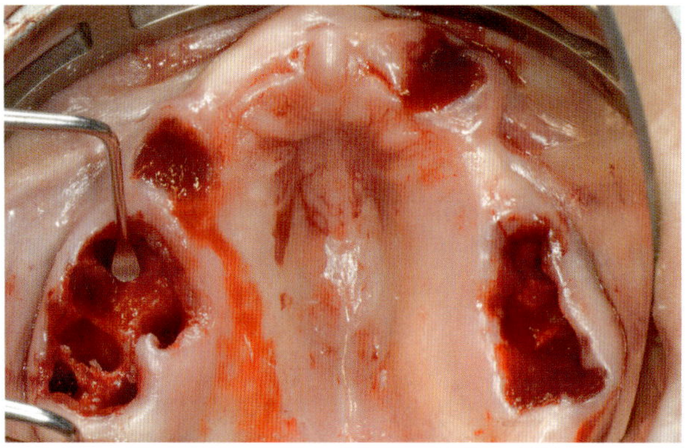

Fig 7-11 Curettage of the socket with a bone curette to remove granulation tissue or loose bone fragments.

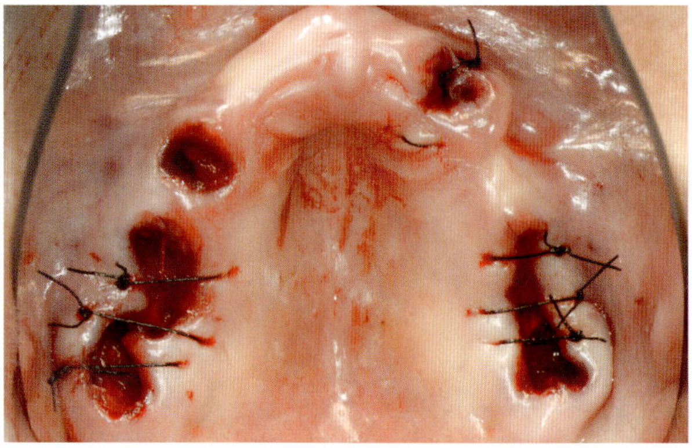

Fig 7-12 After smoothing the sharp bone edges, adaptation of the wound margins is performed with single-button sutures and a horizontal mattress suture.

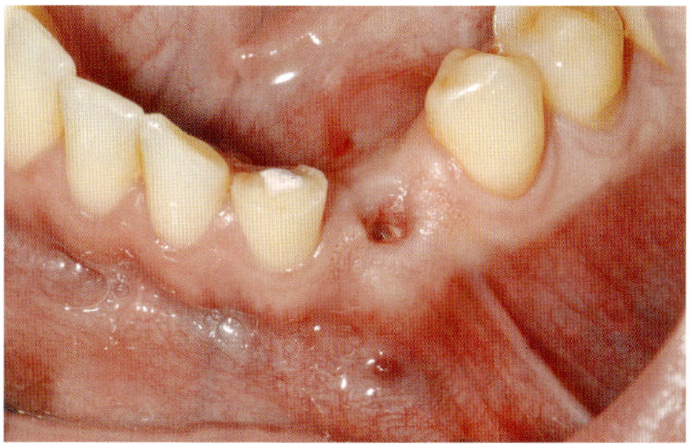

Fig 7-13 Initial clinical situation after anterior tooth trauma with, among other things, root fracture of tooth 33.

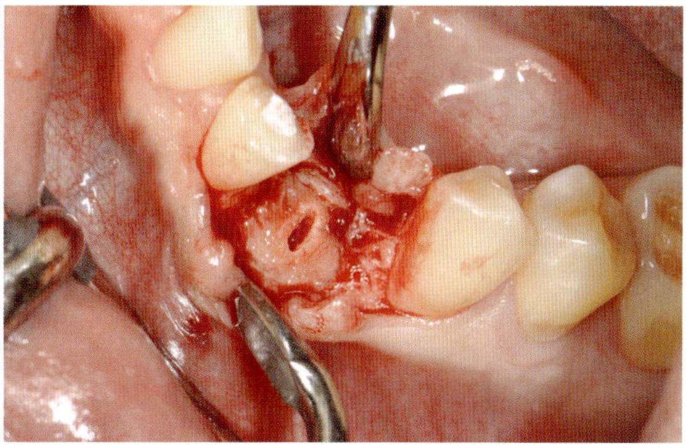

Fig 7-14 Exposure of the root remnant at region 33.

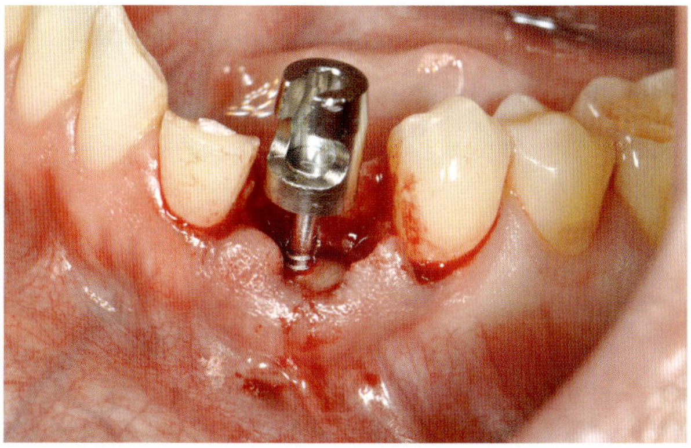

Fig 7-15 After predrilling along the root canal, the lag screw is inserted.

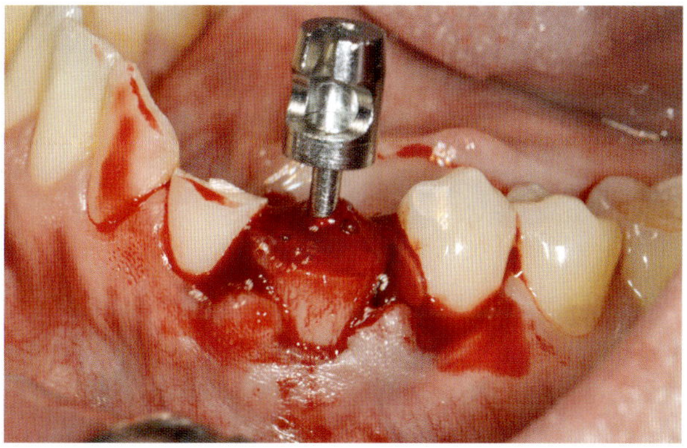

Fig 7-16 Step-by-step removal of the root remnant.

Video 7-2
Minimally invasive removal of tooth 33 with the Benex extraction system.

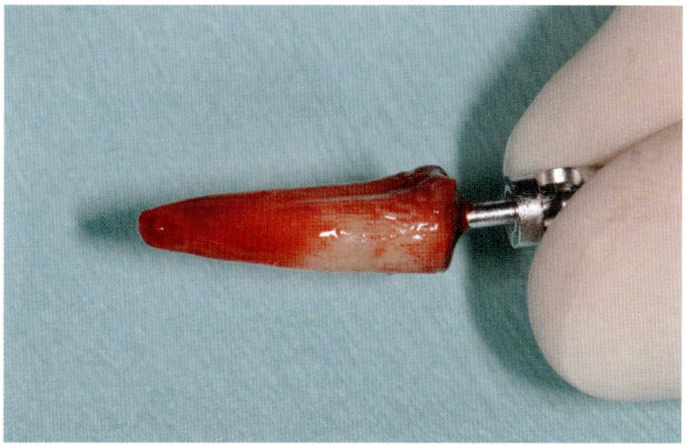

Fig 7-17 Inspection of the removed root residue with inserted lag screw.

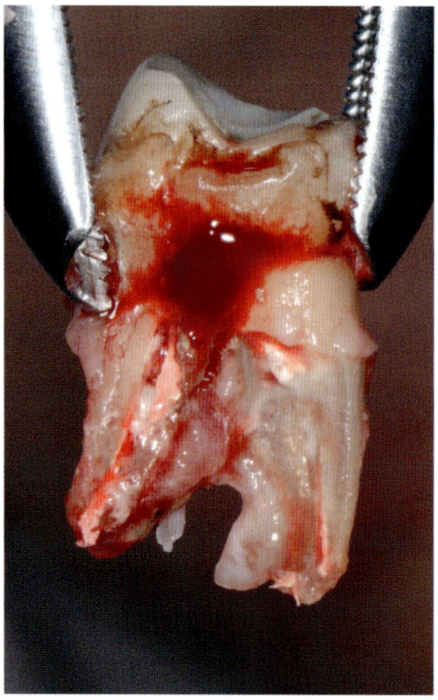

Fig 7-18 Clinical inspection of the removed tooth 27.

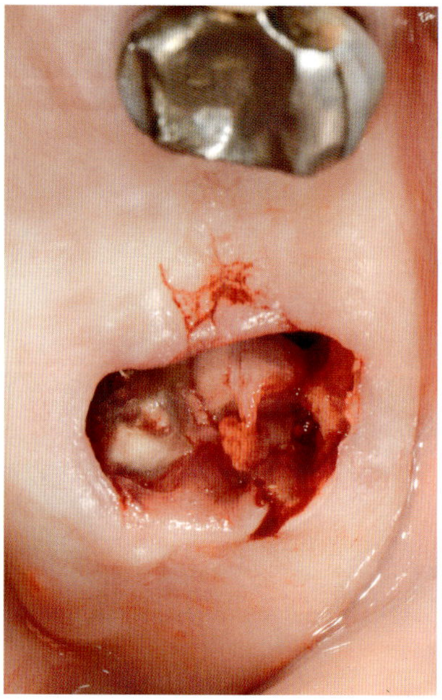

Fig 7-19 The fractured roots are still in situ.

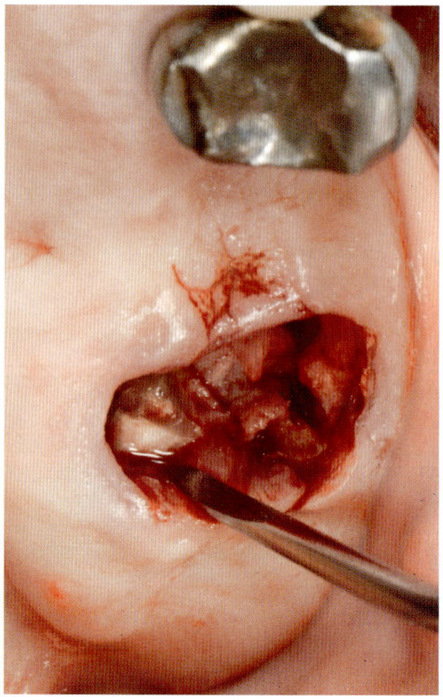

Fig 7-20 Removal of the root remnants with a root elevator.

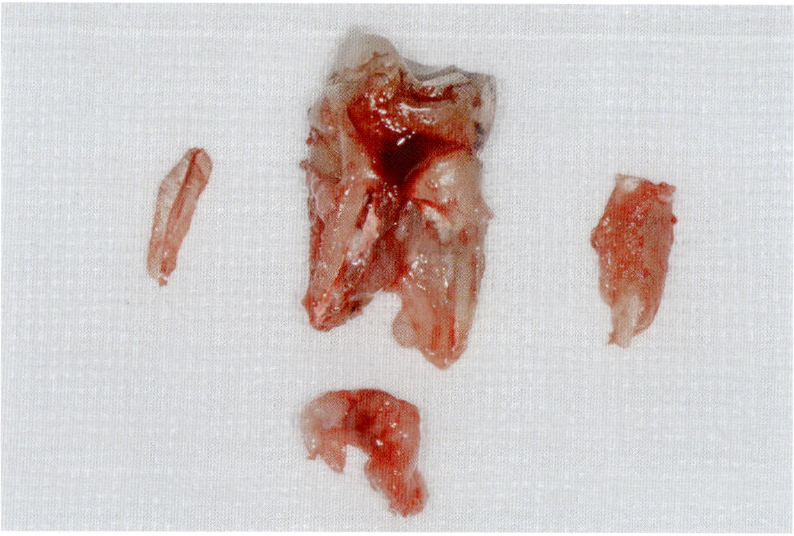

Fig 7-21 Checking the completeness of the tooth.

dinal axis without stretching the alveolar bone and traumatizing the soft tissue. This minimally invasive technique is especially successful when performed in single-rooted teeth with straight roots.

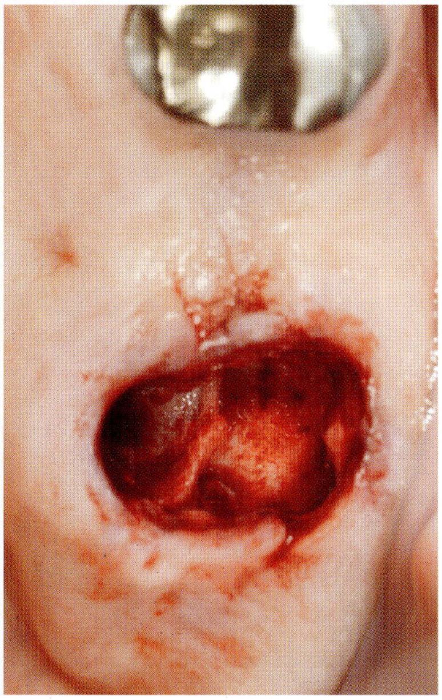

Fig 7-22 Inspection of the alveolar fundus.

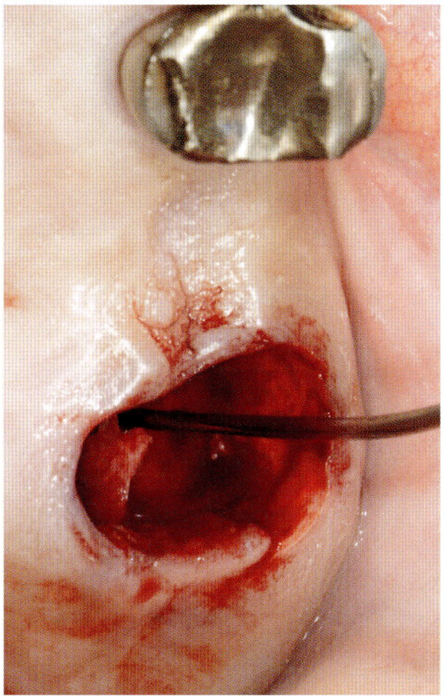

Fig 7-23 Tactile inspection of the continuity of the bony alveolar fundus with a Bowman probe in order to rule out an oroantral communication.

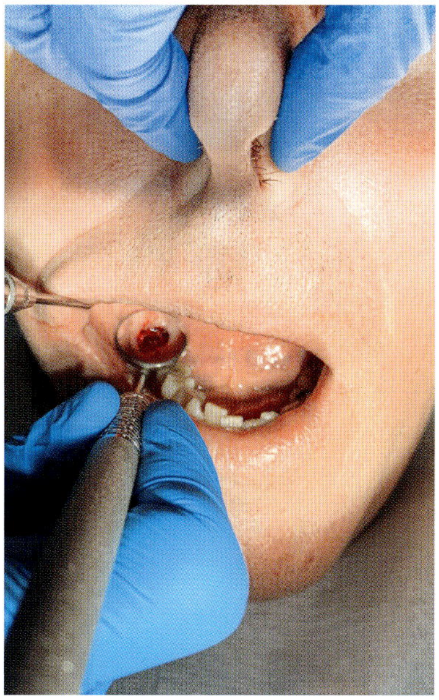

Fig 7-24 If the alveolar fundus is not intact or the findings seem unclear, the nasal blast test is performed.

Wound care and wound closure

After removal of a tooth, it is always checked for completeness (Fig 7-18). The root tips should be palpated to check for any sharp fracture surfaces. If the tooth was separated for removal or if it is fractured (Figs 7-19 and 7-20), the completeness of the tooth must be checked by assembling the tooth fragments (Fig 7-21). If incomplete tooth removal is suspected, the alveolus must be inspected and a radiograph taken, if necessary.

The alveolus is also inspected after complete tooth removal (Fig 7-22). Curettage follows to remove any granulation tissue that may be present, and especially to stimulate bone bleeding. If the roots show a close positional relationship to the maxillary sinus, the bony alveolar fundus is carefully checked tactilely for continuity using a Bowman probe (Fig 7-23), and oroantral communication is ruled out using the nasal blast test (Fig 7-24). The alveolar wall is checked tactilely with the fingers for sharp bone edges, followed, if necessary, by smoothing with a Luer bone rongeur or a rotary instrument under cooling with sterile isotonic saline (osteoplasty). Any tooth or bone fragments are removed by irrigation with sterile isotonic saline. Bidigital compression of the alveolus facilitates soft tissue coverage of the bone wound. In addition, suturing can be performed here to adapt the wound edges. Finally, the alveolus should fill with blood up to the sulcus/marginal epithelium so that a stable coagulum can form.

In certain cases, primary wound closure is performed after tooth removal (e.g. in patients on antiresorptive medication or radiotherapy in the maxillary region).

Postoperative controls and course

A wound check is performed after 1 week at the latest. The wound area is cleaned and disinfected, and any suture material is removed. In the case of primary wound closure, the sutures are removed after 10 days. Depending on the condition of the wound and the patient's condition, further checks may have to be carried out.

Recommended literature

1. Duttenhöfer F, Stricker A, Schmelzeisen R. Zahnentfernung und Osteotomie. In: Gutwald R, Gellrich NC, Schmelzeisen R (Hrsg). Zahnärztliche Chirurgie und Implantologie. Köln: Deutscher Zahnärzte Verlag, 2019.
2. Kreusch T, Lambrecht JT. Die Entfernung nicht retinierter Zähne. In: Lambrecht JT (Hrsg). Zahnärztliche Operationen. Berlin: Quintessenz, 2008.
3. Stricker A, Schmelzeisen R. Zahnentfernung und Osteotomie. In: Gutwald R, Gellrich NC, Schmelzeisen R (Hrsg). Einführung in die zahnärztliche Chirurgie und Implantologie. Köln: Deutscher Zahnärzte Verlag, 2010.
4. Wagner W. Zahnentfernung. In: Schwenzer N, Ehrenfeld M (Hrsg). Zahnärztliche Chirurgie. Stuttgart: Thieme, 2000.
5. Walter C, Schmidt JC, Dietrich T. Minimalinvasive Zahnentfernung mit dem Benex-Extraktionssystem. Quintessenz 2013;64:1–8.

Explantation

8

Sebastian Kühl

Indications

There are many indications for the removal of implants. The classic indication for explantation is peri-implantitis, which cannot be successfully treated either regeneratively or resectively (Fig 8-1). Another indication may be a fractured implant that can no longer be restored (Fig 8-2) or implants that have injured vital neighboring structures (Fig 8-3) or are located in body cavities (Figs 8-4 and 8-5). Another indication for explantation may be incorrect implant positioning if the implant is either positioned too close to neighboring structures (Fig 8-6) or cannot be restored prosthetically due to the unfavorable position and axis (Figs 8-7 and 8-8).

Contraindications

Absolute contraindications usually result from the general medical history when patients are no longer operable due to their general condition (chemotherapy, end-stage tumors, etc). A temporary contraindication may be, for example, temporary triple anticoagulation that will be switched to bi- or monotherapy in the foreseeable future. Similarly, acute (peri-implant) infections may be temporary contraindications. These should be chronicized via disinfectant irrigation and mechanical cleaning, with explantation being performed after conversion to the chronic stage (Fig 8-9).

Specific risks

In the (lateral) mandible, there is a specific risk associated with explantation using trephine burs. In this case, life-threatening bleeding can occur if the sublingual artery ruptures due to the undercut in the lingual region of the jaw (Figs 8-10 and 8-11) or if the incisive artery is injured in the anterior region[1]. Otherwise, the specific risks are similar to those of surgical tooth removal with the general risks of postoperative bleeding, swelling, impaired wound healing or injury to adjacent structures (opened maxillary sinus) as well as postoperative pain.

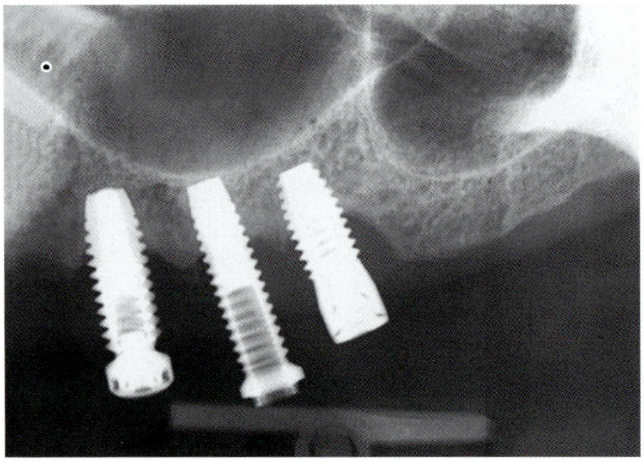

Fig 8-1 All implants show pronounced bone loss due to peri-implantitis and represent a classic indication for explantation.

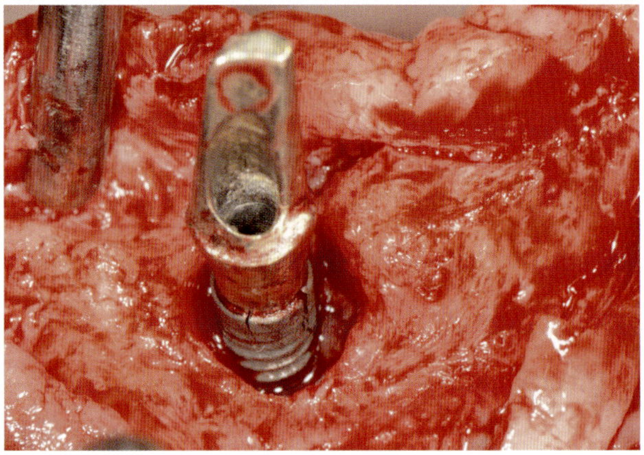

Fig 8-2 Implant fracture with double longitudinal fracture and bone loss around the implant as a result of bacterial contamination of the bone.

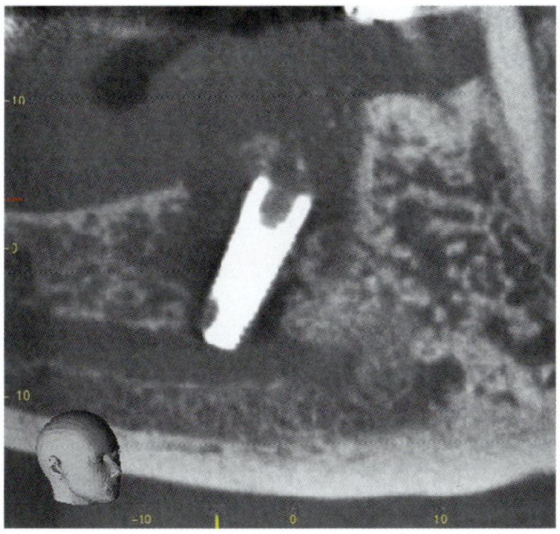

Fig 8-3 Nerve injury due to too deep implant placement is an indication for explantation.

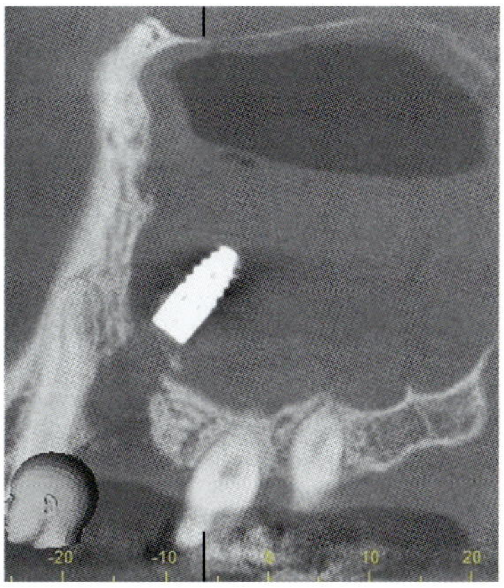

Fig 8-4 Implant dislocated into the maxillary sinus is a clear indication for explantation.

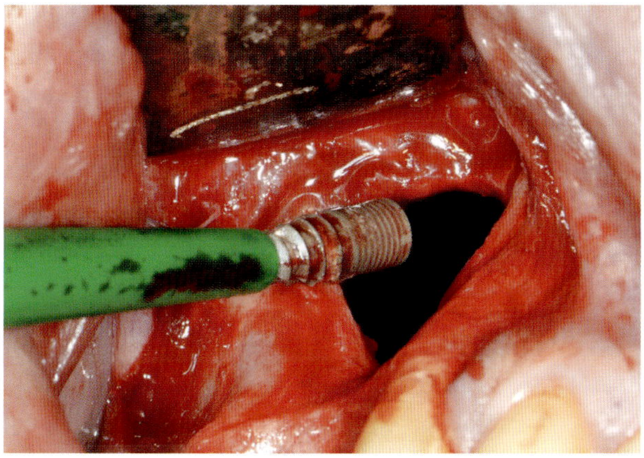

Fig 8-5 Implant removed from the maxillary sinus.

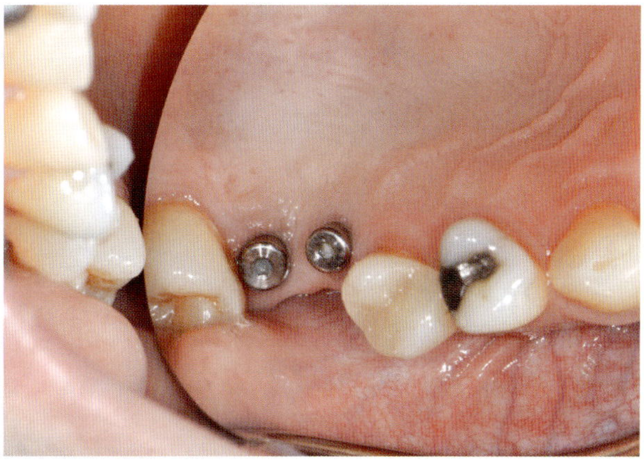

Fig 8-6 Incorrect implant position with pronounced proximity to the neighboring tooth is an indication for explantation.

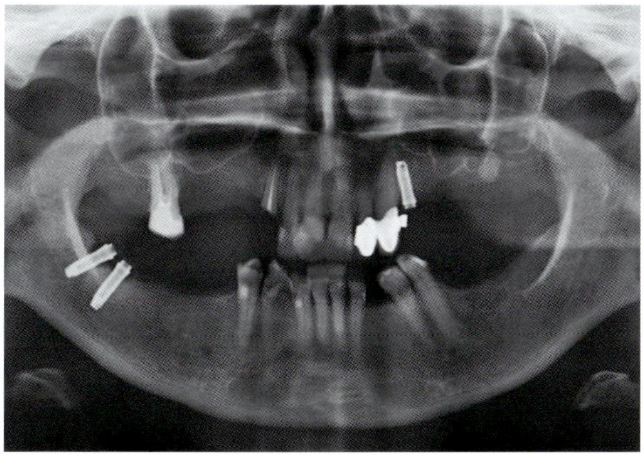

Fig 8-7 Incorrect implant positioning. The posterior implant 47 cannot be restored prosthetically due to the incorrect position; additional visible bone loss due to peri-implantitis.

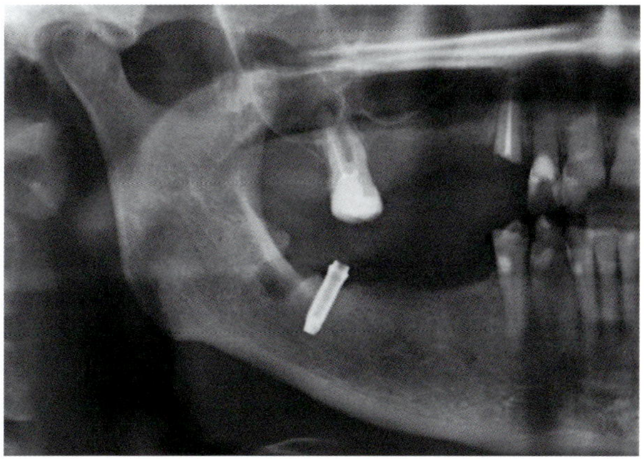

Fig 8-8 Situation after explantation of implant 47 due to incorrect position and peri-implantitis.

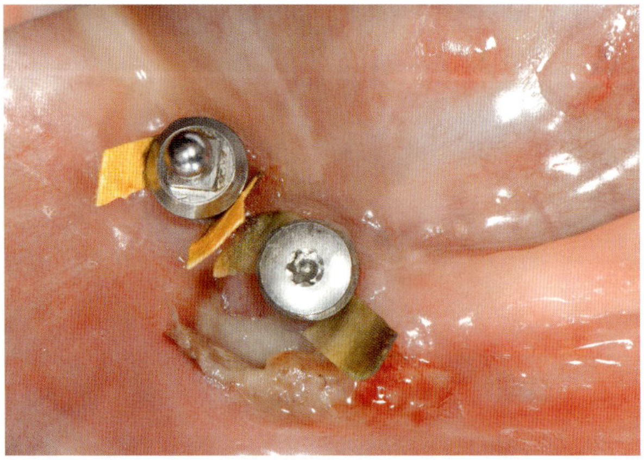

Fig 8-9 Acute infection with pus leakage is a temporary contraindication for explantation. A transition from the acute to the chronic stage should be attempted before explantation.

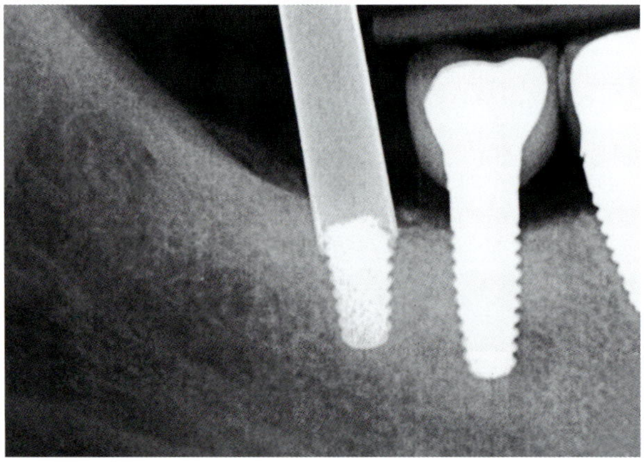

Fig 8-10 A control image taken *alio loco* during an attempt to remove a fractured ceramic implant in the lateral mandible with a trephine drill (see also Fig 8-11).

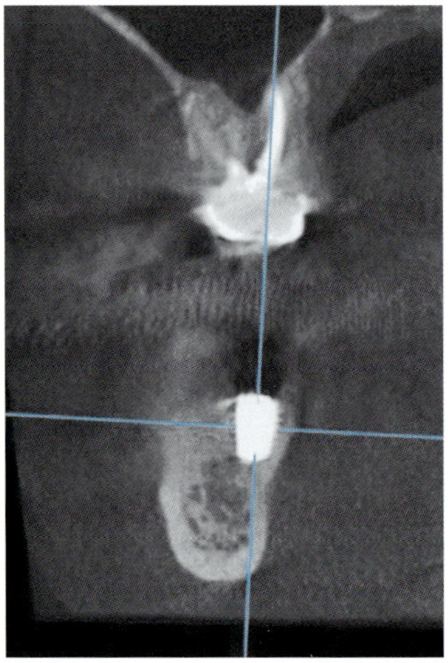

Fig 8-11 Cone beam computed tomography (CBCT) of the same case as in Fig 8-10. Due to the lingual undercut, removal by a trephine drill is associated with the risk of injury to the sublingual artery.

Local anesthesia

This procedure is identical to local anesthesia for surgical tooth removal. In the mandible, a combination of conduction anesthesia and buccal infiltration is usually chosen. In the maxilla, buccal infiltration and palatal conduction anesthesia of either the nasopalatine nerve or the greater palatine nerve are used. Ideally, the local anesthetic should contain a vasoconstrictor to somewhat reduce bleeding intraoperatively and provide a sufficiently long period of anesthesia.

Step-by-step clinical procedure

The clinical procedure depends on the general explantation technique and approach. In principle, explantations should be performed analogously to ankylosed teeth because of the previous osseointegration. In the rarest cases, an implant can be unscrewed or moved with the aid of forceps. Various auxiliary instruments for explantations are available on the market that can reduce or even prevent an osteotomy around the implant. A special explantation set for titanium implants (BTI implant explantation set; Biotechnology, Pforzheim, Germany) has proven successful. Small screws are screwed into the implant to be removed in an anticlockwise direction with a self-tapping thread (Figs 8-12 and 8-13). These self-tapping screws then wedge into the implant so that a special ratchet can then be used to attempt to rotate the implant out of the bone (Video 8-1). This technique should always be attempted initially because it can prevent flaring and osteotomy. If removal is not successful using this explantation set, specific piezo devices can be used to perform a targeted osteotomy around the implant (Figs 8-14 and 8-15). This applies in particular to the removal of ceramic implants, as the BTI system does not work in

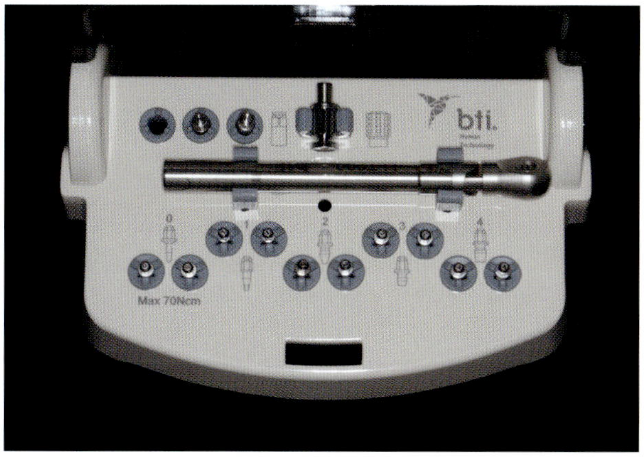

Fig 8-12 The BTI system with self-tapping screws that are inserted counterclockwise into the implant.

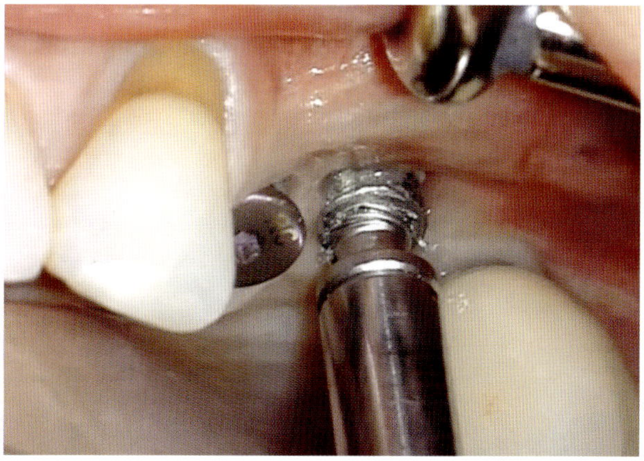

Fig 8-13 The explantation screw of the BTI system wedged in the implant.

Video 8-1
Explantation with the BTI explantation system.

Video 8-2
Explantation with piezosurgery.

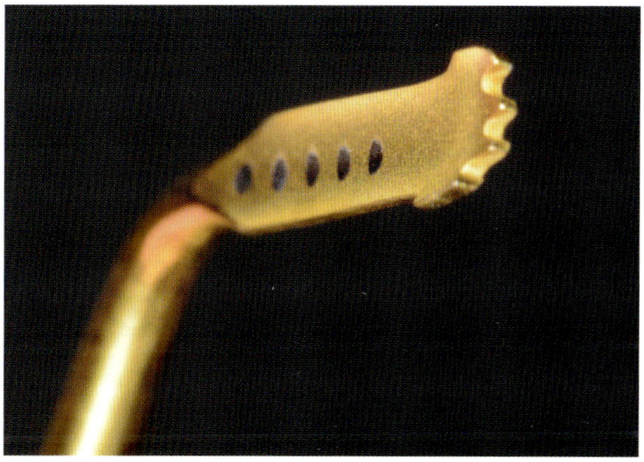

Fig 8-14 Specifically shaped, concave piezosurgical device for targeted and gentle osteotomy around an implant. The black marks are used for depth control.

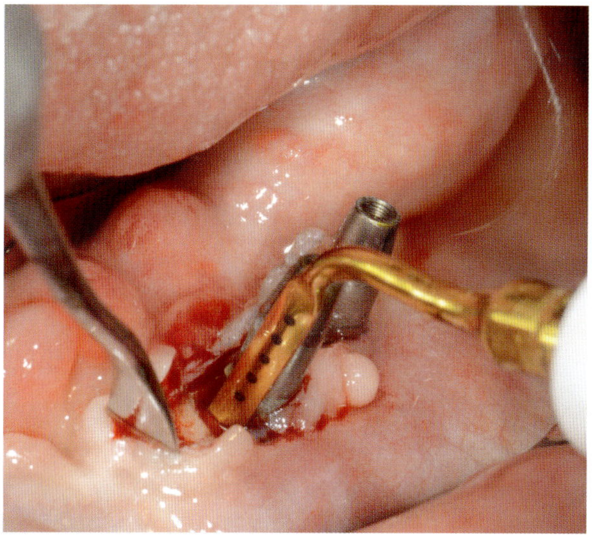

Fig 8-15 Specifically shaped piezosurgical device in clinical use.

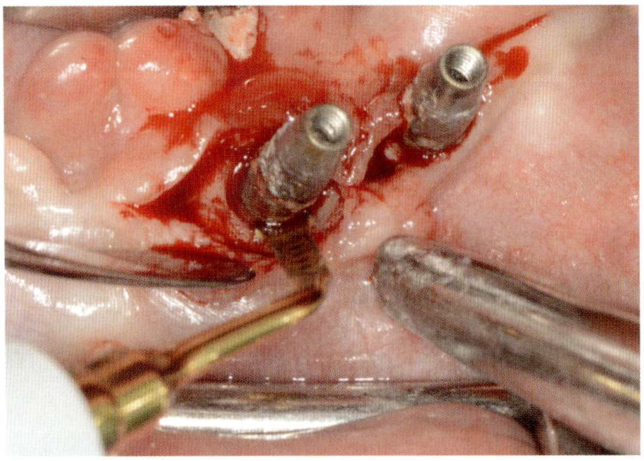

Fig 8-16 Use of the specific piezosurgical devices for gentle osteotomy in a circular manner around the implant.

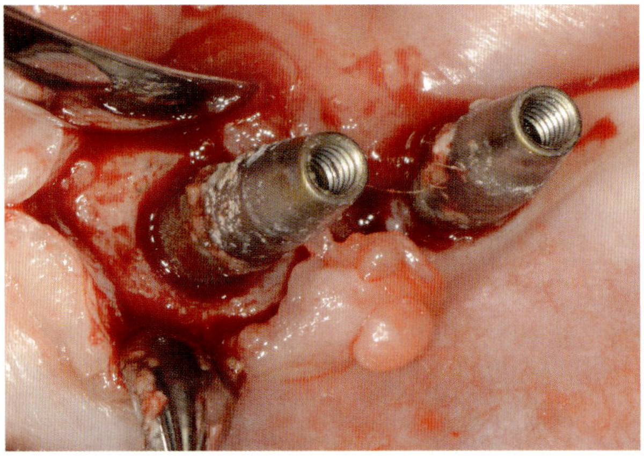

Fig 8-17 Clearly visible gap around the implant after osteotomy with piezosurgery.

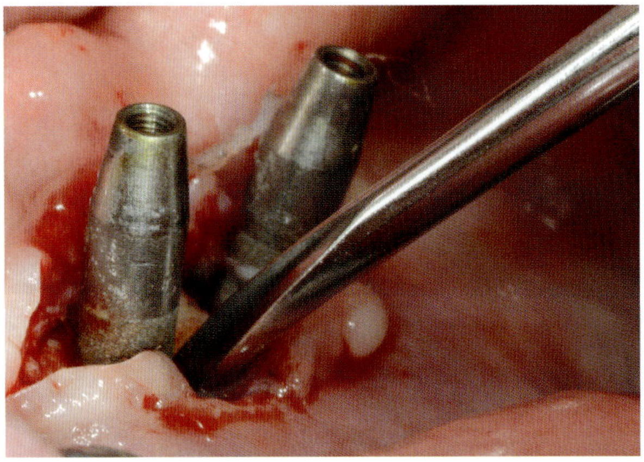

Fig 8-18 The gap created by piezosurgery can be used to mobilize the implant with an elevator.

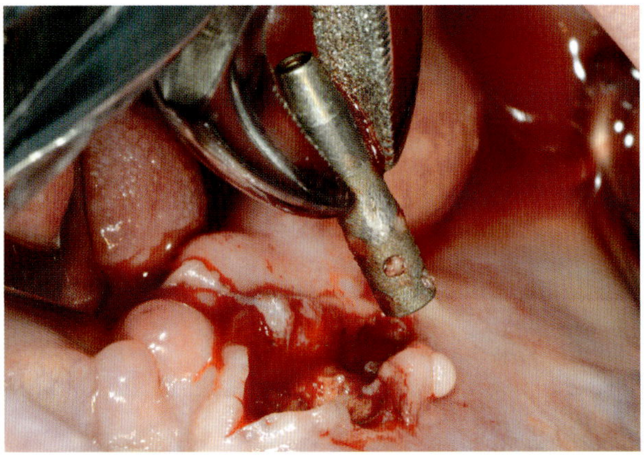

Fig 8-19 After mobilization of the implant by piezosurgery and an elevator, the implant is explanted with forceps.

such cases due to the hardness of zirconium oxide (Fig 8-10, Video 8-2). The specific piezosurgical devices are concave in shape and allow an osteotomy to match the shape of the implant (Fig 8-16). In this way, the peri-implant bone can be weakened, and then the implant can be removed either with the BTI system or with the use of elevators, as for the osteotomy of ankylosed roots (Figs 8-17 and 8-18). Alternatively, the implant can be unscrewed with forceps (Fig 8-19).

If the implant cannot be removed using the methods described above, a mucoperiosteal flap may need to be mobilized in some cases to better control an osteotomy around the implant. Usually, an intrasulcular incision is made around the implant with marginal extension to the two adjacent teeth and vertical relief (Video 8-2). The

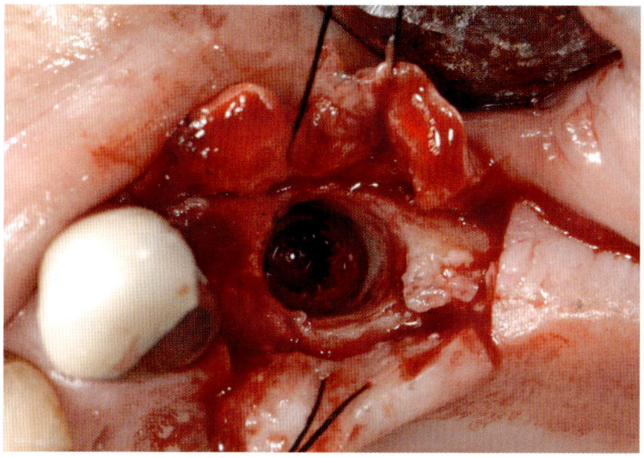

Fig 8-20 Extensive defect during explantation of a reduced-diameter implant using a trephine drill.

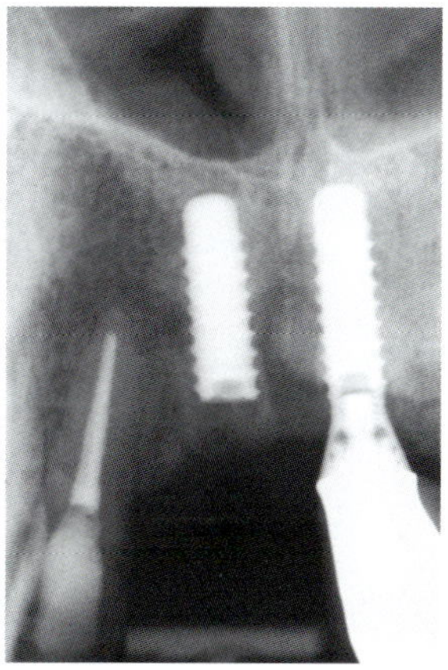

Fig 8-21 Deeply fractured implant 11.

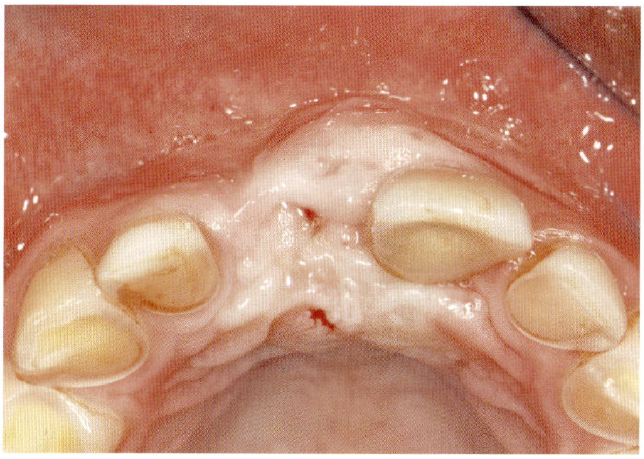

Fig 8-22 Clinical view of region 11 (see Fig 8-21).

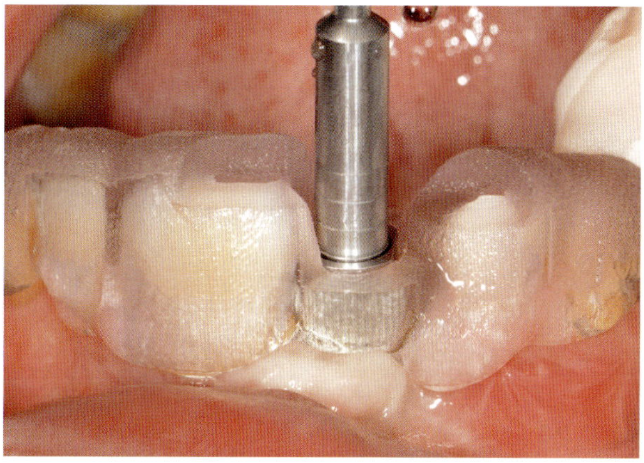

Fig 8-23 A template-guided explantation was planned to achieve targeted explantation without major loss of substance.

better overview then allows piezosurgery for performing a targeted osteotomy around the implant in order to remove it, either with the BTI system, an elevator or forceps. Here it is recommended to work with diamond-coated forceps because the diamond-coating prevents the forceps from slipping due to wedging in the titanium. If piezosurgical equipment is not available, the osteotomy can of course also be performed with rotary instruments, but this is always associated with significantly more bone loss in comparison.

The use of trephine drills is not recommended because they can lead to very large defects, depending on the implant design (Fig 8-20). In the worst case, wedging with the implant can cause fracture of the trephine drill, making explantation much more difficult (Figs 8-24 to 8-32).

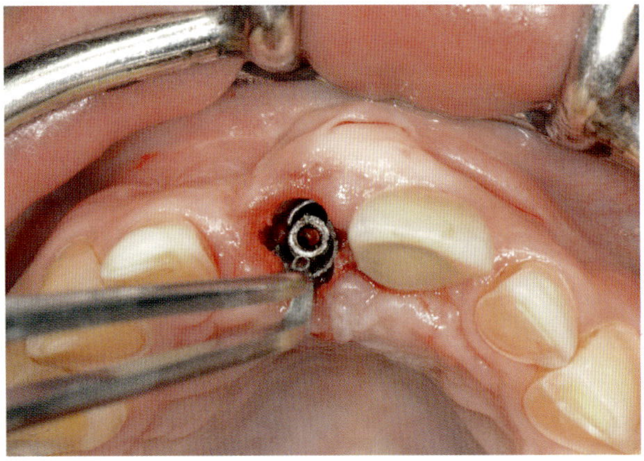

Fig 8-24 Fracture of the trephine drill due to extensive stresses on the implant.

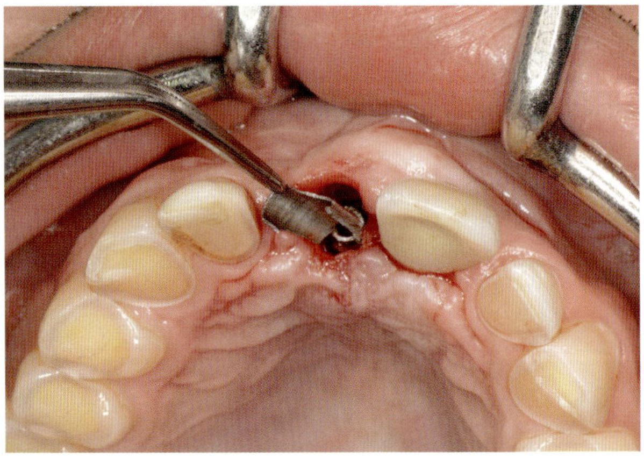

Fig 8-25 Removal of the fractured trephine components.

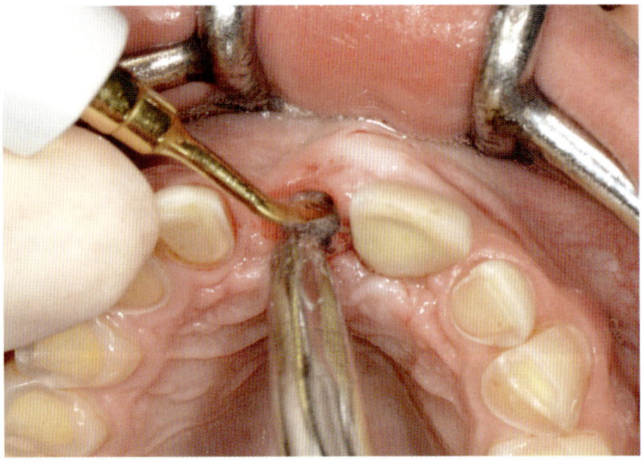

Fig 8-26 Gentle osteotomy by special piezosurgical devices around the fractured implant 11.

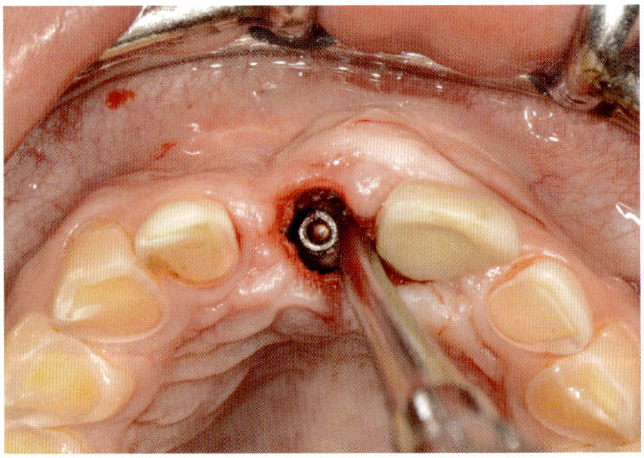

Fig 8-27 After gentle osteotomy with piezosurgery, the implant is mobilized in the mesiodistal direction. No pressure should be applied to the buccal wall.

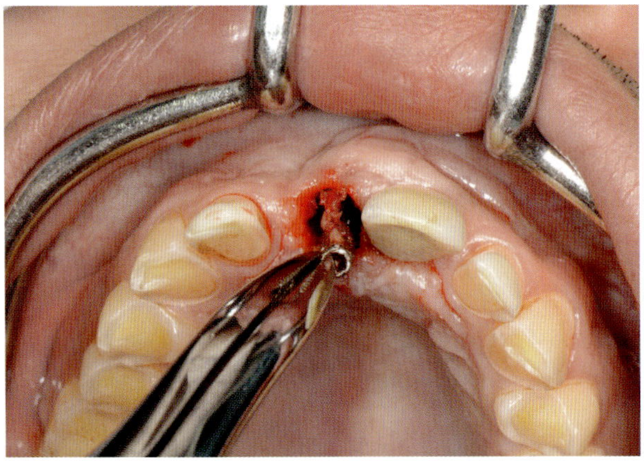

Fig 8-28 After osteotomy with piezosurgery and mobilization by means of elevators, gentle rotation is performed with root-rest forceps.

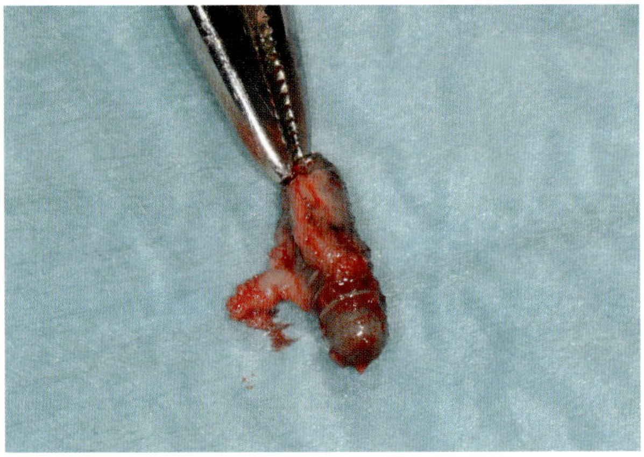

Fig 8-29 Successfully explanted implant.

Wound care and closure

After successful explantation, the "alveolus" should be well curetted. This applies especially if an osteotomy has been performed around the implant. This procedure always results in the scattering of titanium chips, some of which may be infected. These chips should ideally not remain in the bone. The placement of a suture can help to stabilize the coagulum and prevent a wound-healing disorder. A double-loop suture or cross suture (Fig 8-32) has proven successful in this case (see Section 3). Analogous to surgical tooth removal, 4-0 or 5-0 monofilament sutures can be used.

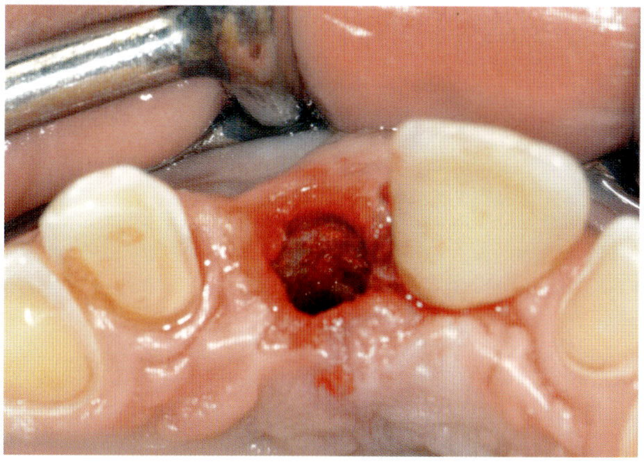

Fig 8-30 By avoiding pressure on the buccal wall, it was possible to preserve it almost completely.

Postoperative controls and course

A postoperative radiograph can be taken to document the course. Depending on the effort and local anatomy (proximity to the nerve), a check should be made on the first or second postoperative day. The suture is usually removed after 1 week. Concomitant antibiotic therapy is not necessary and is required at most due to the patient's individual medical history. Analgesics are prescribed according to need, medical history, and body weight.

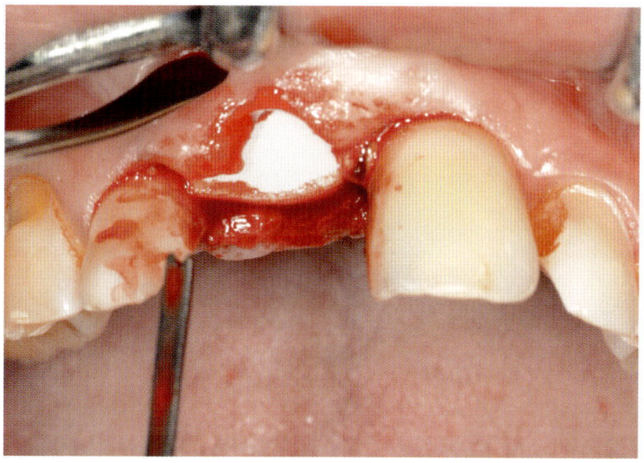

Fig 8-31 Care of the wound: Alveolar stabilization by inserting a collagen membrane after preparation of a buccal and palatal split flap.

Reference

1. Tomljenovic B, Hermann S, Filippi A, Kühl S. Life-threatening hemorrhage associated with dental implant surgery: a review of the literature. Clin Oral Implants Res 2016;27:1079–1084.

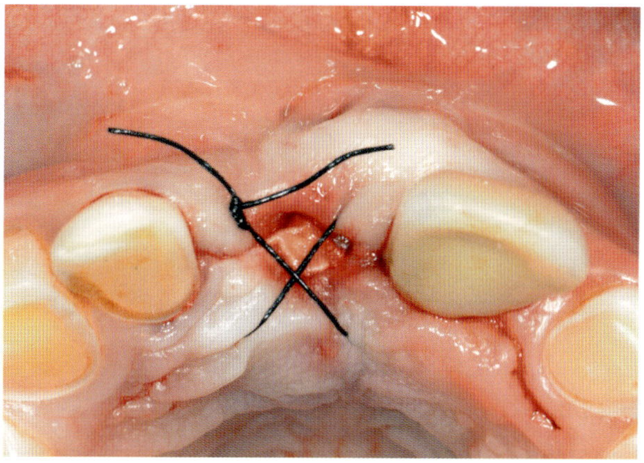

Fig 8-32 Double-loop suture over the membrane to stabilize the coagulum.

Surgical tooth removal

9

Sebastian Kühl

Indications

Surgical tooth removal is indicated either for impacted and/or displaced teeth (Figs 9-1 and 9-2) or when a tooth cannot be removed conventionally with forceps or elevators due to other conditions. Classically, these are teeth with an ankylosed root where fracture of the crown occurs when removal is attempted or, more generally, persistent root remnants (Figs 9-3 and 9-4). However, surgical tooth removal may also be indicated when a multirooted tooth with divergent roots should be removed in the most non-invasive way possible, especially in the region of the maxillary first molars (Fig 9-4).

Contraindications

Absolute contraindications usually result from the general medical history, when patients are no longer operable due to their general condition (chemotherapy, terminal tumors, etc). A temporary contraindication may be, for example, temporary triple anticoagulation that will be switched to bi- or monotherapy in the foreseeable future. Similarly, acute (apical or pericoronal) infections may be considered a temporary contraindication, as adequate depth of anesthesia may not be achieved during surgery. In these cases, disinfecting rinses, mechanical cleansing or drainage should be used to achieve chronicity of the inflammatory process prior to surgical tooth removal.

Specific risks

Specific risks result from the general medical history (underlying diseases and medications) and the local anatomy, since surgical tooth removal always involves an (intraalveolar) osteotomy, which may injure neighboring structures such as the lingual nerve and the mental nerve or the maxillary sinus mucosa. Depending on the degree of ankylosis, heat may also be generated due to lack of irrigation at the tip of the drill, resulting in heat necrosis. Compared with nonsurgical tooth removal, surgical tooth removal therefore results in significantly more postoperative complications in terms of wound healing disorders (ostitis), which manifest primarily in the mandible (Figs 9-5 to 9-7)[2]. Furthermore, an increased risk of bleeding must be expected due to the osteotomy.

Local anesthesia

This is identical to local anesthesia in surgical wisdom tooth removal. In the mandible, a combination of conduction anesthesia and buccal infiltration is usually selected. In the maxilla, buccal infiltration and palatal conduction anesthesia of either the nasopalatine nerve or the greater palatine nerve are used. Ideally, the local anesthetic should contain a vasoconstrictor to somewhat reduce severe bleeding intraoperatively and to achieve a sufficiently long period of anesthesia.

Very highly displaced maxillary canines occupy a special position (Fig 9-1). It is not uncommon for the root tips to extend far dorsally into the maxillary sinus or cranially toward the floor of the nose. In such cases, it may not be possible to achieve sufficient local anesthetic depth with conventional local anesthesia (buccal and palatal), so that either additional intranasal anesthesia should be used, or intubation anesthesia should be planned in advance.

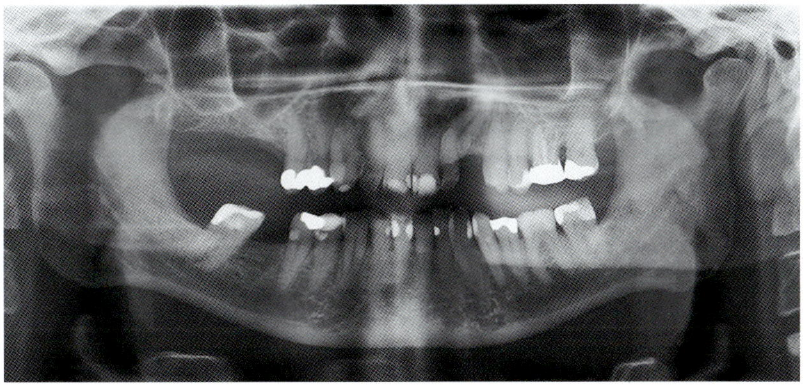

Fig 9-1 Retained and displaced canine (tooth 23) is an indication for surgical tooth removal.

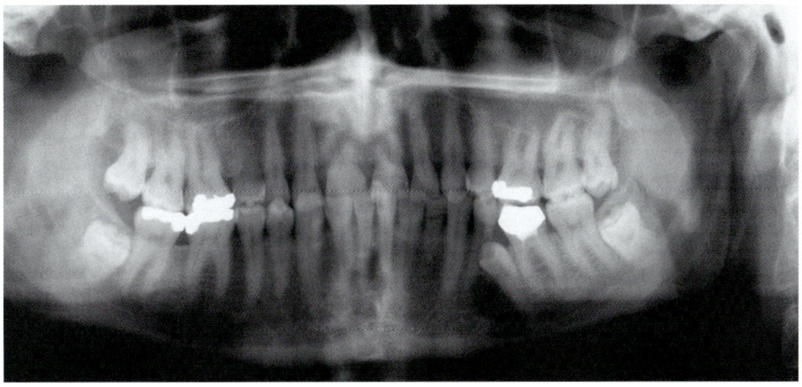

Fig 9-2 Retained and displaced premolar (tooth 35) is an indication for surgical tooth removal.

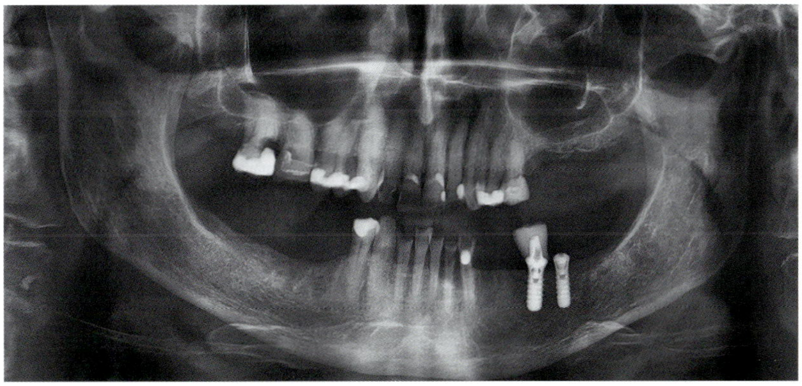

Fig 9-3 Panoramic radiograph of an 85-year-old female patient. No periodontal gap is visible on the mandibular anterior teeth, which may indicate ankylosis.

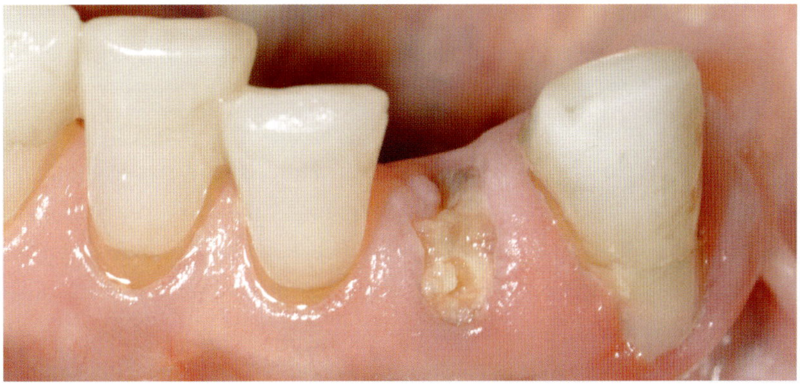

Fig 9-4 Clinical situation (see Fig 9-3) after attempting removal of tooth 32 with forceps. A crown fracture occurred due to the ankylosis. Subsequently, the tooth had to be surgically removed.

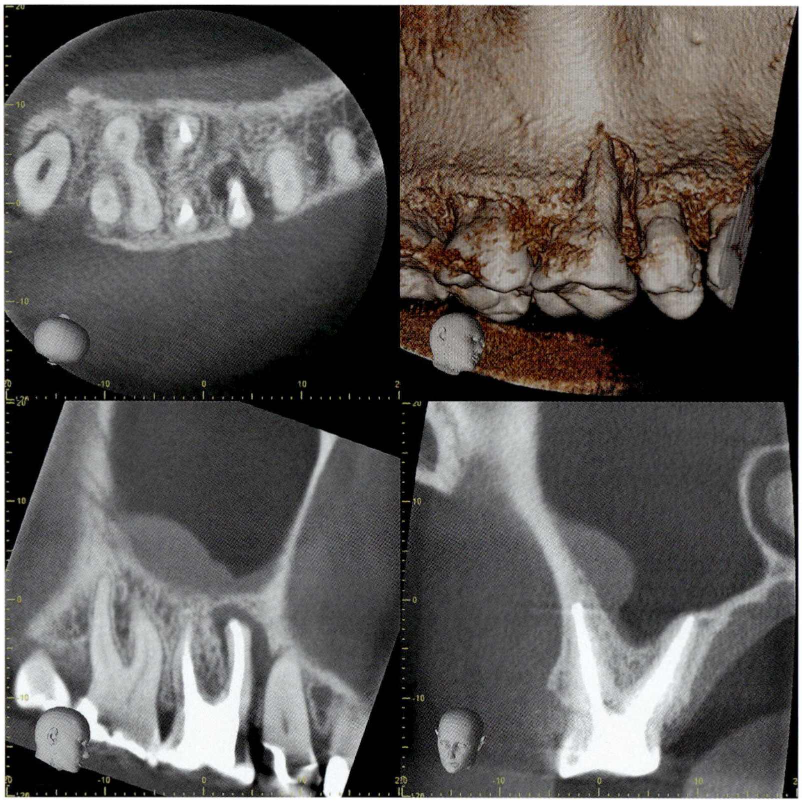

Fig 9-5 The roots in region 16 are splayed in a V-shape. To reduce the trauma to the surrounding bone, an intraalveolar osteotomy with separation of the individual roots is indicated.

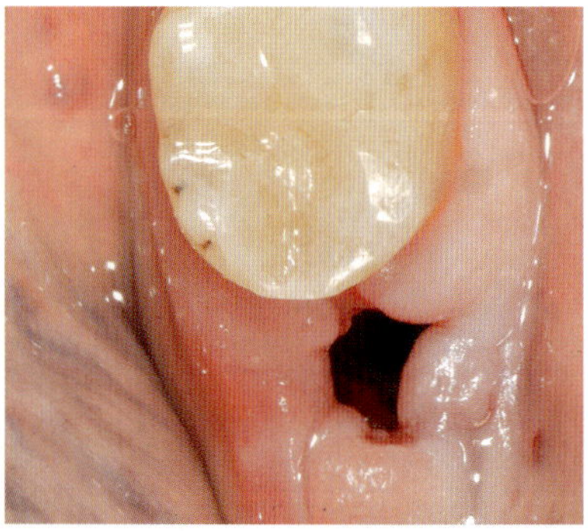

Fig 9-6 Wound infection after intraalveolar osteotomy.

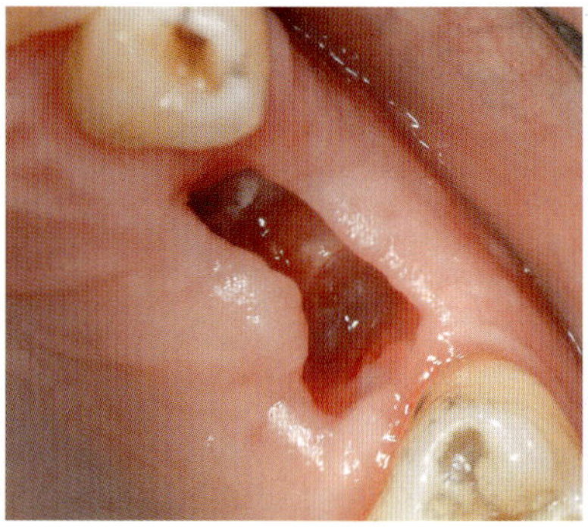

Fig 9-7 *Ostitis circumscripta/ alveolitis sicca* with visible exposed bone.

Step-by-step clinical procedure

Intraalveolar osteotomy: single-rooted teeth

In the past, various textbooks have usually described surgical tooth removal with the formation of a vestibular mucoperiosteal flap and osteotomy of the buccal bone wall. Studies on the structural changes of the alveolus after tooth removal could show that different resorption patterns can occur, and that the buccal wall is especially fragile to resorption processes due to its morphology (bundle bone)[1]. The formation of a flap and osteotomizing the buccal wall can actually be considered obsolete today, with very few exceptions (e.g. in the region of a mandibular or maxillary second molar with poor visibility and otherwise limited access to a deeply retained, fractured root apex).

Modern intraalveolar osteotomy attempts to remove a root without forming a mucoperiosteal flap, while primarily sparing the buccal bone. The goal is to create space for elevators to mobilize a root by selectively separating the root in combination with minimal osteotomy of the alveolar bone (Figs 9-8 to 9-12). In this technique, the use of magnifying glasses in combination with a light source matched to them is very helpful.

The procedure begins by separating the crown at the gingival level to expose the root (Fig 9-8). Either a Lindemann bur or diamond bur can be used here. As soon as osteotomy is performed in the bone, a Lindemann bur should

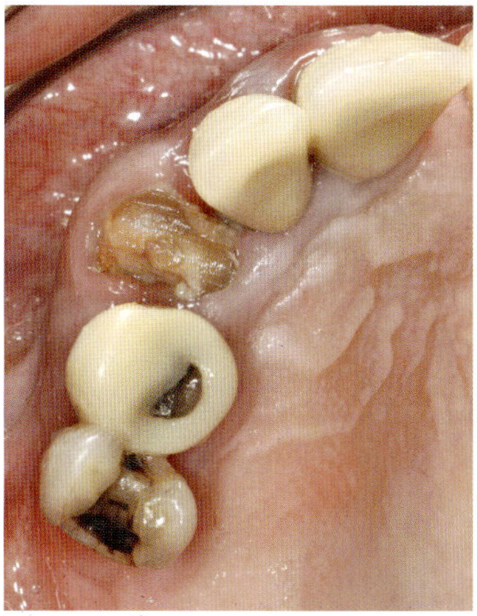

Fig 9-8 Intraalveolar osteotomy of a maxillary canine with ankylosis. After separating the crown, osteotomy is performed either mesially or distally with a Lindemann bur to create space.

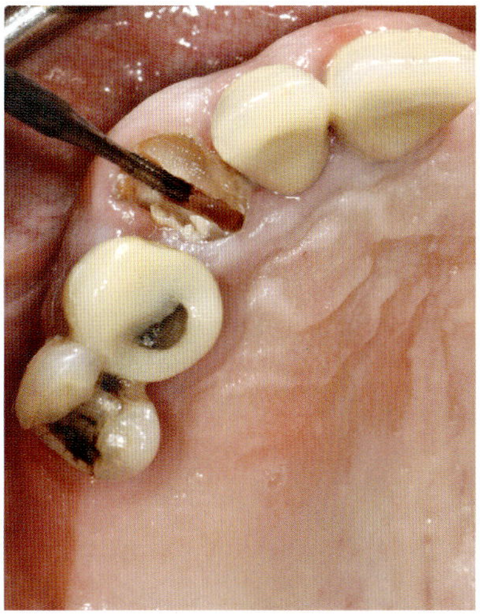

Fig 9-9 Separation of the root using a Lindemann bur in the bucco-oral direction in order to exert as little force as possible on the buccal wall with the elevator.

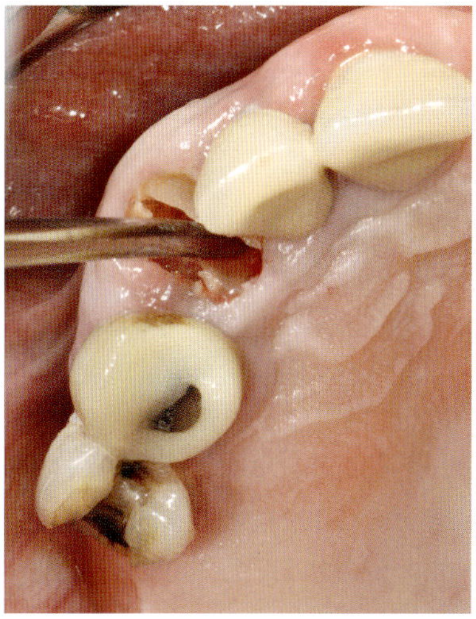

Fig 9-10 After separation, the root is selectively fractured by elevators. If part of the root is then removed, space is created to allow the root to move into this gap.

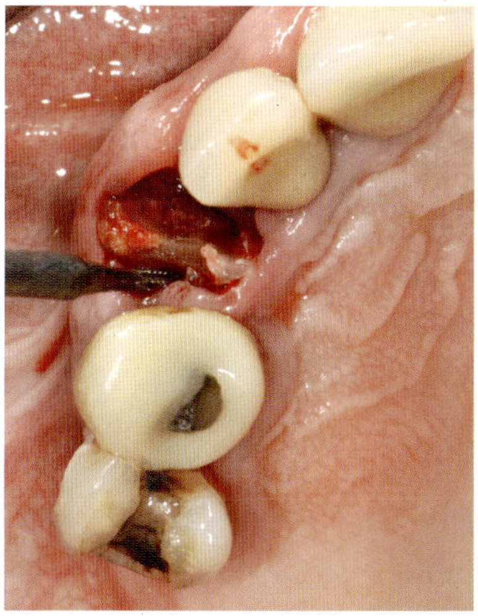

Fig 9-11 Osteotomy distally with a Lindemann reamer to mobilize the root mesially into the previously created space.

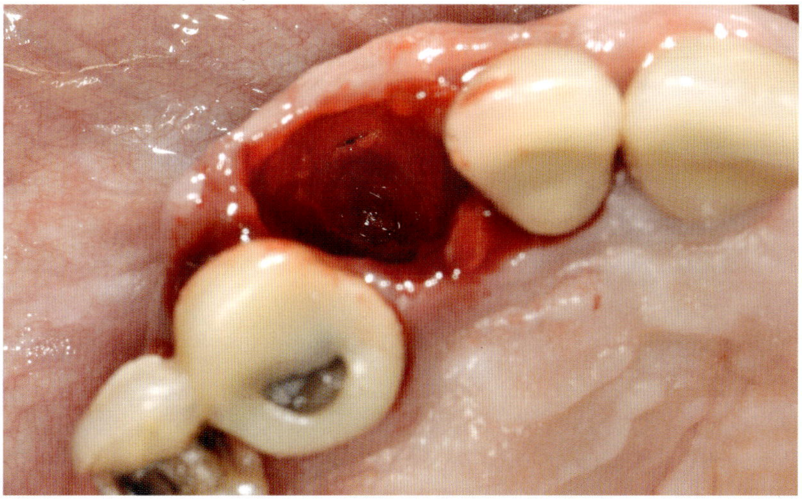

Fig 9-12 Intraalveolar osteotomy preserved the buccal lamella almost intact.

be used, since lower speeds are used here compared with diamond burs, and the sterile isotonic saline solution can have a positive effect on avoiding wound-healing disorders. After setting down the crown, the root is separated into two parts (Fig 9-9). It is recommended to design the separation in a bucco-oral orientation and to separate the root into a mesial and distal part (Fig 9-9). An elevator can then be used to break the root into two parts. Bucco-oral separation prevents force from being applied to the very fragile buccal wall, thus better protecting it

(Fig 9-10). Once part of the root has been mobilized and removed, an (intraalveolar) osteotomy is performed on the opposite side to create a gap between the remaining root and the alveolus (Fig 9-11). This gap, in turn, serves to allow the root to move by means of elevators. If the root does not move, the osteotomy must be widened and, if necessary, the opposite bone around the root must also be further weakened. The less bone that is osteotomized, the lower the postoperative complication rates and the better the postoperative healing (Fig 9-12).

Intraalveolar osteotomy: multirooted teeth

Here, too, it is important to try to surgically remove the tooth without forming a mucoperiosteal flap and with maximum protection of the buccal alveolar wall. Particularly in the region of the maxillary first molars, divergent root processes can occur, which are formed in a regular V-shape (Fig 9-5, Video 9-1). In these cases, the use of forceps without separating the roots results in a larger bone wound. Analogous to the procedure for single-rooted teeth, the crown is first separated using a Lindemann bur or diamond bur (Fig 9-13, Video 9-1). The roots can then be separated from each other depending on their number and course (Fig 9-14, Video 9-1). Subsequently, each individual root can be mobilized with elevators (Deppeler) so that, ideally, the buccal wall can be completely spared (Figs 9-15 and 9-16). The same procedure can be followed in the mandible, taking the anatomy into consideration. After the crown has been set down, the roots are usually separated in the bucco-oral direction (Video 9-2). Diamond burs should only be used "in the tooth" in this case as well, since they can lead to a wound-healing disorder in rapidly rotating contra-angle handpieces without sterile saline solution if they are used for osteotomy. In the bone region, it is advisable to switch to slowly rotating instruments or alternatively to ultrasonic attachments, such as piezosurgery, to be able to osteotomize with sterile isotonic saline. Here, too, the first step is to try to remove one of the two roots after separation to create sufficient space for the mobilization of the opposite root. If one of the two roots cannot be moved, further separation of the root is performed and, if necessary, another osteotomy. In addition to the use of elevators, finer osteotomes such as special root lifters can also be used.

Surgical removal of impacted and displaced teeth

In contrast to intraalveolar osteotomy, the formation of a mucoperiosteal flap cannot be avoided in retained and displaced teeth. The incision should be performed in such a way that the flap provides sufficient visibility and can be extended, and that the wound edges do not overlap the osteotomy defect (Video 9-3). After preparation of a mucoperiosteal flap, the crown should be visualized via osteotomy up to the largest circumference with a ball bur or a Lindemann bur under irrigation with sterile isotonic saline. Following the osteotomy, initial mobilization is performed to assess whether the tooth can be mobilized in principle or to get an impression of the extent of ankylosis. Initial mobilization by means of an elevator is followed by decapitation in the area of the cementoenamel junction. This creates space and provides a good view of the root. To mobilize the root, it (or part of it) is separated with a Lindemann bur. An elevator (Deppeler) can then be used to blast the root, and the looser fragments are removed with forceps or root remnant forceps. An elevator can then be used to try to move the root into the space created. It may be necessary to create a small osteotomy between the root and the directly adjacent bone beforehand so that there is room for the elevator to mobilize. By careful rotational movements, the root can then be moved into the area of least resistance. The more ankylosed

Video 9-1 Surgical tooth removal with intraalveolar osteotomy of a maxillary first molar (video identical to Video 7-1).

Video 9-2 Surgical tooth removal with intraalveolar osteotomy of a mandibular first molar.

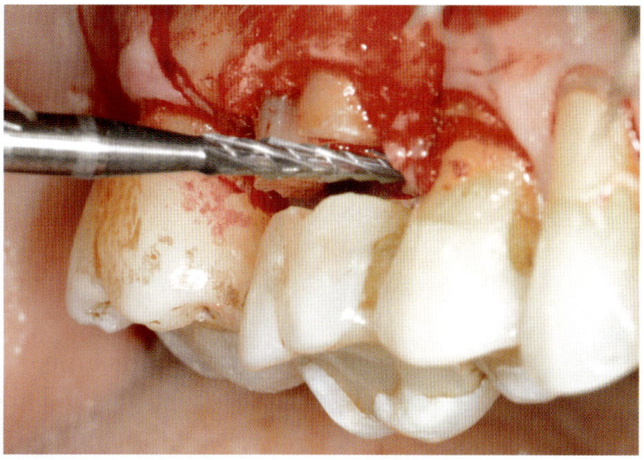

Fig 9-13 Removal of the crown using a Lindemann bur.

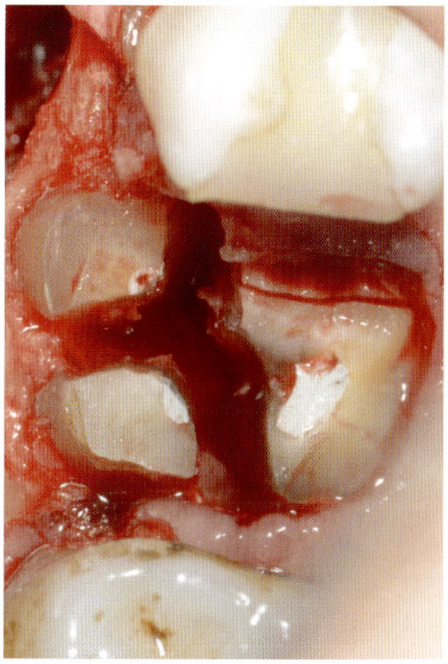

Fig 9-14 Roots separated by a Lindemann bur.

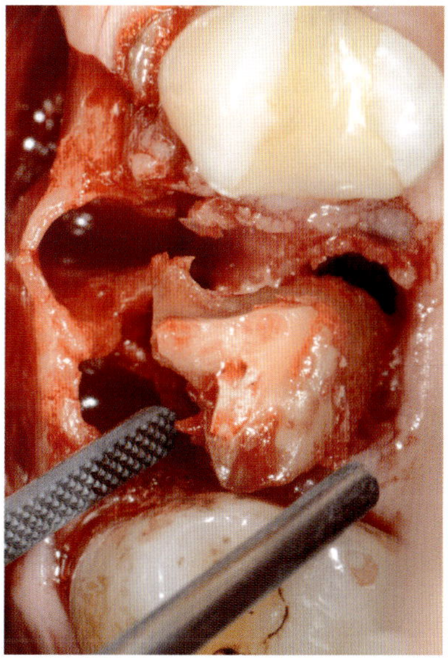

Fig 9-15 After mobilization of the roots by elevators, the individual roots can be removed with forceps or tweezers.

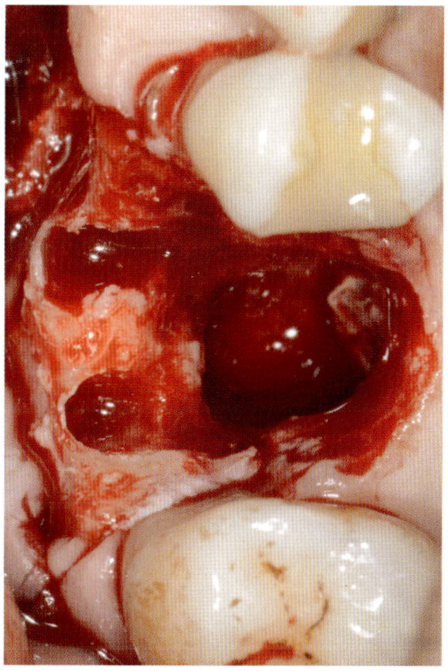

Fig 9-16 Preservation of the buccal wall by separation and removal of the individual roots.

a root is, the deeper the separation and osteotomy around the root should be. The removed root is checked for completeness. After curettage and irrigation, the surgical area can be filled with collagen fleece, especially in larger defects. In addition to stabilizing the coagulum, the soft tissue is also stabilized and prevented from collapsing, especially on the palate in the case of impacted canines. A stent made preoperatively serves to protect the wound in the first few days postsurgery, especially during food intake (soft food). In addition, this can also be used as a stent in patients under anticoagulation (Video 9-3, patient on ASA 300). Provided the stent has been

Video 9-3 Surgical removal of a retained and displaced canine 13.

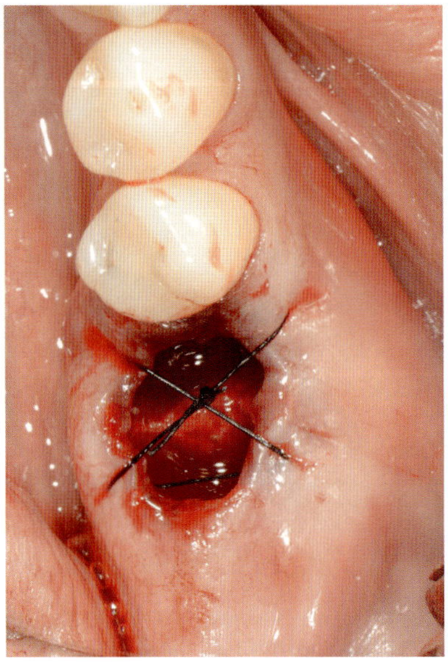

Fig 9-17 Offset double-loop suture: A double uninterrupted single-knot suture creates a cross in the center. The deeper the punctures are placed in the direction of the vestibule, the more pressure can be applied to the alveolus (see also Videos 9-1 and 9-2).

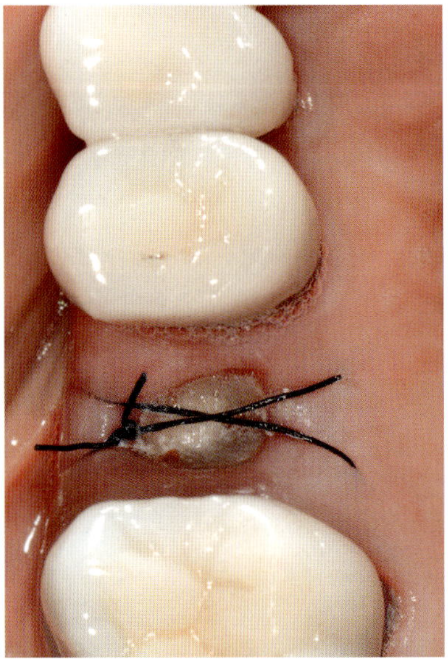

Fig 9-18 Double-loop suture to stabilize the collagen cone inserted to stabilize the coagulum.

"hollowed out" in the area of surgery, the reservoir can be used to hold dental adhesive pastes or temporary relining materials, making the stent even more efficient in terms of hemostasis or wound healing.

Wound care and closure

After surgical tooth removal, at least one situation suture should be applied compared with simple tooth removal. This should ideally stabilize the coagulum and, if possible, exert pressure on the alveolus to prevent secondary bleeding. These requirements are particularly fulfilled by a double-loop or cross suture (Fig 9-17, Videos 9-1 and 9-2). This is essentially a continued, double single-knot suture. The deeper the punctures are made in the direction of the vestibule, the more pressure can be applied specifically to the wound. In addition, due to the cross that forms, an insert into the alveolus, for example, in the form of collagen fleece cones, can be well stabilized and secured against premature slipping out (Fig 9-18). The basic prerequisite for the insertion of a foreign material (bone substitute or collagen fleece) into the socket is the clinically verified absence of pus during the procedure.

Postoperative controls and course

A postoperative radiograph may be performed to ensure that all tooth fragments have been removed. This is particularly useful in patients undergoing focal restoration prior to, for example, radiotherapy, valve replacement or antiresorptive therapy, when it was not possible to clearly ensure intraoperatively that all tooth portions had been removed. Depending on the effort and local anatomy (proximity to the nerve), a check should be made on the first or second postoperative day. The suture is usually removed after 1 week. Concomitant antibiotic therapy is not necessarily required and depends on the individual patient's medical history. Analgesics are prescribed according to need, medical history, and body weight.

References

1. Araújo MG, Lindhe J. Dimensional ridge alterations following tooth extraction. An experimental study in the dog. J Clin Periodontol 2005;32:212–218.
2. Blum IR. Contemporary views on dry socket (alveolar osteitis): a clinical appraisal of standardization, aetiopathogenesis and management: a critical review. Int J Oral Maxillofac Surg 2002;3:309–317.

Surgical removal and coronectomy of wisdom teeth

10

Marc Joos, Fabio Saccardin,
Dorothea Dagassan-Berndt, Andreas Filippi,
Sebastian Kühl

Surgical removal of wisdom teeth

Indications

Compared with other oral surgical procedures, surgical wisdom tooth removal carries the risk of more serious complications such as permanent sensory disturbances at the inferior alveolar nerve or lingual nerve. Therefore, when establishing the indication, the expected benefits must outweigh the risks, especially when prophylactic removal is involved.

The classic indication for wisdom tooth removal is recurrent acute or chronic pericoronitis (Fig 10-1). If left untreated, this can lead to abscessation, pericoronal bone loss or follicular cysts. If acute pericoronitis is present, the infection must first be chronicized by local antiseptic measures before surgical tooth removal. Furthermore, wisdom tooth removal is also indicated in cases of caries, attachment loss, and resorption of the adjacent teeth (Fig 10-2) as well as for prosthetic-surgical reasons (e.g. in the context of a planned crown lengthening procedure) or for orthodontic reasons. In addition, wisdom tooth removal may be necessary as part of a focal restoration or in the case of pericoronal pathologies (e.g. follicular cyst, odontogenic keratocyst).

Prophylactic wisdom tooth removal is recommended, especially before the age of 25, when occlusal placement is no longer expected due to displacement or the degree of retention. However, prophylactic wisdom tooth removal should not involve a close anatomical positional relationship between the root and the mandibular canal with the vascular nerve cord contained therein, which carries the risk of damage to these vital structures. Likewise, based on the general medical history, there should also not be a high risk of general medical complications (hemorrhagic diathesis, infectious diseases, antiresorptive drugs, radiotherapy, immunosuppression, etc).

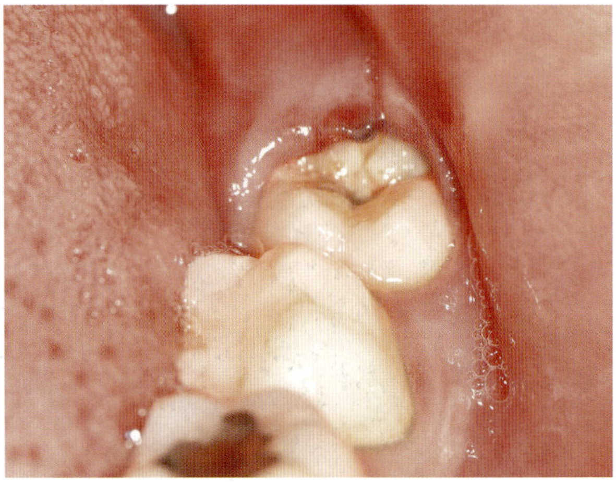

Fig 10-1 The classic indication for wisdom tooth removal is recurrent pericoronitis, shown here with swelling and redness of the gingiva and mucosa.

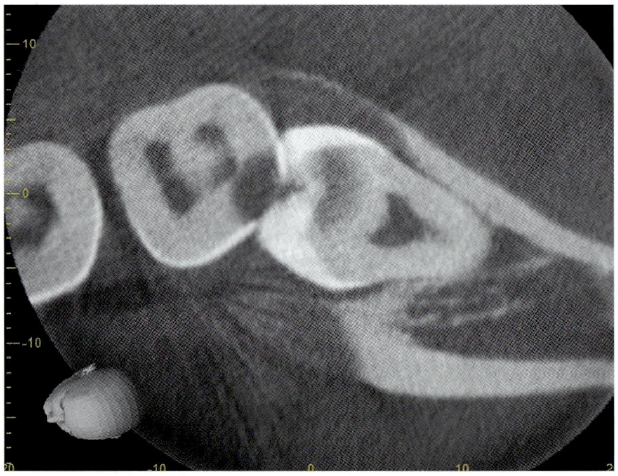

Fig 10-2 Cone beam computed tomography (CBCT) shows caries on the wisdom tooth and the molar in front of it.

Contraindications

The absolute contraindications usually result from the medical history, when patients are currently inoperable or inoperable due to their general medical condition (ongoing chemotherapy, end-stage tumor, etc).

A temporary contraindication may be the short-term use of medication such as temporary triple anticoagulation that could be switched to bi- or monotherapy in the foreseeable future. Similarly, acute pericoronitis is a temporary contraindication. This can be chronicized with antiseptic irrigation in combination with the local application of anti-inflammatory preparations or drains. In pregnant women, elective wisdom tooth removals should only be performed in the second trimester, if at all.

A reason for leaving wisdom teeth in place can be the replacement of non-preservable molars in the same quadrant (orthodontic placement) or in other quadrants (tooth transplantation). At the very least, this option should be discussed with the patient (Figs 10-3 to 10-10). Basically, a symptomless wisdom tooth without any pathology, with a complex degree of retention and displacement as well as a close positional relationship to the important anatomical structures, should be considered as a (at least temporary) contraindication for surgical removal

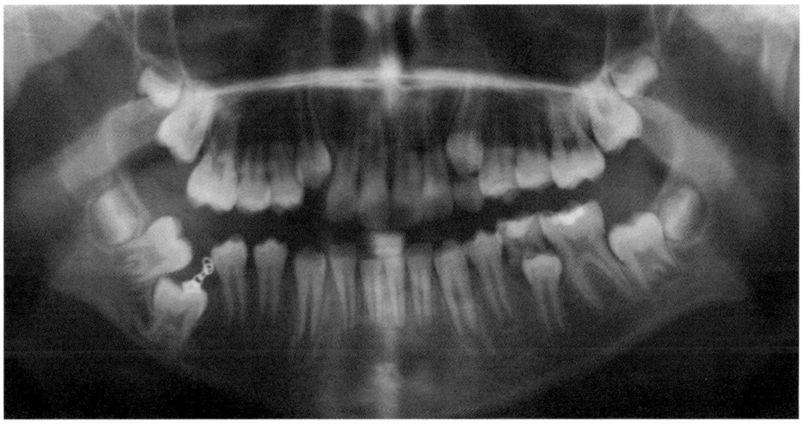

Fig 10-3 Initially, an attempt was made to orthodontically align tooth 46. However, since this was unsuccessful, its surgical removal and the subsequent orthodontic alignment of teeth 47 and 48 was planned. The indication for the removal of wisdom tooth 48 was therefore no longer present.

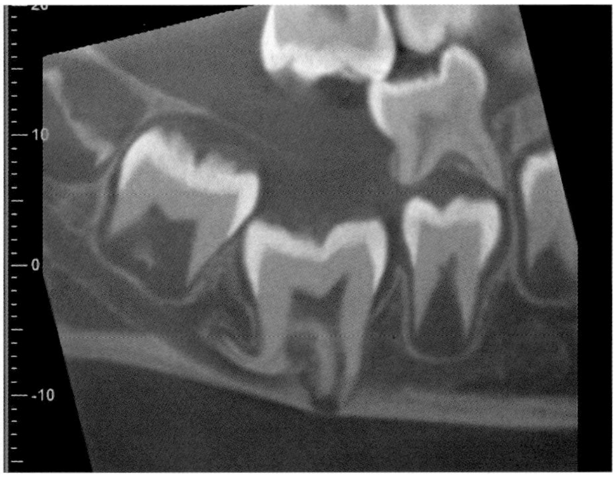

Fig 10-4 Tooth 46 shows a close positional relationship to the mandibular canal. In addition, the distal and mesiolingual roots are curved distally.

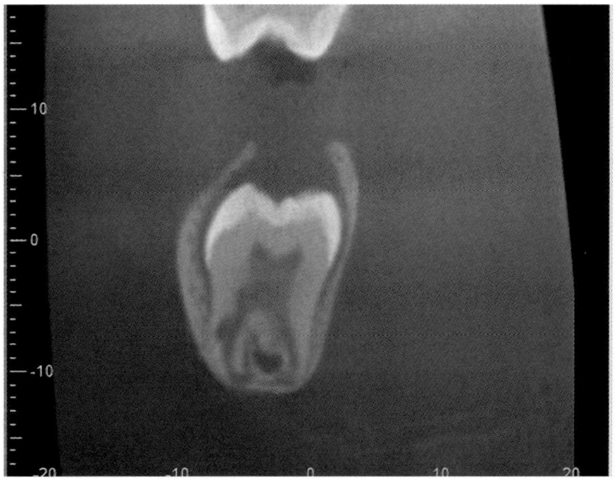

Fig 10-5 In the region of the mesiolingual root, the mandibular canal runs interradicularly.

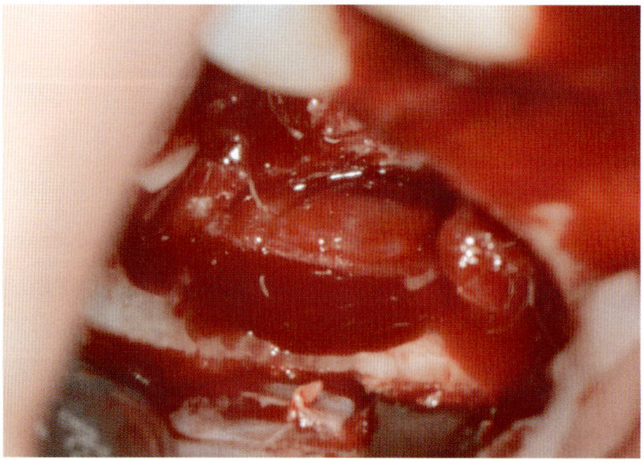

Fig 10-6 Intraoperative view of the vascular nerve cord of the mandibular canal after removal of tooth 46.

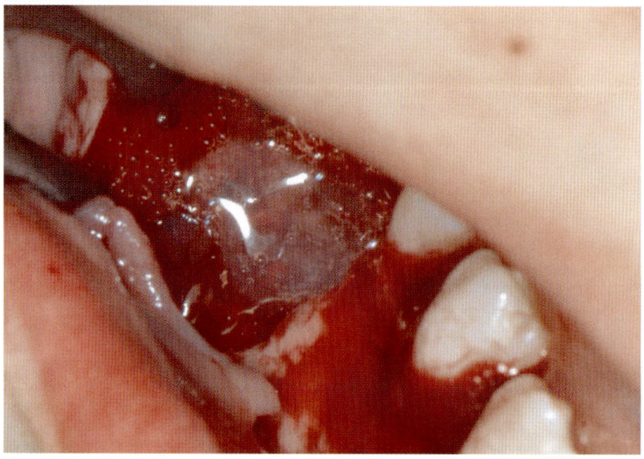

Fig 10-7 The exposed vascular nerve cord of the mandibular canal is covered with fibrin glue for protection.

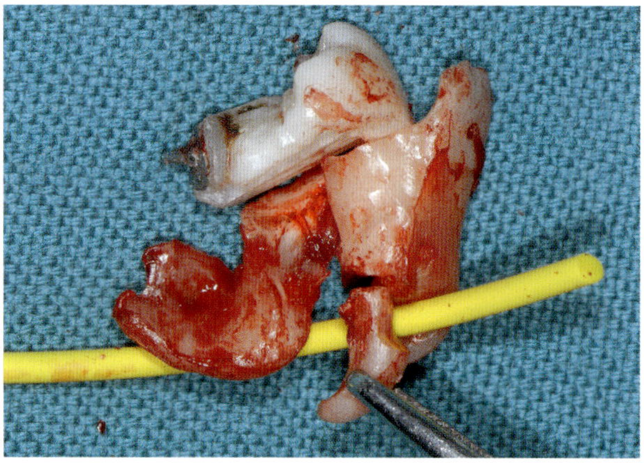

Fig 10-8 Checking the completeness of the removed tooth 46: The course of the vascular nerve cord is also shown for illustration.

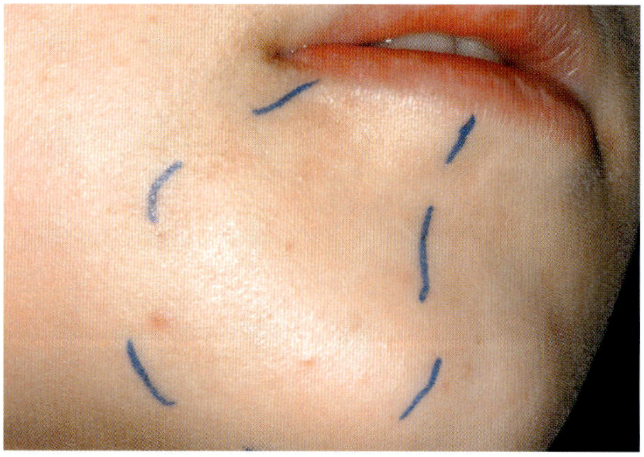

Fig 10-9 Temporary hypesthesia in the region of the inferior alveolar nerve.

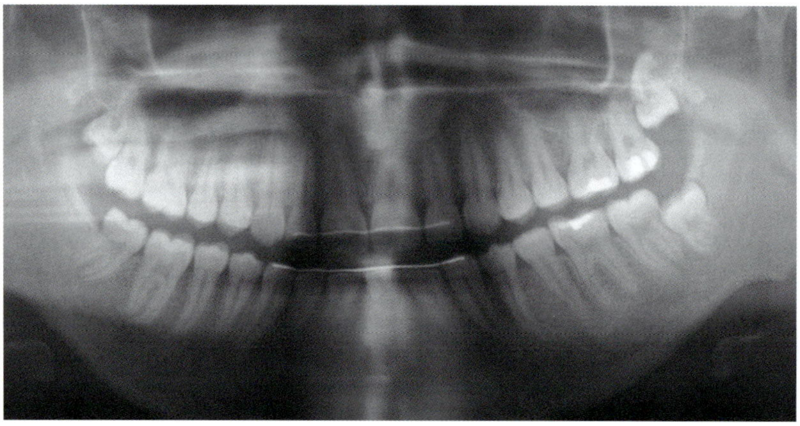

Fig 10-10 After completion of the treatment, teeth 47 and 48 are aligned. In a further step, wisdom teeth 18, 28, and 38 can be removed.

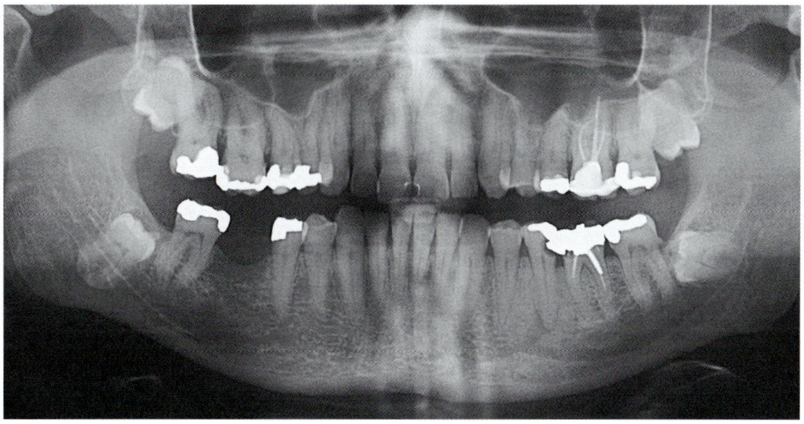

Fig 10-11 Contraindication for wisdom tooth removal: The patient is already elderly and asymptomatic, radiologically no pathologies are visible, and the surgical removal of tooth 48 carries the risk of damaging the inferior alveolar nerve.

due to the high intra- and/or postoperative risk of complications (Fig 10-11).

Specific risks

Specific risks include lesions on adjacent neural structures (inferior alveolar nerve, lingual nerve, buccal nerve) and opening of the maxillary sinus. Other risks include intraoperative (especially in the presence of a retromolar canal) (Fig 10-12) and postoperative bleeding, ostitis, wound healing disorders, swelling, and postoperative pain. In addition, the entire tooth (or teeth) as well as root portions may be dislocated into the surrounding tissue, e.g. into the maxillary sinus (Figs 10-13 to 10-16), the sublingual lodge or other regions (Figs 10-17).

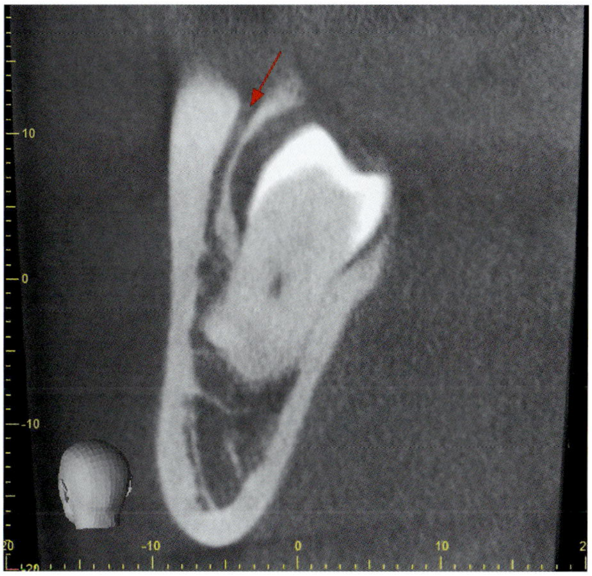

Fig 10-12 CBCT shows a buccally running retromolar canal (arrow) in close positional relation to the wisdom tooth crown.

Local anesthesia

In the maxilla, sufficient depth of anesthesia can usually be achieved by block anesthesia at the greater palatine nerve and by buccal infiltration anesthesia in the wisdom tooth region. The local anesthetic should contain an epinephrine supplement of 1:200,000 to somewhat reduce intraoperative bleeding and achieve sufficient anesthetic duration. In the mandible, block anesthesia of the inferior alveolar nerve and lingual nerve, and infiltration of the buccal nerve is performed. In addition, infiltration anesthesia buccally of the wisdom tooth to be removed is an option.

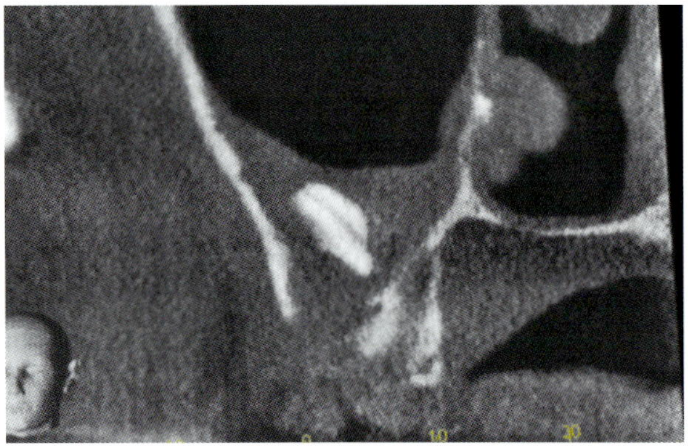

Fig 10-13 Root remnant dislocated into the maxillary sinus.

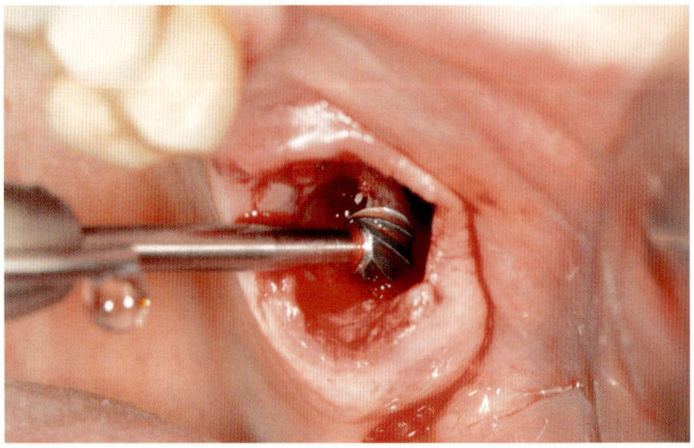

Fig 10-14 Access to the dislocated root remnant is widened by osteotomy (osteotomy of the bone septum).

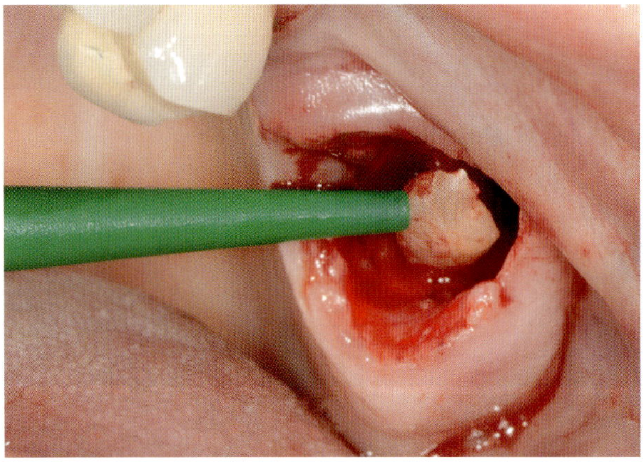

Fig 10-15 The root remnant can then be removed by a fine suction tip. This reduces the risk of displacing the tooth fragment further into the maxillary sinus.

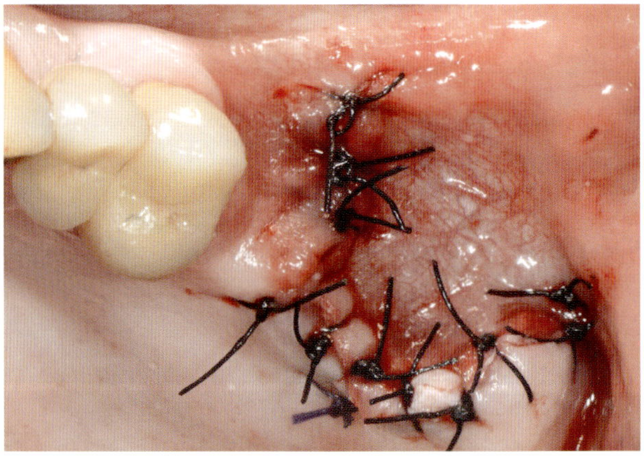

Fig 10-16 After removal of the root remnant, the maxillary sinus was closed here with a buccal flap according to Rehrmann.

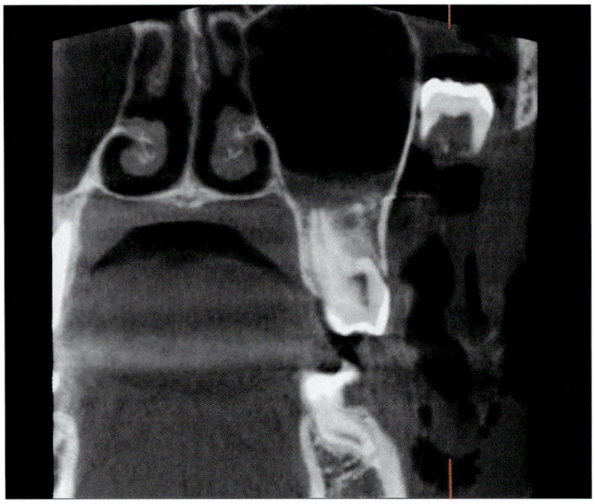

Fig 10-17 During the attempted tooth removal, tooth 28 was dislocated under the zygomatic arch.

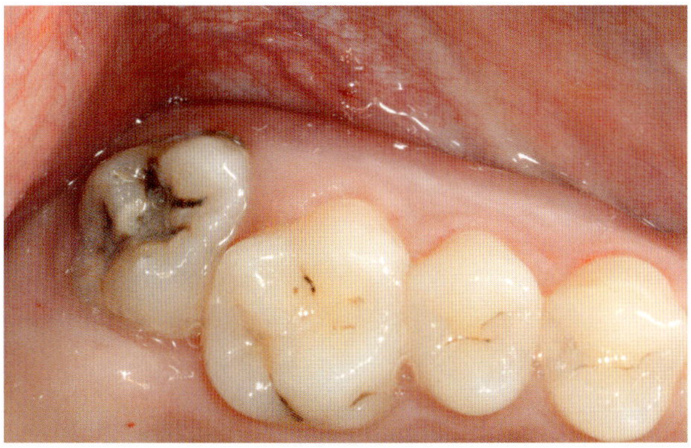

Fig 10-18 Initial clinical situation with planned removal of the impacted and displaced tooth 18 and the carious and buccally displaced tooth 17.

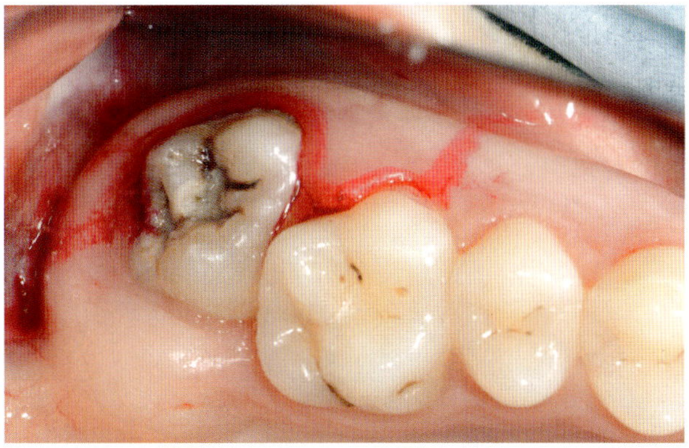

Fig 10-19 The vertical incision has been drawn here on tooth 16 due to the additional extraction of tooth 17. If only tooth 18 had been planned for extraction, the releasing incision would be located in the same way at tooth 17.

Step-by-step clinical procedure

Maxilla

The surgical procedure depends primarily on how the wisdom tooth is positioned in the dental arch and whether or not it is erupted. In the case of impacted wisdom teeth, a vertical incision is made mesially at the line angle of the second molar to relieve the tension. The higher a wisdom tooth is displaced, the further mesially the vertical releasing incision should be located (at the line angle of the first molar). Starting from the vertical releasing incision at the second molar, an intrasulcular incision is made buccally, and the incision is then continued on the distal alveolar ridge or maxillary tuberosity 1 to 2 cm further, depending on the situation (Figs 10-18 and 10-19).

This is followed by mobilization of a buccal mucoperiosteal flap (Fig 10-20). Fine raspatories are particularly suitable for this purpose (e.g. the Glickman raspatory; see Section 2). After mobilization of the mucoperiosteal flap, a buccal osteotomy is usually required to create a gap between the crown of the impacted wisdom tooth and the bone at the second molar (Figs 10-21 and 10-22), but also to expose the largest circumference of the tooth crown. If the crown of the wisdom tooth to be removed does not have bone coverage, removal may be possible without osteotomy. Decapitation or separation of wisdom teeth in the maxilla is very rarely necessary and should be avoided, if possible. Tooth removal is performed carefully (sparing the maxillary tuberosity) with a fine, angulated Deppeler elevator (Figs 10-23 and 10-24). The tooth roots are then inspected and checked for completeness. Remaining portions of the tooth follicle are removed with a bone curette or a Luer bone rongeur. Sharp bone edges are smoothed with rotary instruments under cooling with sterile isotonic saline. This is followed by careful probing of the alveolar fundus with a Bowman probe and the nasal blast test to rule out a possible oroantral communication (see Section 11). Before closure, the wound area is extensively irrigated with sterile isotonic saline to remove any remaining bone chips or tooth splinters.

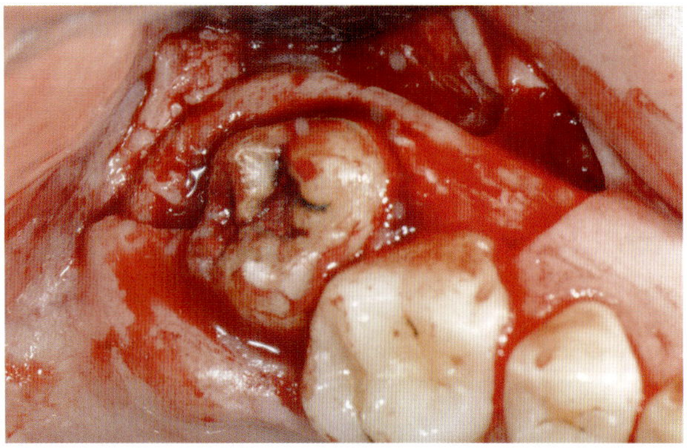

Fig 10-20 After the incision, the buccal mucoperiosteal flap is mobilized.

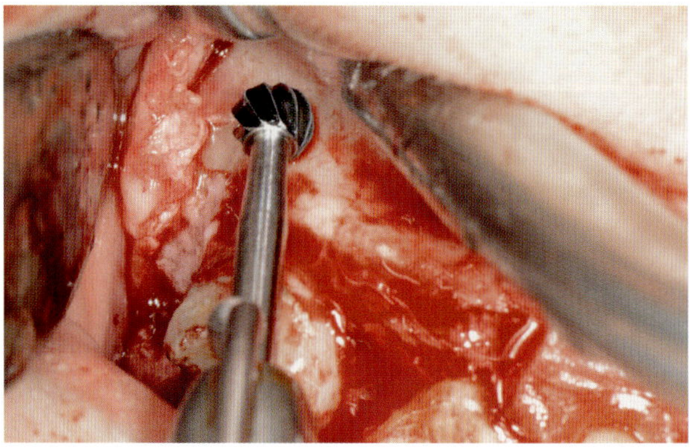

Fig 10-21 Buccal osteotomy with a large rose bur.

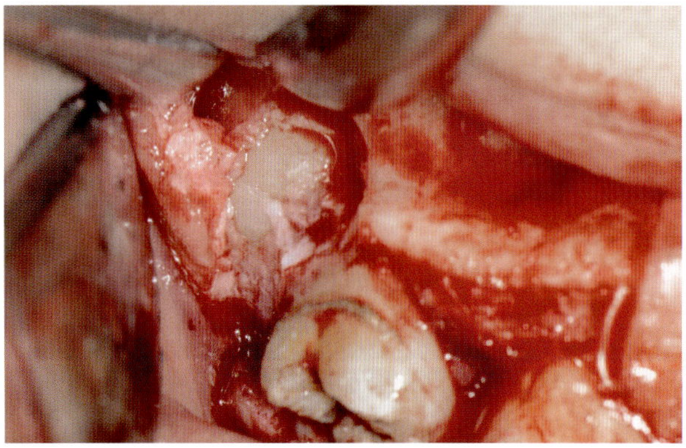

Fig 10-22 Visualization of the largest circumference of tooth 18 after osteotomy.

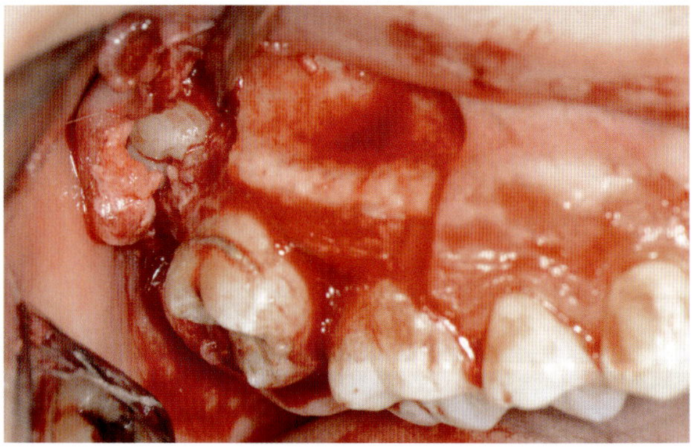

Fig 10-23 Tooth 18 can now be mobilized and removed with a narrow, angulated Deppeler elevator.

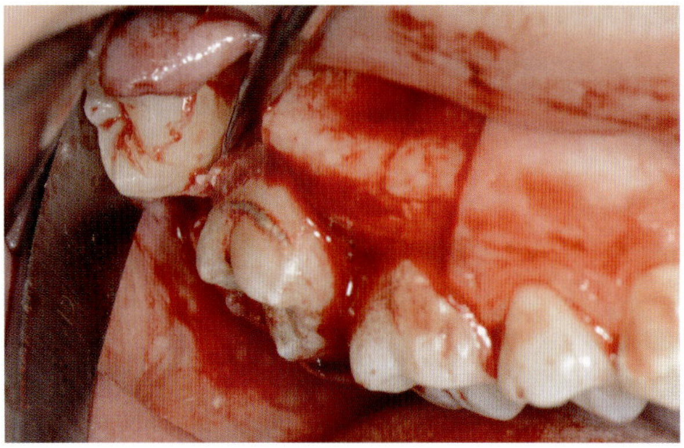

Fig 10-24 To prevent dorsal dislocation, a raspatory can be inserted between the tooth and the soft tissue.

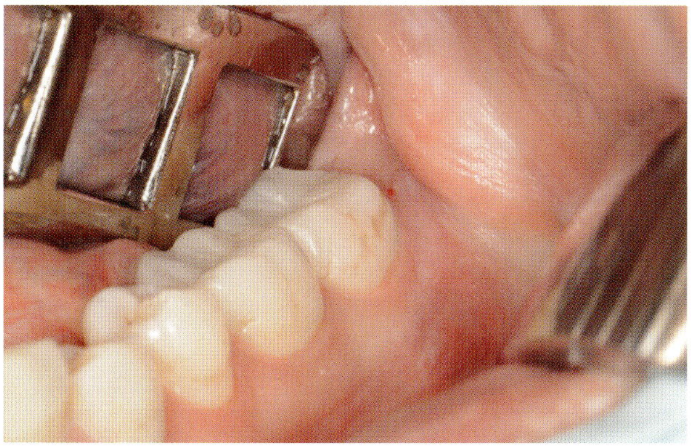

Fig 10-25 Initial clinical situation in the posterior mandible before surgical removal of wisdom tooth 38.

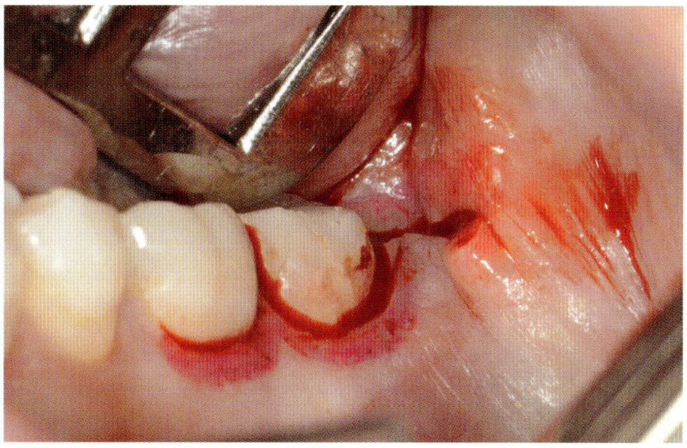

Fig 10-26 The incision is made buccally intrasulcularly and the releasing incision is directed distobuccally.

Mandible

The surgical procedure in the mandible, analogous to the maxilla, depends on the position of the wisdom tooth in the dental arch and the type of retention and dislocation. A buccal intrasulcular incision is made from the first to the second molar. It must be noted that distal to the second molar, the lingual nerve runs along the alveolar ridge toward the floor of the mouth in approximately 20% of cases[2]. Therefore, the releasing incision should be made from the distobuccal cusp of the second molar or, in the case of partially retained teeth, from the distobuccal portion of the exposed crown of the wisdom tooth in the direction of the vestibule (Video 10-1). Therefore, the releasing incision has a distobuccal direction and is oriented to the ascending branch of the mandible (Figs 10-25 and 10-26). A buccal mucoperiosteal flap is prepared with fine raspatories in a mesiodistal direction (Fig 10-27, Video 10-2). Lingually, care must be taken to guide the raspatory strictly subperiosteally when mobilizing the soft tissue, and mobilization is only carried out as far as is necessary for inserting an instrument to protect the lingual nerve (e.g. a Williger/Partsch raspatory or a Davis brain spatula; see Section 2) (Fig 10-28). The soft tissue distal to the second molar is not infrequently fused with the tooth follicle of the impacted wisdom tooth. Mobilization of the soft tissue may be difficult as a result. In order to place a lingual raspatory to protect the lingual nerve, it is recommended to first prepare the mucoperiosteal flap in the direction of the ascending branch of the mandible and then carefully mobilize the mucoperiosteal flap distal to the impacted wisdom tooth on a bony support in a lingual direction. The tooth follicle usually detaches from the overlying soft tissue so that the raspatory can then be inserted lingually. In the buccal region, a Wilde retractor is preferable to a Langenbeck retractor for holding the mobilized soft tissue (see Section 2) (Video 10-3), as it is much gentler on the soft tissue (less hematoma formation). This is followed by the osteotomy with rotating instruments of different diameters

Video 10-1 Incision guidance during surgical removal of a mandibular wisdom tooth.

Video 10-2 Mobilization of the buccal mucoperiosteal flap.

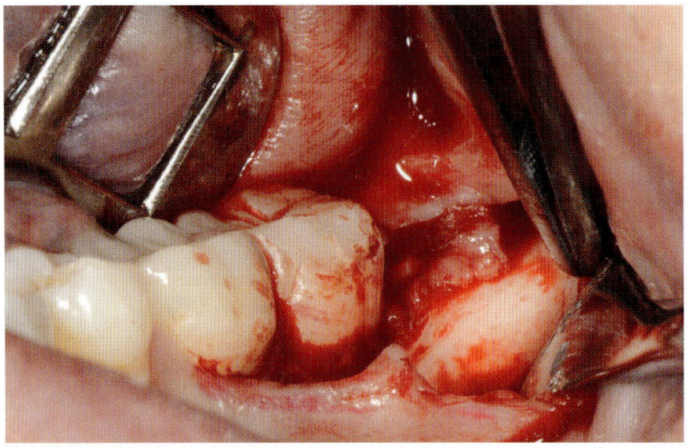

Fig 10-27 After preparation of the buccal mucoperiosteal flap, a Wilde retractor is inserted.

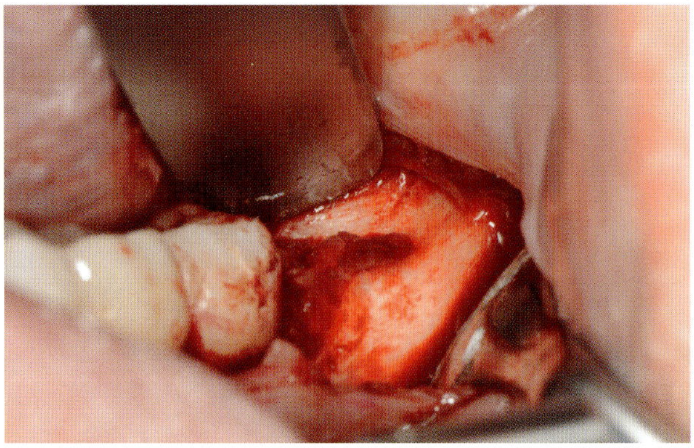

Fig 10-28 In the lingual region, a Davis brain spatula is inserted to protect the lingual nerve.

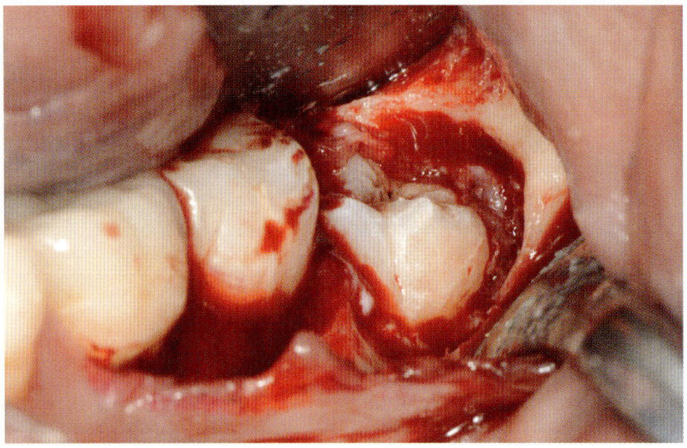

Fig 10-29 Visualization of the tooth crown through the osteotomy.

Video 10-3 Wilde retractor.

Video 10-4 Osteotomy.

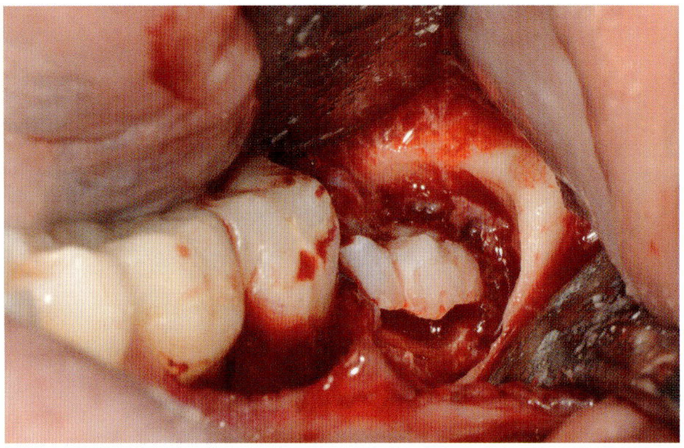

Fig 10-30 Decapitation is performed while protecting the lingual portions.

Video 10-5 Further osteotomy with a Lindemann bur.

Video 10-6 Removal of the crown.

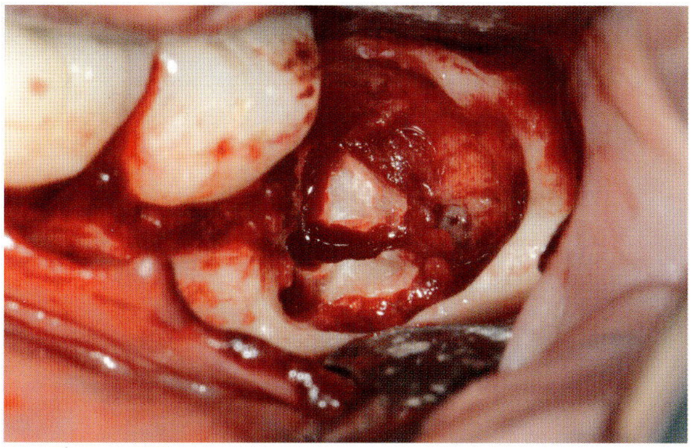

Fig 10-31 Separation of the roots according to the anatomy: here with the buccal and lingual root.

Video 10-7 Removal of the tooth crown.

Video 10-8 Separation of the roots.

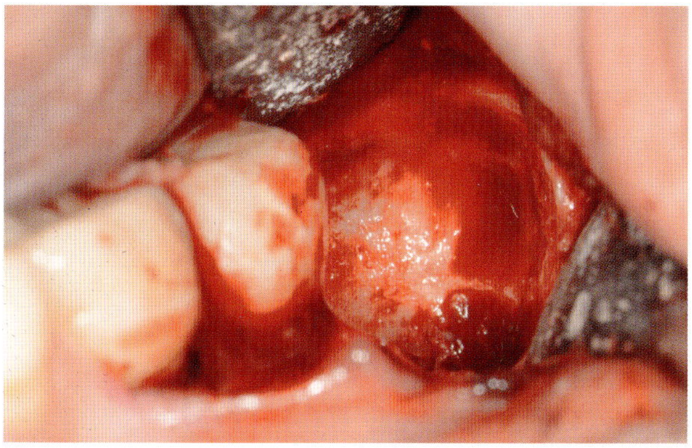

Fig 10-32 Checking the alveolus after removal of the roots in toto.

Video 10-9 Removal of the distal root.

Video 10-10 Removal of the mesial root.

to expose the tooth crown (Fig 10-29). For better control of the rotating instrument, the osteotomy is performed with a pulling motion from lingual to buccal or from distal to mesial (Videos 10-4 and 10-5). The crown should be exposed at least buccally to the cementoenamel junction (CEJ), and then, if necessary, the dental crown should be separated from the rootstock with a Lindemann bur and cleanly set down with a an elevator (Fig 10-30, Video 10-6). Removal of the tooth crown (Video 10-7) is followed, if necessary, by separation of the roots according to the root anatomy (Fig 10-31, Video 10-8). Finally, the remaining root portions are mobilized with an elevator, and remnants of the tooth follicle are removed with a Luer bone rongeur (Fig 10-32, Videos 10-9 and 10-10). Sharp bone edges are smoothed with rotary instruments (Video 10-11) and followed by irrigation with sterile isotonic saline to remove any remaining bone chips or tooth splinters.

Video 10-11 Smoothing of sharp bone edges.

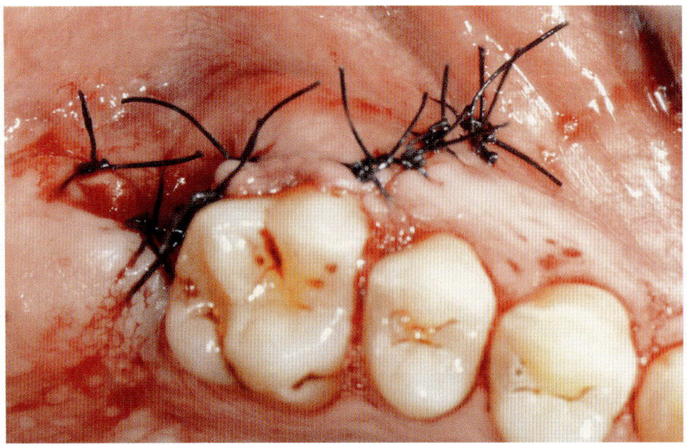

Fig 10-33 Maxilla: reduction of the mucoperiosteal flap and fixation with sutures.

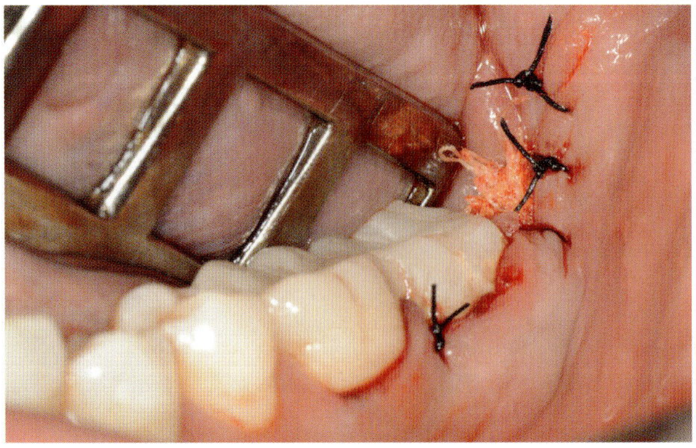

Fig 10-34 Mandible: semi-open wound closure with insertion of an iodoform strip as drainage.

Video 10-12 Wound closure and insertion of an iodoform drain.

Wound care and closure

The mucoperiosteal flap is reduced and fixed with 3-0 or 4-0 sutures (Figs 10-33 and 10-34). In the mandible, distal to the second molar, a double-loop suture can prevent the flap from slipping cranially and ensure a tight dentogingival closure to avoid increased probing depths distal to the second molar postoperatively (see Section 3). Mobilized interdental papillae can be fixed with vertical mattress sutures (see Section 3). Releasing incisions are typically treated with single-button sutures (see Section 3). In the mandible, the wound care of choice is a semi-open wound closure with a short iodoform strip as a drain for 2 days (Video 10-12); in the maxilla, primary wound closure is performed. If the maxillary sinus is opened (see Section 11) after removal of erupted or partially retained wisdom teeth, soft tissue closure is performed if there are no signs of sinusitis (Fig 10-16).

Postoperative controls and course

A postoperative panoramic radiograph is indicated only in special situations (e.g. if remaining tooth fragments are suspected). Depending on the individual situation, a check-up can be performed on the first or second postoperative day. The drainage in the mandible is typically removed 2 days after wisdom tooth removal. The sutures are usually removed after 1 week. It is generally not necessary to prescribe an antibiotic unless dictated by the individual patient history or surgical course. Analgesics are prescribed according to need, medical history, and body weight (see Section 14). Preoperative administration of a one-shot dosage of cortisone can significantly reduce postoperative morbidity and should be considered on a case-by-case basis[1] (see Section 14).

Recommended literature

1. Acham S, Klampfl A, Truschnegg A, Kirmeier R, Sandner-Kiesling A, Jakse N. Beneficial effect of methylprednisolone after mandibular third molar surgery: A randomized, double-blind, placebo-controlled split-mouth trial. Clin Oral Investig 2013;17:1693–1700.
2. Bailey E, Kashbour W, Shah N, Worthington HV, Renton TF, Coulthard P. Surgical techniques for the removal of mandibular wisdom teeth. Cochrane Database Syst Rev 2020;7:1–162.
3. Kiesselbach JE, Chamberlain JG. Clinical and anatomic observations on the relationship of the lingual nerve to the mandibular third molar region. J Oral Maxillofac Surg 1984;42:565–567.
4. Kunkel M, Fritz U, Pistner H, et al. S2k-Leitlinie: Operative Entfernung von Weisheitszähnen. AWMF-Registernummer: 007-003. Stand: August 2019.
5. Lambrecht JT, Hoffmeister B. Operative Entfernung retinierter und verlagerter Zähne. In: Lambrecht JT (Hsrg). Zahnärztliche Operationen. Berlin: Quintessenz, 2008.
6. Lambrecht JT, von Planta M (Hrsg). Zahnärztliche Risikopatienten. Berlin: Quintessenz, 2018.

Coronectomy

Indications

The indication is debatable for the avoidance of inevitable damage to the inferior alveolar nerve by surgical wisdom tooth removal, i.e. in the case of the interradicular course of the mandibular canal with contact to the wisdom tooth root, or in the case of complete encirclement of the mandibular canal by the wisdom tooth roots (Figs 10-35 to 10-38), which occurs in less than 4% of cases[4].

As a general rule, the indication for coronectomy should be very narrow and strict. Under no circumstances should it lead to inexperienced practitioners failing to remove mandibular wisdom teeth completely, and uncritically leaving in place roots or root portions.

Contraindications

Contraindications exist if the wisdom tooth does not have a close anatomical positional relationship to the mandibular canal in the CBCT. In this case, complete tooth removal must be attempted.

Other contraindications are: profound caries, pulp necrosis or discomfort from pulpitis around the wisdom tooth; high-risk patients (chemotherapy, HIV infection, diabetes mellitus, antiresorptive medication, long-term steroid treatment, radiotherapy in the head and neck region, etc); and failed complete tooth removal.

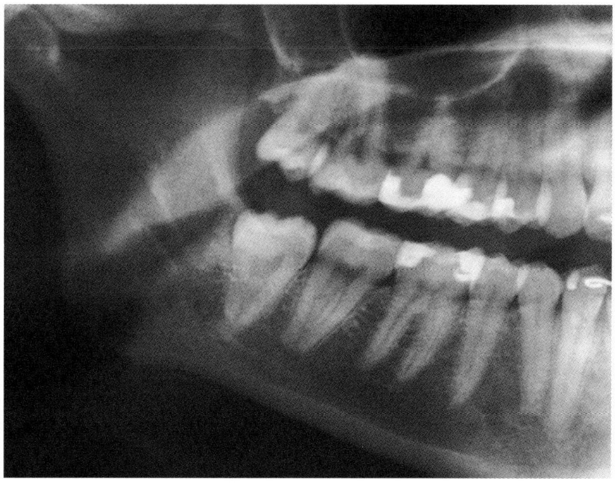

Fig 10-35 Partially retained and decayed tooth 48 in a 32-year-old generally healthy patient. Based on the preoperative panoramic radiograph, radiographic superimposition of tooth root 48 with the inferior border of the mandibular canal was evident. A CBCT was obtained for further clarification.

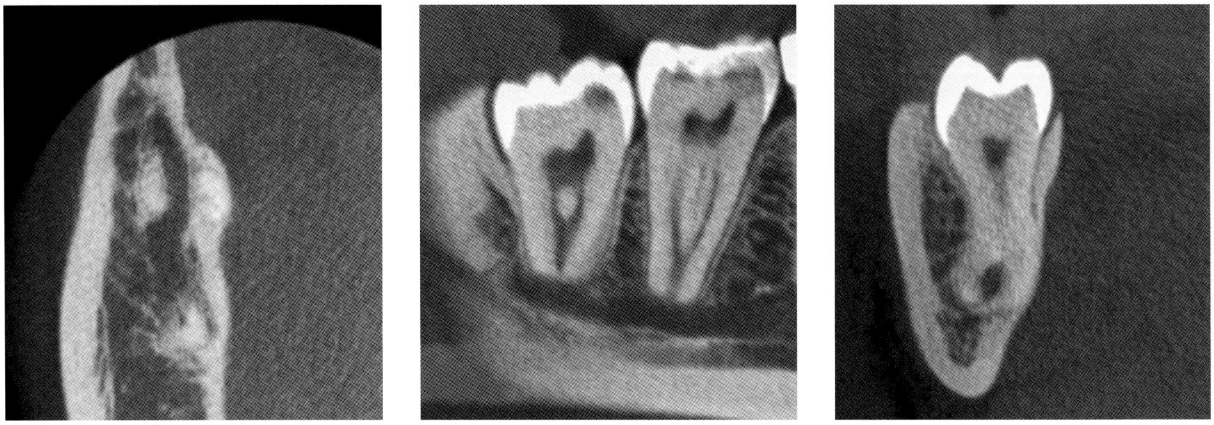

Figs 10-36 to 10-38 On the basis of the CBCT, a complete enclosure of the mandibular canal by the two-rooted tooth 48 can be seen. Interradicularly, the bony boundary of the mandibular canal could not be traced throughout. Due to the increased risk of nerve lesion, both complete removal and coronectomy were discussed with the patient. The patient opted for the latter procedure.

Specific risks

- Intraoperative mobilization of the rootstock by instruments (in 2% to 38% of cases)[1,5],
- Second surgical intervention due to postoperative complications (less than 5% of cases)[2,5], e.g. wound dehiscence without complete epithelialization, discomfort from pulpitis or pulp necrosis (pain symptoms resemble ostitis, which is usually recurrent), migration of the root with connection to the oral cavity,
- The risk of ostitis (less than 12% of cases) or wound infection (in 1% to 5.8% of cases) is not increased and is equivalent to that of complete tooth removal[1,3,5].

Local anesthesia

- Block anesthesia on the inferior alveolar nerve, lingual nerve, and buccal nerve.

Step-by-step clinical procedure

Initially, analogous to surgical wisdom tooth removal, an intrasulcular incision is made from the mesial third of the mandibular first molar to the wisdom tooth, with distobuccal release at a 45-degree angle over the ascending ramus of the mandible (Figs 10-39 and 10-40). A mucoperiosteal flap is then mobilized from the buccal side. On the lingual side, the mucoperiosteal flap can be minimally mobilized and a Davis brain spatula or wide raspatory can be used to protect the lingual nerve (Fig 10-41). Osteotomy follows under constant cooling with sterile isotonic saline to expose the crown of tooth 48 to the CEJ (Fig 10-42). A sharp surgical bur is then used to create a predetermined breaking point for decapitation (Fig 10-43). It is recommended that the rotating instrument penetrates approximately two-thirds of the vestibulo-oral width of the tooth crown to avoid injury to the lingual soft tissue. Then, for decapitation, an elevator is guided to the created predetermined breaking point and rotated, and the dental crown is cleanly set down (Figs 10-44 and 10-45). The patient must be informed of the corresponding crack-

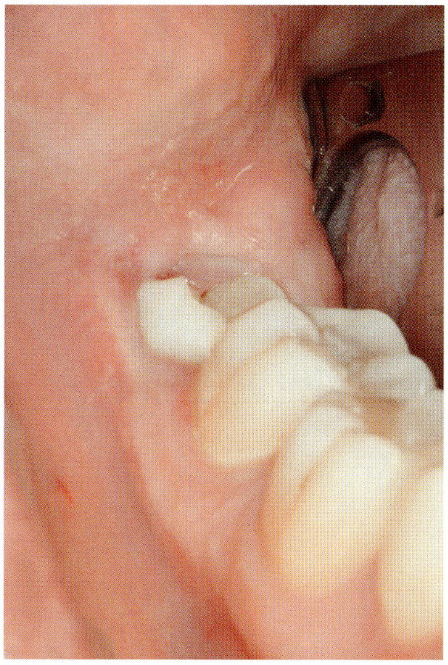

Fig 10-39 Initial clinical situation: Leaving the partially retained tooth 48 in place would sooner or later have led to progressive caries and/or pericoronitis. Coronectomy would no longer have been possible in the presence of pulp necrosis.

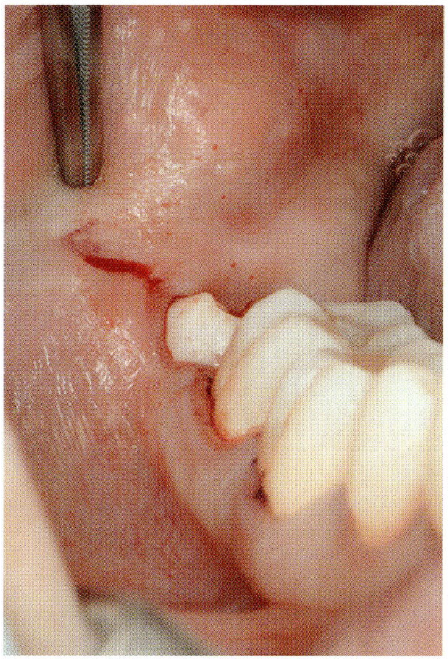

Fig 10-40 After the intrasulcular incision starting at the mesial third of tooth 46 in the direction of tooth 48 with a distobuccal releasing incision at a 45-degree angle over the *ramus ascendens* of the mandible.

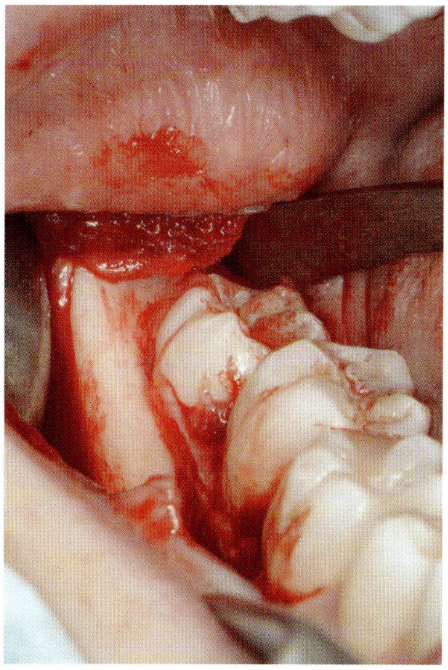

Fig 10-41 After preparation of the buccal mucoperiosteal flap, the soft tissue is minimally mobilized on the lingual side and a Williger raspatory is inserted to protect the lingual nerve.

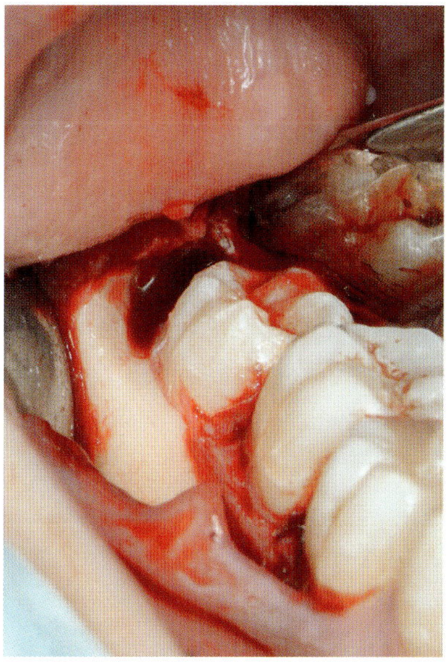

Fig 10-42 The osteotomy exposes the crown of tooth 48 to the cementoenamel junction (CEJ).

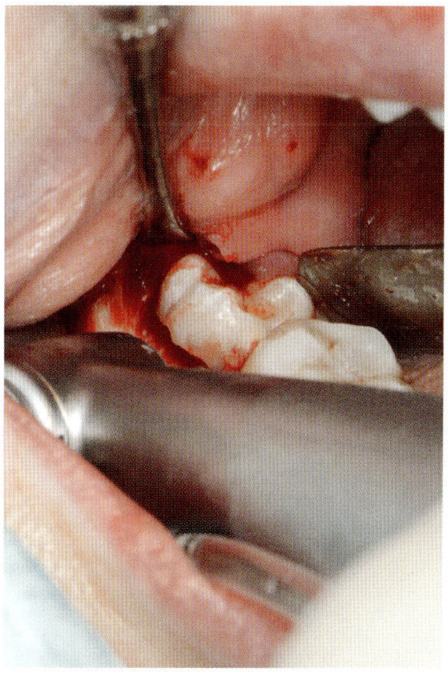

Fig 10-43 A separator is used to create a predetermined breaking point for the elevator at the level of the CEJ (decapitation).

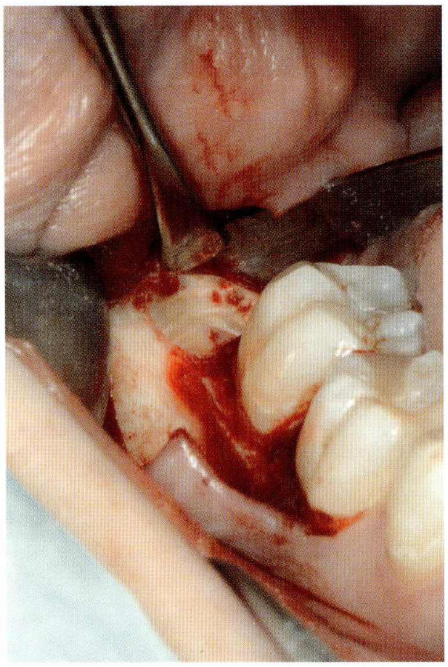

Fig 10-44 Situation after the crown has been removed. The root canal must not be mobilized.

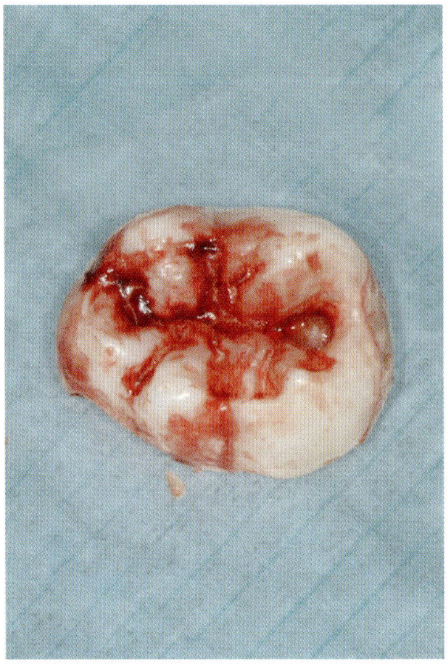

Fig 10-45 Crown of tooth 48 after decapitation.

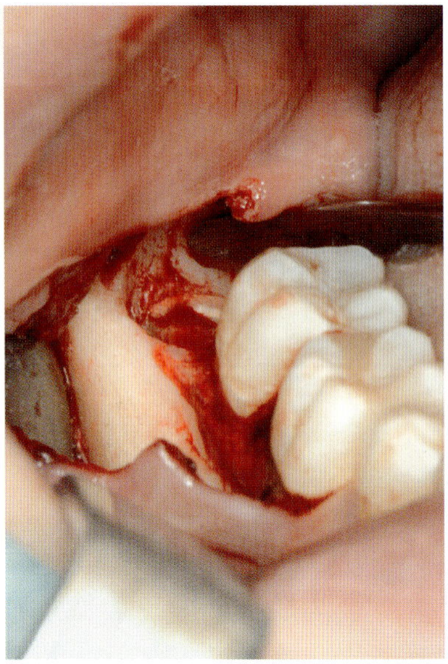

Fig 10-46 The rootstock is reduced 3 to 4 mm below the bone level with a diamond bur. All enamel must be removed in this process.

ing sound shortly beforehand. The rootstock must not be mobilized under any circumstances during decapitation. If the rootstock exhibits increased mobility after decapitation, complete removal of the roots must be performed due to the increased risk of infection. The follicular tissue can then be removed with a Lucas bone curette or a Luer bone rongeur. The rootstock is then reduced in height together with the pulp it contains (analogous to pulp amputation in partial pulpotomy) with a diamond roller or ball at high speed at least 3 mm below the surrounding bone level (Fig 10-46). Here, the deeper the better. However, perforation in the area of lingual bone retraction must be avoided. Sufficient marginal bone coverage lingually must be ensured. Furthermore, no enamel portions must remain (Fig 10-47). No further treatment is required with regard to the pulp.

Wound care and closure

After osteoplasty and careful irrigation with sterile isotonic saline (to remove bone chips below the mucoperiosteal flap), this flap is reduced. For primary wound closure in partially retained or even completely erupted teeth, the mucoperiosteal flap margins must be appropriately deepithelialized with a scalpel. Wound closure is performed at the distobuccal releasing incision with single-button sutures, and in the papilla area between the first and second molars with a vertical mattress suture (3-0 or 4-0 non-resorbable sutures) (Fig 10-48). Distal to the second molar, a double-loop suture is suitable.

After the surgical procedure or a few days later, a hemifacial panoramic radiograph (Fig 10-49) is taken to record the status quo. This is considered a reference image for further radiologic imaging of the region. This is followed by the postoperative workup (see Section 15). Med-

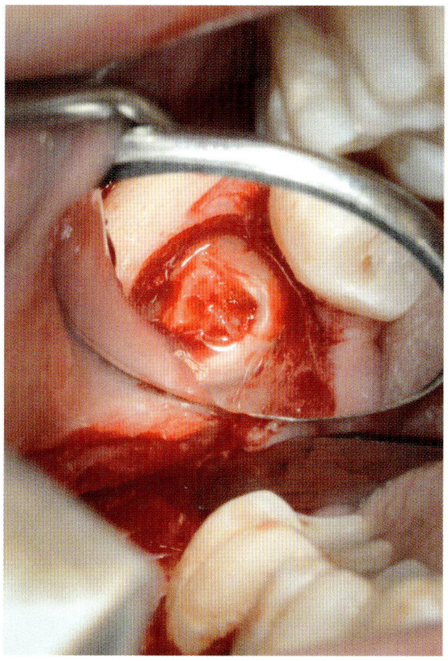

Fig 10-47 Rootstock left in place from occlusal (photo via dental mirror). The resected pulp needs no further treatment.

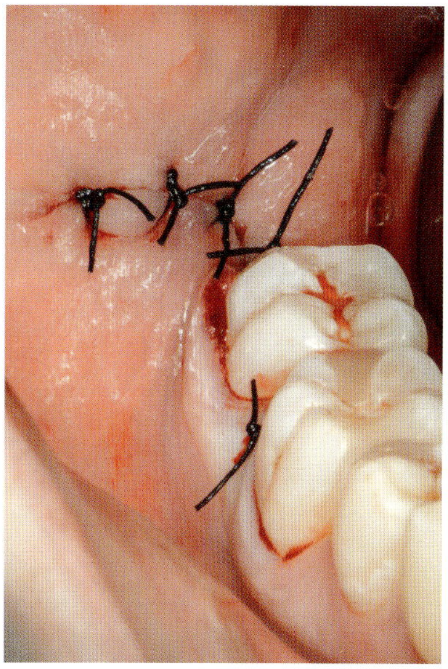

Fig 10-48 Primary wound closure with single-button sutures in the area of the distobuccal releasing incision and a vertical mattress suture at papilla 46/47.

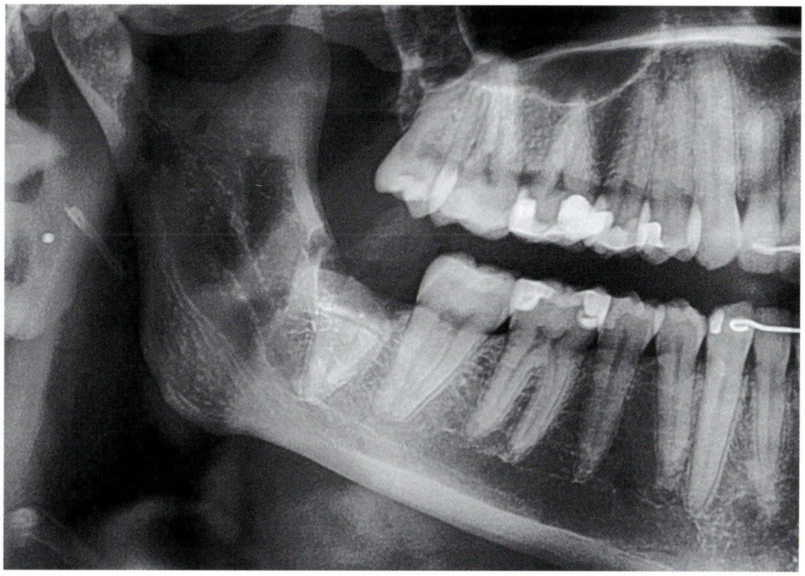

Fig 10-49 Radiologic control with a hemifacial panoramic radiograph: The left rootstock is 3 mm subcrestal.

ications include analgesic (if needed), antiseptic, a cooling bag for swelling prophylaxis, and reserve swabs. Antibiotic is not obligatory and is recommended in the literature only in case of preoperative pericoronitis.

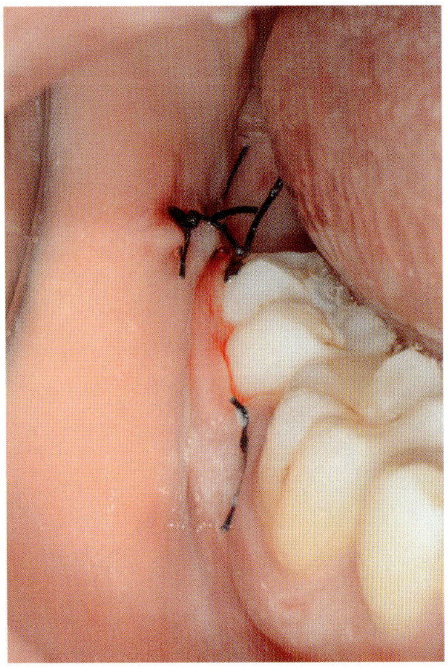

Fig 10-50 Situation 2 days post-operatively after disinfection.

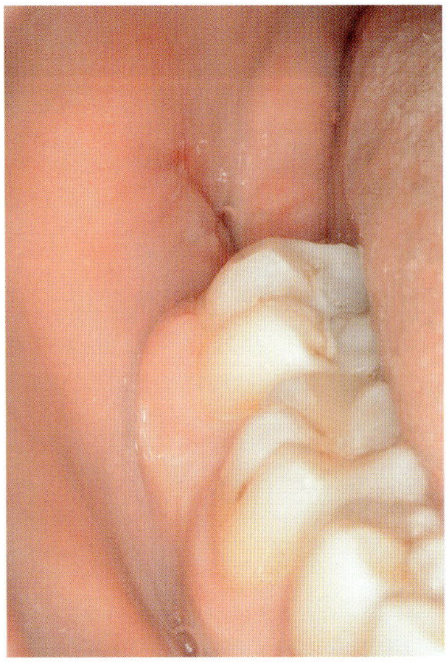

Fig 10-51 Situation 10 days post-operatively after suture removal.

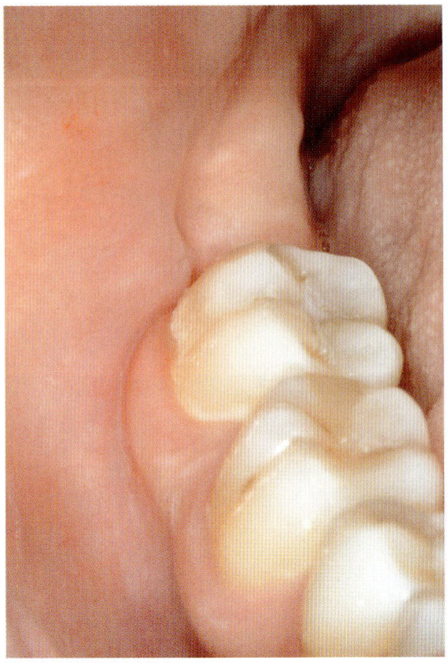

Fig 10-52 Clinical control after 6 months: Small scarring retraction in the area of the incision.

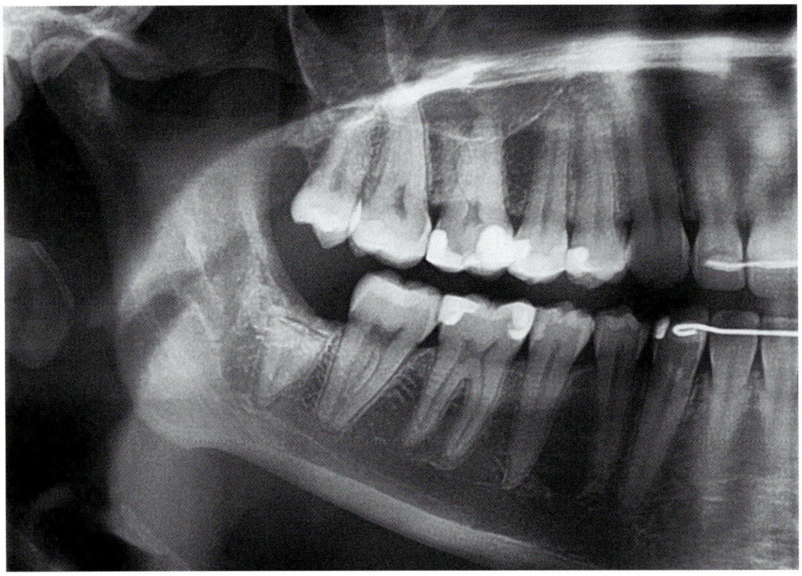

Fig 10-53 Radiologic control after 6 months: Reossification cranial to the root at region 48.

Postoperative controls and course

The first control is performed on the second postoperative day. The wound is disinfected with an antiseptic and the sufficiency of the primary wound closure is checked (Fig 10-50). The sutures are removed 10 days postoperatively (Fig 10-51). The next clinical and radiologic follow-up check should be performed after 6 to 12 months (Figs 10-52 and 10-53), and annually thereafter.

If complications occur postoperatively, such as wound dehiscence or complaints due to pulpitis or the migration of the root with connection to the oral cavity, a second surgical procedure usually involving complete removal of the rootstock will be necessary.

References

1. Cilasun U, Yildirim T, Guzeldemir E, Pektas ZO. Coronectomy in patients with high risk of inferior alveolar nerve injury diagnosed by computed tomography. J Oral Maxillofac Surg 2011;69:1557–1561.
2. Hatano Y, Kurita K, Kuroiwa Y, Yuasa H, Ariji E. Clinical evaluations of coronectomy (intentional partial odontectomy) for mandibular third molars using dental computed tomography: a case-control study. J Oral Maxillofac Surg 2009;67:1806–1814.
3. Leung YY, Cheung LK. Safety of coronectomy versus excision of wisdom teeth: A randomized controlled trial. Oral Surg Oral Med Oral Pathol Oral Radiol Endod 2009;108:821–827.
4. Maglione M, Costantinides F, Bazzocchi G. Classification of impacted mandibular third molars on cone-beam CT images. J Clin Exp Dent 2015;7:224–231.
5. Renton T, Hankins M, Sproate C, McGurk M. A randomised controlled clinical trial to compare the incidence of injury to the inferior alveolar nerve as a result of coronectomy and removal of mandibular third molars. Br J Oral Maxillofac Surg 2005;43:7–12.

Closure of opened maxillary sinuses

11

Fabio Saccardin, Sebastian Kühl

In tooth extractions, apicectomies (apical surgery), and cyst operations in the maxillary posterior region, there is the risk of an unphysiologic connection between the oral cavity and the maxillary sinus, so-called oroantral communication (OAC). This is due to the close anatomical positional relationship of the tooth roots. In this context, the individual teeth have different incidences with regard to a maxillary sinus opening when teeth are removed: first molar 0.6%, second molar 0.5%, third molar 0.3%, second premolar 0.2%, and first premolar and canine 0.1%[11]. If an OAC remains untreated over a longer period of time, this can lead to maxillary sinusitis due to germ colonization from the oral flora. Under certain circumstances, epithelialization occurs inside the junction and an oroantral fistula (OAF) develops.

Prior to any oral surgery in the maxillary posterior region, a preoperative single tooth radiograph or panoramic radiograph must be performed to assess the risk of an OAC. Radiographic projection of the root tips into the maxillary sinus or extensive periradicular pathology increase the risk in this regard. The patient must be informed about this potential complication preoperatively (see Section 5). In addition, the preoperative condition of the maxillary sinus should be reviewed anamnestically, clinically, and radiologically. In acute sinusitis, patients often report headache, sensation of pressure/discomfort in the infraorbital region, maxillary sinus weather sensitivity, toothache in several maxillary posterior teeth, increasing pain intensity when bending down, concussion pain when climbing stairs, obstructed nasal breathing or fever as part of the history. In chronic sinusitis (> 3 months), the same symptoms may occur, but usually with less intensity; in some cases, patients are asymptomatic. On clinical examination, palpation and percussion tenderness in the canine fossa, infraorbital foramen or laterofacial maxillary sinus wall are typical of the presence of sinusitis. Radiologically, this is usually manifested by a thickening of the Schneiderian membrane or by complete maxillary sinus shadowing of varying density (empyema in purulent sinusitis). If the radiologic findings are unclear in this regard and do not match the medical history or clinical findings, it is recommended to perform cone beam computed tomography (CBCT)[9].

If a tooth has been completely removed in the maxillary posterior region, a standard operating procedure (Fig 11-1) always follows to exclude an OAC. Initially, the osseous alveolar fundus is carefully checked for continuity using a Bowman lacrimal probe (Fig 11-2). If the alveolar fundus is not intact or the findings appear unclear, the Valsalva maneuver follows (Fig 11-3). The patient's nose is held closed with the fingers and the patient is instructed to allow pressure to build up in the nasal cavity (as in blowing the nose). If an OAC is present, air will audibly escape into the oral cavity with a hissing or whistling sound, and occasionally bubbles will be observed. However, if the Schneiderian membrane is radiologically thickened or exhibits polyp-like changes, the Valsalva maneuver may also be falsely negative due to the valve effect. In these cases, the reverse Valsalva maneuver (Fig 11-4) must be performed. Here, the patient closes the mouth and inflates the cheeks. If an OAC is present, the patient will not be able to do this because the pressure will cause the air to escape into the maxillary sinus or the nasal cavity, respectively. At this point, it should be mentioned that failure to recognize or even ignoring a present OAC is considered a treatment not performed *lege artis*.

If an OAC is diagnosed by inspection, probing or the Valsalva maneuver, the condition of the maxillary sinus is decisive for any further procedure. If the maxillary sinus is clear, soft tissue closure is performed directly. However, if there are anamnestic, clinical or radiologic signs of sinusitis, or if there is spontaneous secretion/pus

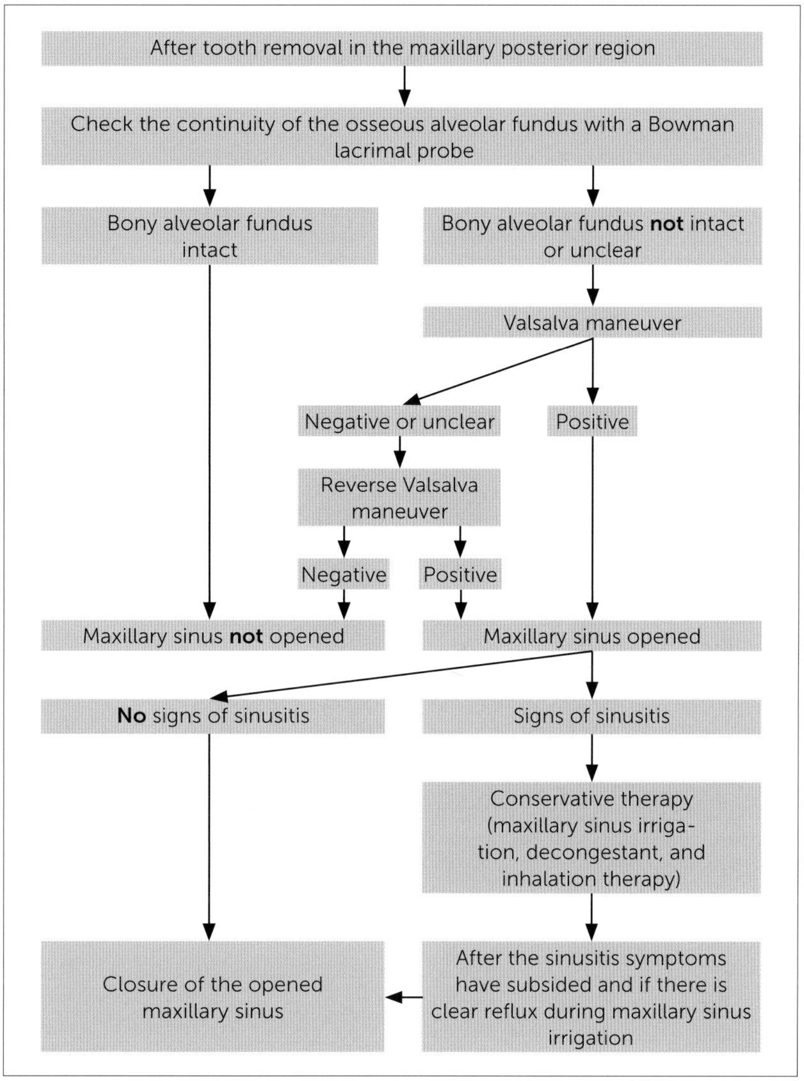

Fig 11-1 Standard operating procedure after tooth removal in the maxillary posterior region to exclude or treat OAC or OAF.

discharge (empyema) via the OAC, immediate soft tissue closure must not be performed even in the case of a small perforation. In this case, a two-stage procedure should be chosen. This means that the sinusitis must first be chronicized by conservative therapy before soft tissue closure can be performed.

Conservative therapy for sinusitis consists of daily transalveolar sinus irrigation with a blunt irrigation cannula (e.g. with a peripheral venous catheter as an attachment) and heated, sterile isotonic saline solution (Figs 11-5 to 11-7). Decongestant nasal drops are also prescribed. This is intended to facilitate exudate drainage via the *ostium naturale*. Adjuvant inhalation therapy with water vapor (essential oils, chamomile, saline aerosols as additives) can be performed: Heat application promotes blood flow, which has an anti-inflammatory effect.

The use of antibiotics (aminopenicillin possibly with beta-lactamase inhibitor; clindamycin in case of penicillin allergy) is recommended in the literature only in case of acute exacerbation of sinusitis or abscess with the tendency to spread[9,14].

Only after the sinusitis symptoms have subsided, and providing there is clear reflux during maxillary sinus irrigation, can soft tissue closure of an OAC/OAF be performed under perioperative antibiotic administration and a decongestant.

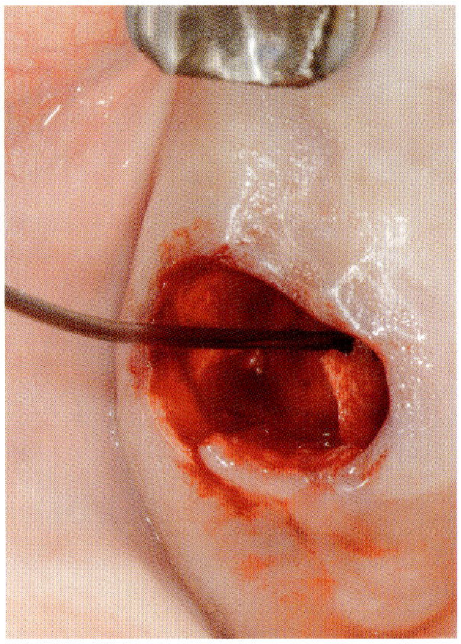

Fig 11-2 Tactile check of the continuity of the bony alveolar fundus with a Bowman lacrimal probe.

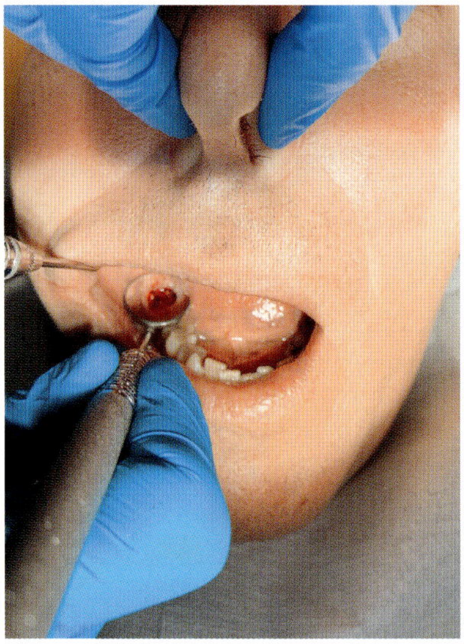

Fig 11-3 In the Valsalva maneuver, the patient's nose is held closed with the fingers and pressure is built up in the nasal cavity on command.

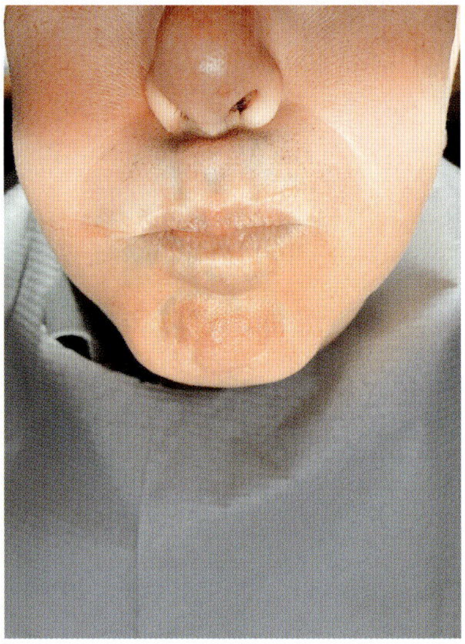

Fig 11-4 In the reverse Valsalva maneuver, the patient must close the mouth and inflate the cheeks.

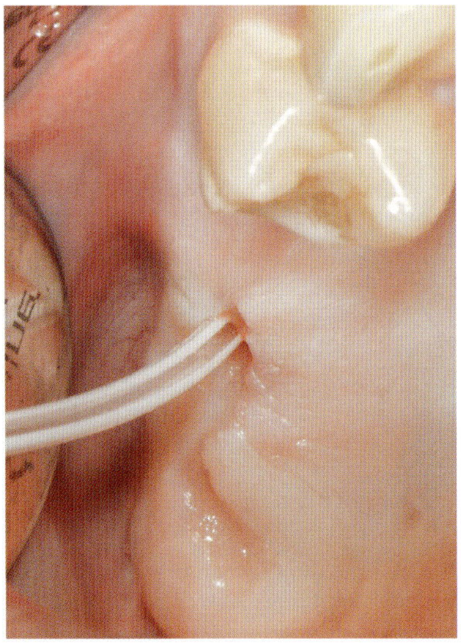

Fig 11-5 Transalveolar maxillary sinus irrigation with a peripheral venous catheter.

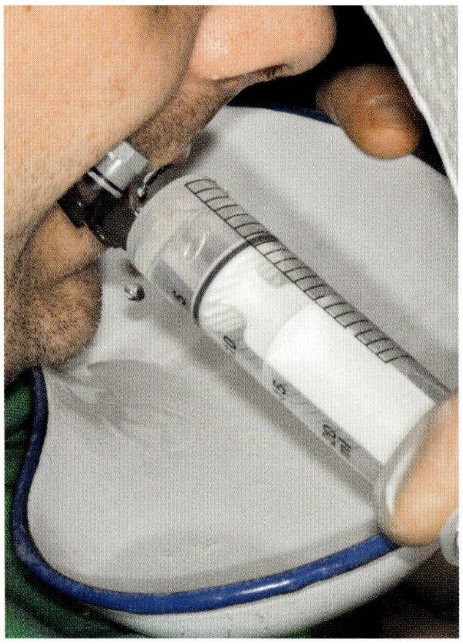

Fig 11-6 During maxillary sinus irrigation, the patient should lean forward while blowing the nose.

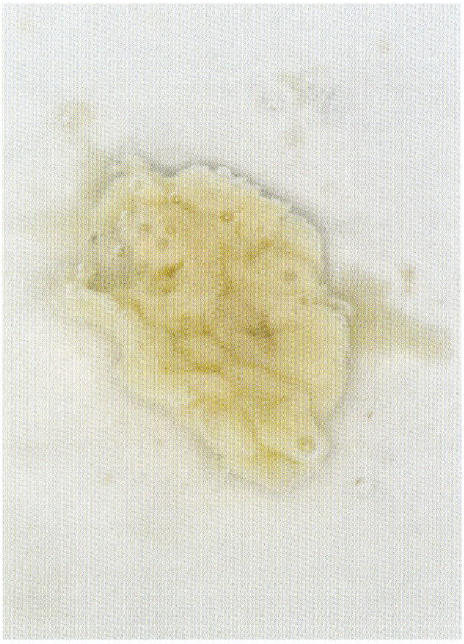

Fig 11-7 Turbid reflux during transalveolar maxillary sinus irrigation (purulent sinusitis).

Rehrmann buccal flap

Indications

- OAC/OAF (without signs of sinusitis),
- Flap technique of choice for soft tissue closure of a wound area in patients on antiresorptive medication (bisphosphonates, denosumab, tyrosine kinase inhibitors, etc) or after radiotherapy has been performed (> 40 Gray).

Contraindications

- Signs of acute sinusitis (temporary) (Figs 11-8 to 11-14).

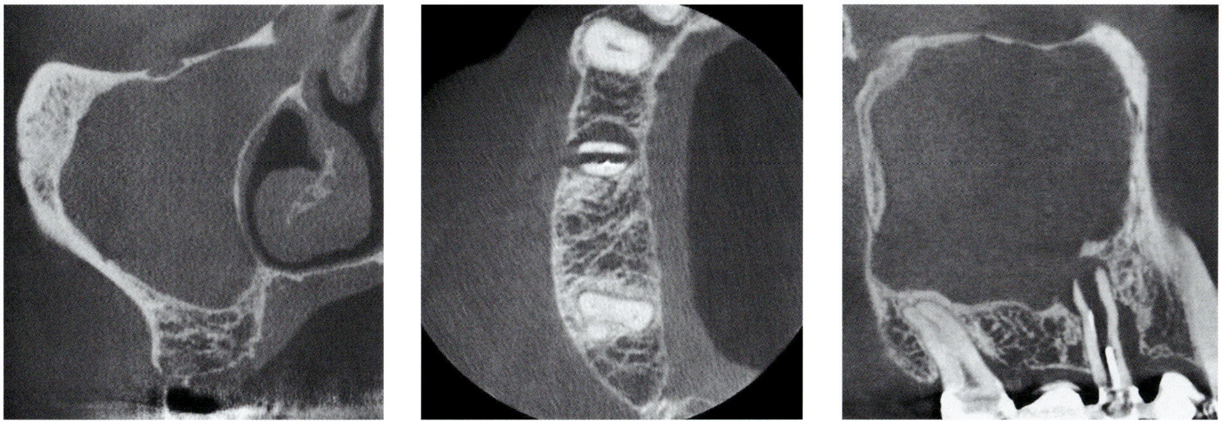

Figs 11-8 to 11-10 A 79-year-old patient complained of unilateral sinusitis symptoms. On the basis of the preoperative CBCT, the longitudinally fractured abutment tooth 15 was visible as a dentogenic focus, which led to the complete shadowing of the right maxillary sinus. The *ostium naturale* was occluded and thus the ventilation or drainage of the maxillary sinus was no longer guaranteed.

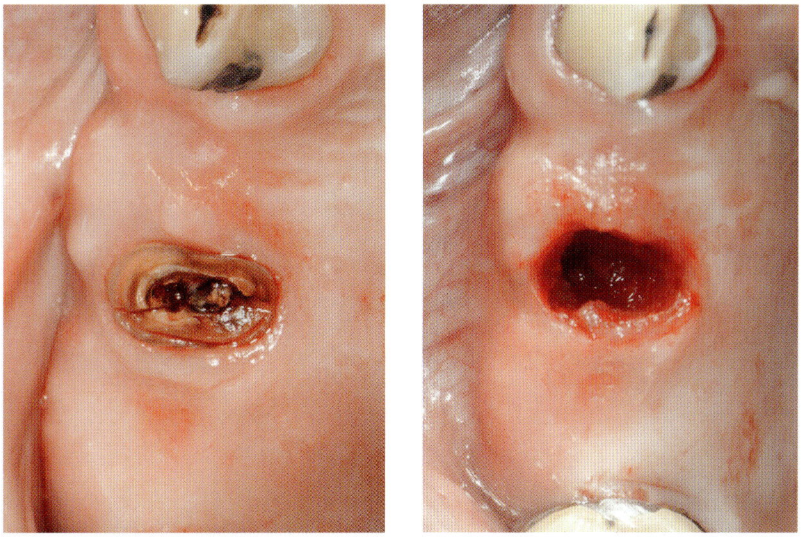

Figs 11-11 and 11-12 An OAC due to the removal of tooth root 15 was expected on the basis of the preoperative CBCT. This was followed by conservative therapy for sinusitis.

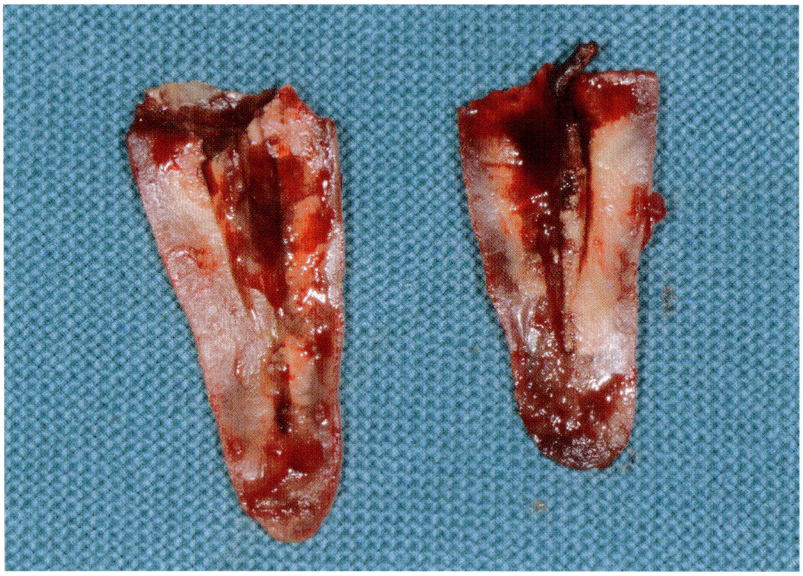

Fig 11-13 Longitudinally fractured tooth root 15 ex vivo.

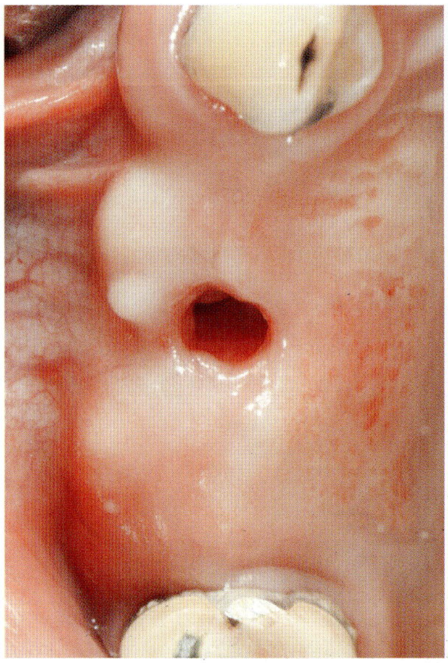

Fig 11-14 Preoperative situation after resolving the sinusitis: The OAC has meanwhile become an OAF.

Specific risks

- Injury to the parotid duct.

Local anesthesia

If necessary, the already anesthetized surgical area for soft tissue closure must be extended intraoperatively by additional conduction anesthetics on the infraorbital nerve and the greater palatine nerve or infiltration anesthetics on the adjacent teeth.

Step-by-step clinical procedure

For the buccal trapezoidal flap, two vertical releasing incisions are initially made mesially and distally to the alveolus and OAC/OAF, respectively (Figs 11-15 and 11-16). The incision is always made from apical to the adjacent tooth position tangential to the alveolus and not to the line angle of the adjacent tooth. In this way, the coronal displacement of the trapezoidal flap can avoid postoperatively exposed bone areas or recessions on the gingiva or periodontal pockets. It is also important to ensure that the base of the flap is sufficiently wide to guarantee adequate flap vascularization. In the course of the releasing incision, the parotid duct must be spared. In case of doubt, this is exposed with the narrowest Bowman lacrimal probe. Subsequently, the trapezoidal mucoperiosteal flap can be lifted from its bony base with a narrow raspatory (Fig 11-17).

For tension-free closure, a new scalpel blade is used to slit the periosteum at the base of the flap (Fig 11-18). The incision at the periosteum is then spread or stretched with dissecting scissors or a wide raspatory to lengthen the trapezoidal flap (Fig 11-19).

If necessary, a sharp bone edge of the buccal alveolar wall is smoothed by osteoplasty (Fig 11-20). At this point at the latest, the epithelium of the fistula tract (in the case of an OAF) or the marginal and sulcular epithelium (in the case of an OAC) as well as epithelial portions at the end of the flap must be removed with scissors or a scalpel in a minimally invasive manner, since otherwise epithelialized wound edges lying against

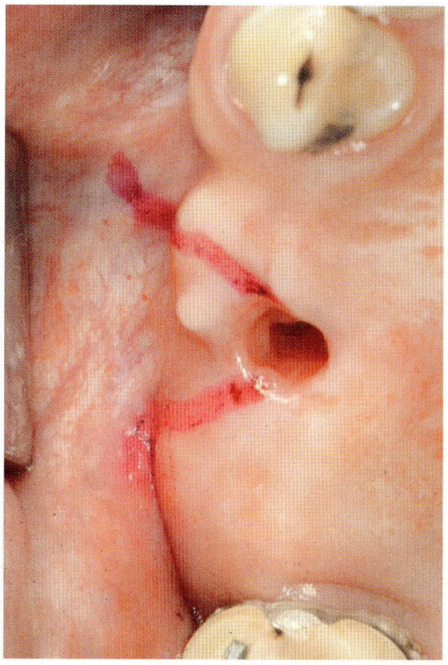

Fig 11-15 Initial intraoperative situation with marked incision line (Castellani solution).

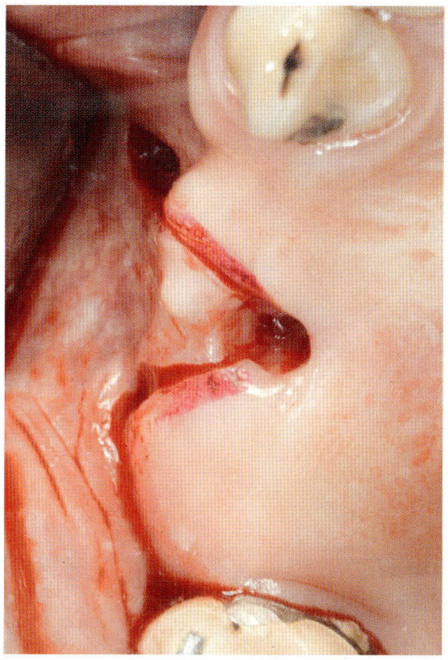

Fig 11-16 Two vertical releasing incisions mesial and distal to the OAF form the trapezoidal flap.

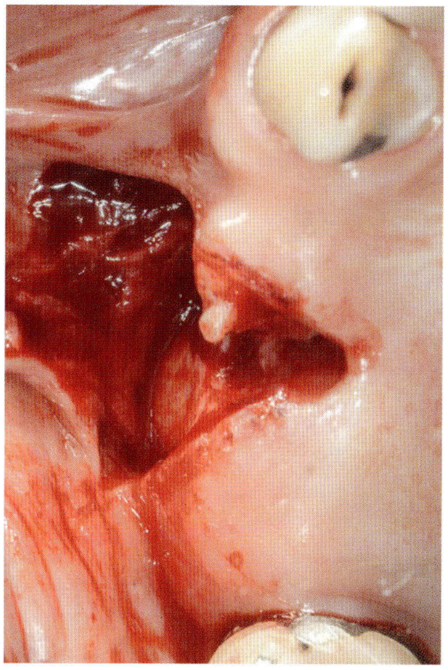

Fig 11-17 After mobilization of the trapezoidal flap using a narrow raspatory.

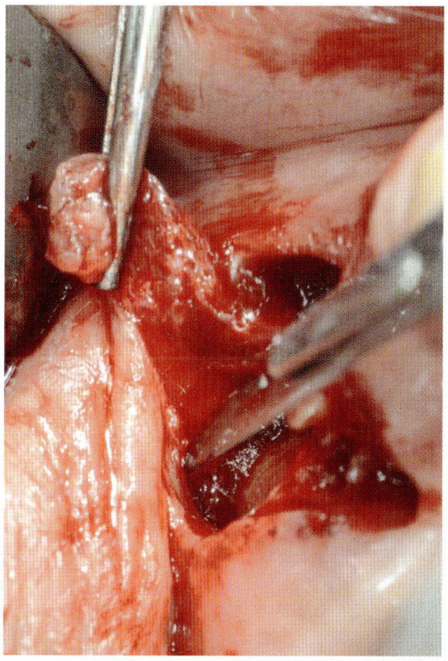

Fig 11-18 The periosteal slit at the base of the flap is made with a new scalpel blade.

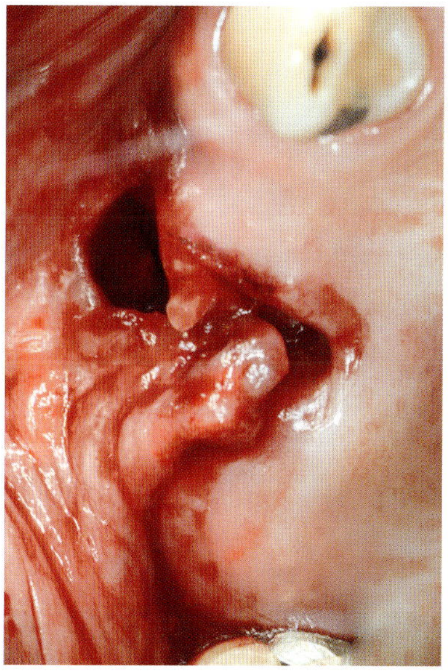

Fig 11-19 The now extended trapezoidal flap allows tension-free closure.

each other will not lead to primary wound healing (Fig 11-21). The now extended flap is adapted from palatal to palatal without tension using one to two horizontal mattress sutures on the periosteum (3-0 or 4-0 resorbable sutures) (Figs 11-22 to 11-24). The incision margins are then tightly closed with several single-button sutures (3-0 or 4-0 non-resorbable sutures) (Fig 11-25).

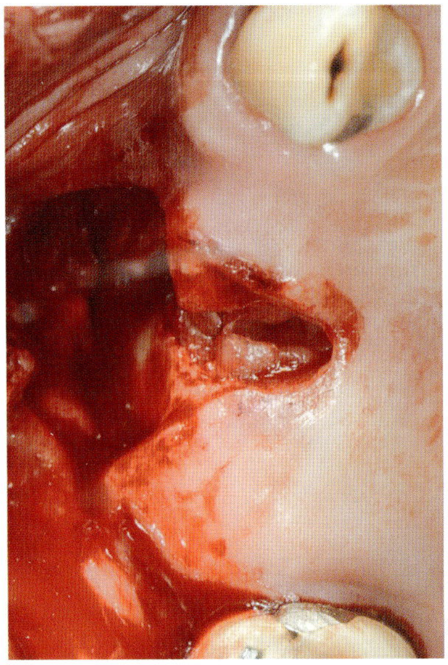

Fig 11-20 After removal of the sharp bone edge at the buccal alveolar wall by a minimal osteoplasty.

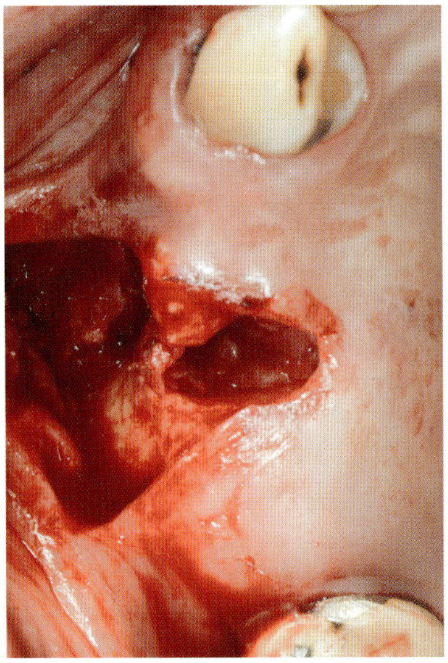

Fig 11-21 After removal of the fistula tract by a circular incision and curettage.

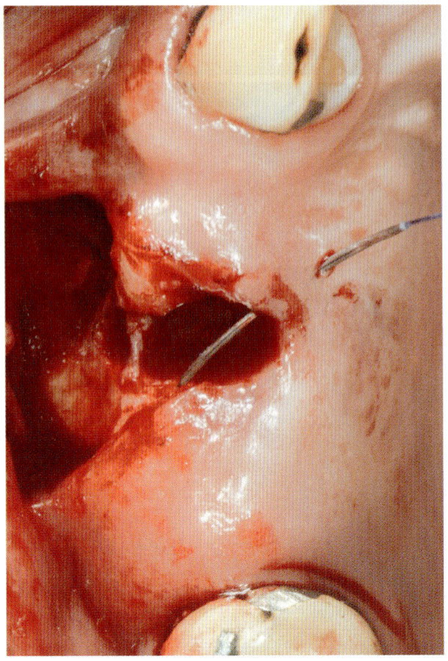

Fig 11-22 The first puncture for the horizontal mattress suture is made from palatal.

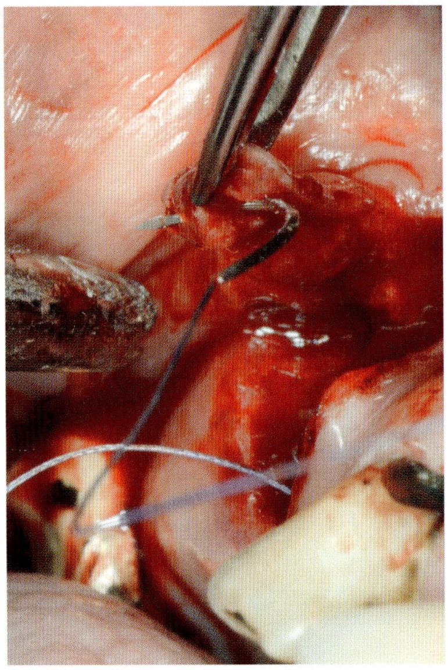

Fig 11-23 The needle is then passed through the periosteum of the trapezoidal flap.

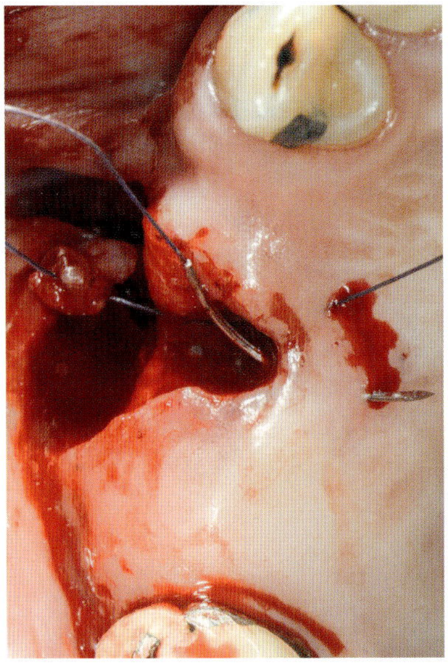

Fig 11-24 Finally, the palatal back stitch is made for the horizontal mattress suture. The trapezoidal flap can now be adapted palatally.

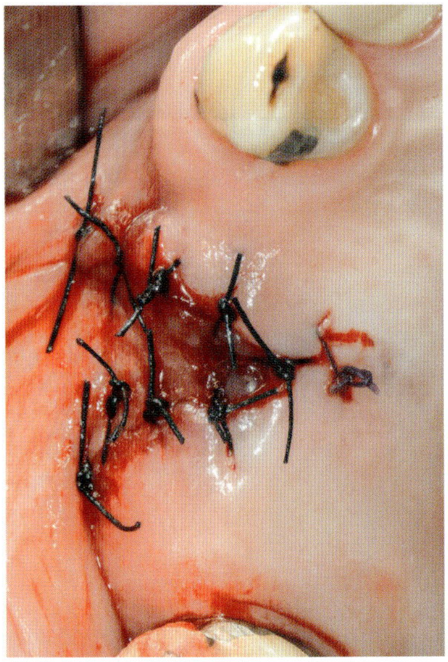

Fig 11-25 Tight closure by several single-button sutures.

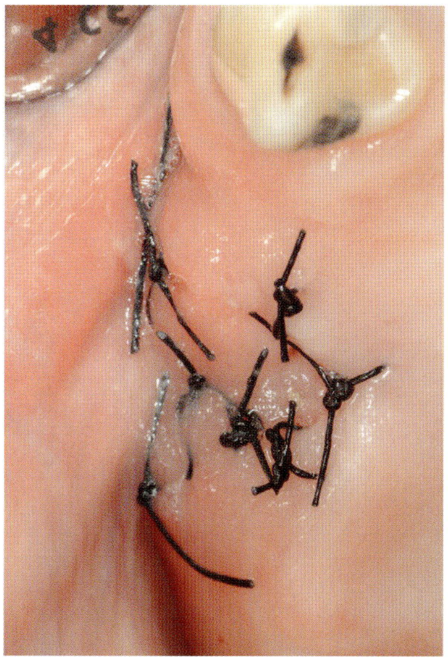

Fig 11-26 Wound situation 10 days postoperatively.

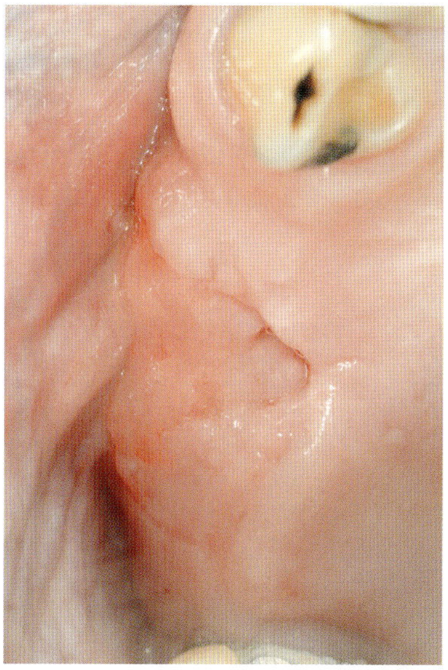

Fig 11-27 Wound situation after suture removal.

Wound care

- Medication: analgesic, antiseptic, decongestant (for a maximum of 7 days), inhalation therapy, antibiotic (not obligatory),
- Cooling bag for swelling prophylaxis and reserve swabs,
- Patient information: The patient should not build up pressure in the maxillary sinus for 10 days or blow the nose and keep the mouth open when sneezing so as to avoid tearing open the wound and the formation of emphysema in the soft tissue. Furthermore, the patient should be informed about possible blood or bloody mucus discharge from the nose or pharynx (signs of maxillary sinus drainage).

Postoperative controls and course

- The first control is performed on the second postoperative day. At this time, the wound is disinfected with an antiseptic, and flap vascularization is checked,
- The sutures are removed after 10 to 14 days at the earliest (Figs 11-26 and 11-27),
- If there are no complications, the next clinical check is performed after 3 to 4 months. If postoperative sinusitis is suspected, further imaging is indicated.

Advantages

- Simple closure technique.

Disadvantages

- Shift of the mucogingival border or loss of keratinized gingiva,
- Flattening of the vestibule (caveat: denture wearers),
- Bone loss due to osteoplasty at the buccal bone lamella.

Modified palatal split flap

Indications

- OAC/OAF (without signs of sinusitis),
- Preservation of keratinized gingiva (e.g. for subsequent implant placement).

Contraindications

- Signs of acute sinusitis (temporary) (Fig 11-28 to 11-32).

Specific risks

- Hemorrhage in the event of injury to the palatal artery.

Local anesthesia

- If necessary, the already anesthetized surgical area for soft tissue closure must be extended intraoperatively by additional conduction anesthetics on the infraorbital nerve and the greater palatine nerve or infiltration anesthetics on the adjacent teeth.

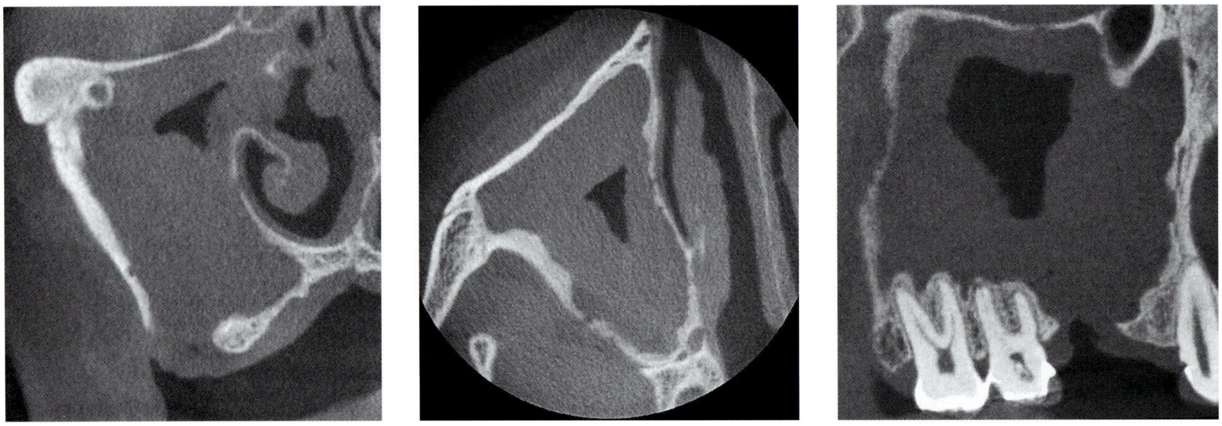

Figs 11-28 to 11-30 On the basis of the preoperative CBCT, an OAF with a severely thickened Schneiderian membrane was recognizable in a 36-year-old patient, which resulted in occlusion of the *ostium naturale*.

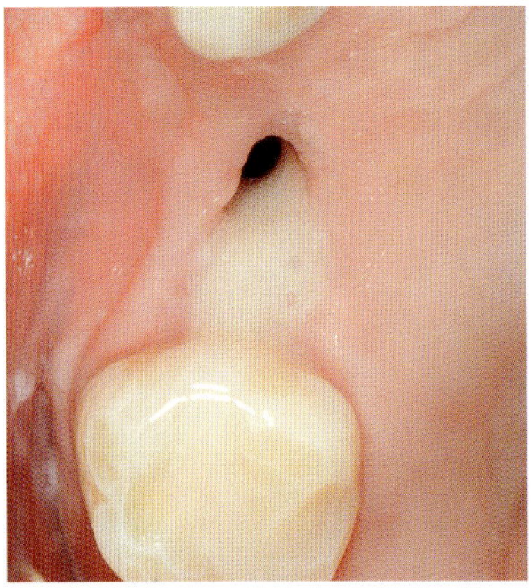

Fig 11-31 Clinical situation: The 36-year-old patient showed an OAF with pus discharge (purulent sinusitis).

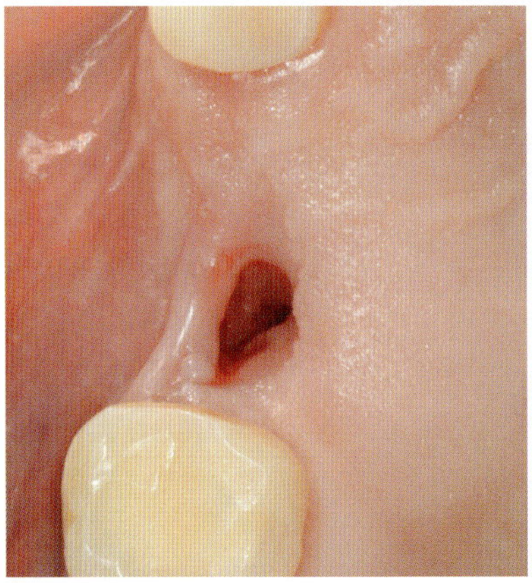

Fig 11-32 Preoperative situation after the sinusitis was resolved by conservative therapy.

Step-by-step clinical procedure

Initially, a paramarginal incision is made on the palate, usually the length of two adjacent teeth, and a vertical releasing incision is made corresponding to the width of the alveolus/OAF in the mesiodistal direction (Video 11-1). In addition, a circular incision is made to remove the fistula epithelium (in the case of an OAF) or the marginal and sulcular epithelium (in the case of an OAC) (Figs 11-33 and 11-34).

The palatal split flap can then be formed (Fig 11-35): The superficial flap consists of the epithelium and subepithelial connective tissue of the mucosa (mucosal flap), and the deeper flap consists of the subepithelial connective tissue and periosteum (connective tissue flap). A minimum thickness of 1 mm should be maintained for the mucosal flap.

After mobilization of the mucosal flap, a second shorter paramarginal incision is made apical to the vertical incision, parallel to the first, and including only the connective tissue flap. The course of the palatal artery must be considered. If necessary, the incision site can be punctured with a cannula to exclude a possible crossing with the blood vessels.

With the aid of a raspatory, the palatal connective tissue flap, including the periosteum, can then be detached from its bony base and rotated by 90 degrees (Fig 11-36). In so doing, the connective tissue flap is pushed under the mobilized mucoperiosteal bridge palatal at the alveolus/OAF (Fig 11-37), which provides additional stabilization and nutrition of the flap.

To fix the connective tissue flap buccally, the formation of a split flap buccal at the alveolus/OAF is performed with the scalpel to below the mucogingival border. The mesial and distal corners of the connective tissue flap are then fixed with two vertical mattress sutures (4-0 resorbable sutures) and pushed into the recipient bed (buccal split flap).

Video 11-1 Maxillary sinus coverage with modified palatal split flap.

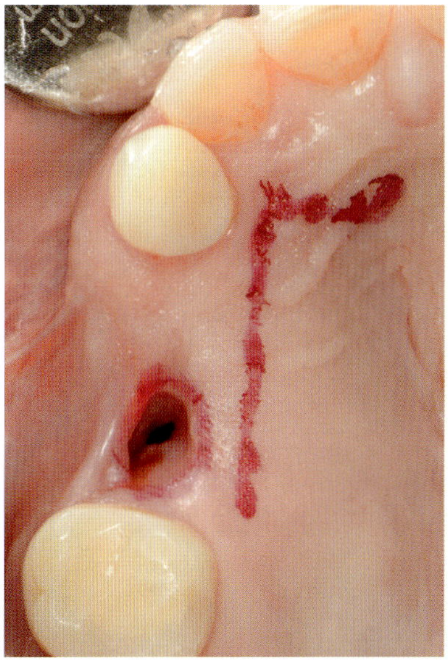

Fig 11-33 Initial intraoperative situation with incision marked (Castellani solution).

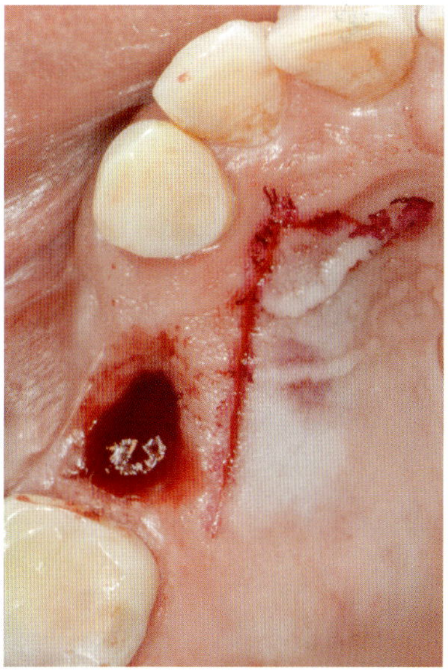

Fig 11-34 Paramarginal incision in the palatal at region 15 to 13 with a vertical releasing incision at region 13, then a circular incision around the OAF.

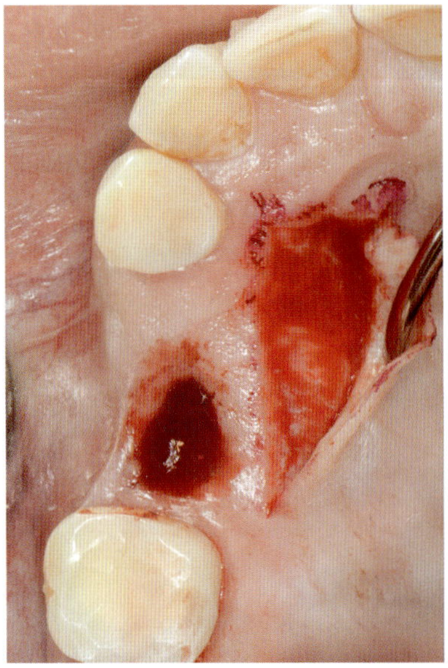

Fig 11-35 Formation of a palatal split flap (mucosal flap) considering a minimum thickness of 1 mm. The mucoperiosteal bridge is left palatal to the OAF.

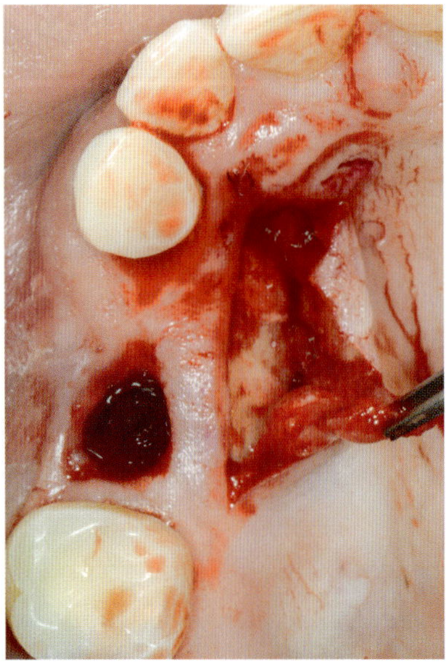

Fig 11-36 After the second shorter paramarginal incision at region 13 to 14, which runs apically of the vertical incision parallel to the first paramarginal incision, the connective tissue flap can be mobilized with a raspatory.

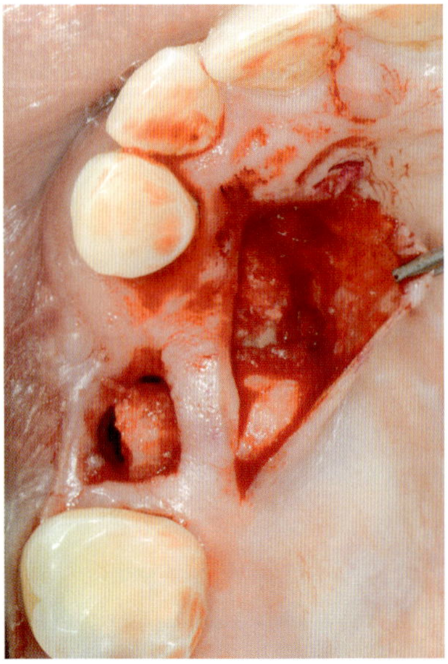

Fig 11-37 The connective tissue flap is then pushed under the palatal mucoperiosteal bridge of region 15. In order to fix it in place, a split flap is formed buccally at region 15 with the scalpel to below the mucogingival border.

A collagen cone can be inserted at the palatal harvest site to stabilize the blood coagulum. The palatal mucosal flap is then reduced again and fixed with single-button sutures (3-0 or 4-0 resorbable sutures). Additional single-button sutures or double-loop sutures (3-0 or 4-0 non-resorbable sutures) at region 16 are used to stabilize the wound margins (Fig 11-38).

Wound care

- Medication: analgesic, antiseptic, decongestant (for a maximum of 7 days), inhalation therapy, antibiotic (not obligatory),
- Cooling bag for swelling prophylaxis and reserve swabs,
- Patient information: The patient should not build up pressure in the maxillary sinus for 10 days or blow the nose and keep the mouth open when sneezing so as to avoid tearing open the wound and the formation of emphysema in the soft tissue. Furthermore, the patient should be informed about possible blood or bloody mucus discharge from the nose or pharynx (signs of maxillary sinus drainage).

Postoperative controls and course

- The first control is performed on the second postoperative day. At this time, the

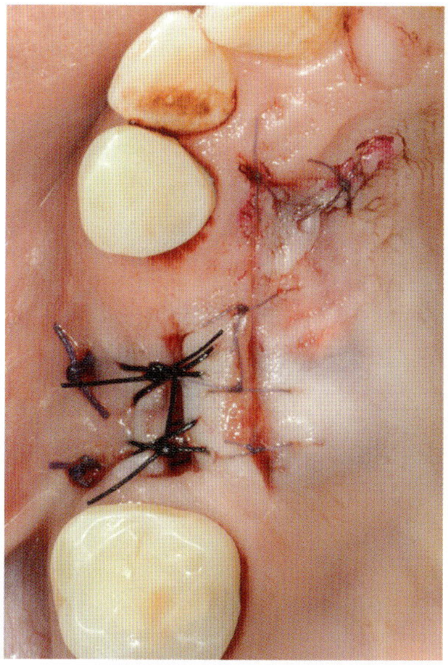

Fig 11-38 The connective tissue flap is then fixed in the buccal split flap with two vertical mattress sutures, and the palatal mucosal flap is repositioned and fixed with single-button sutures. Additional sutures at region 16 are used to stabilize the wound edges.

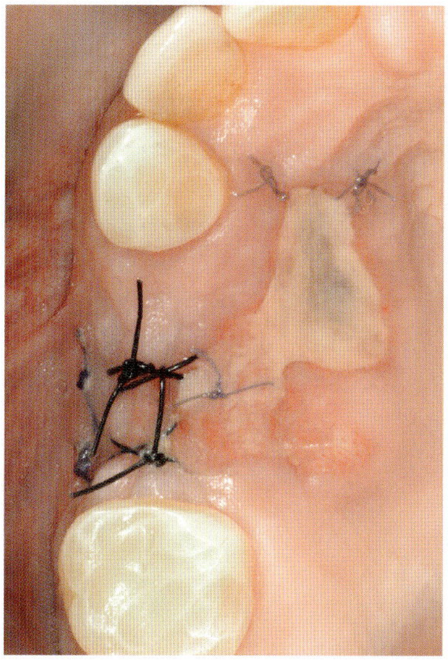

Fig 11-39 Wound situation 10 days postoperatively.

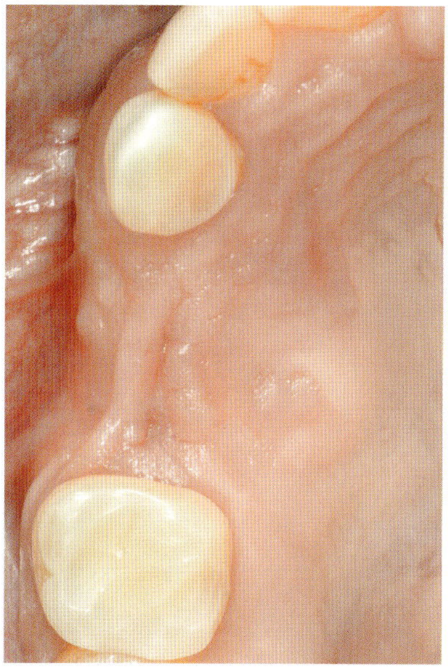

Fig 11-40 Clinical situation after 3 months.

wound is disinfected with an antiseptic and flap vascularization is checked,

- The sutures are removed postoperatively after 10 to 14 days at the earliest (Fig 11-39),
- If there are no complications, the next clinical check is performed after 3 to 4 months (Fig 11-40). If postoperative sinusitis is suspected, further imaging procedures are indicated.

Advantages

- High success rate > 95%[6],
- No displacement of the mucogingival border or loss of keratinized gingiva,
- No flattening of the vestibule,
- No exposed bone area postoperatively,
- The elastic/flexible flap allows easy adaptation,
- Additional stabilization and nutrition of the flap by the mucoperiosteal bridge.

Disadvantages

- Demanding technique,
- Intra- and postoperative risk of injury or rupture of the palatine artery.

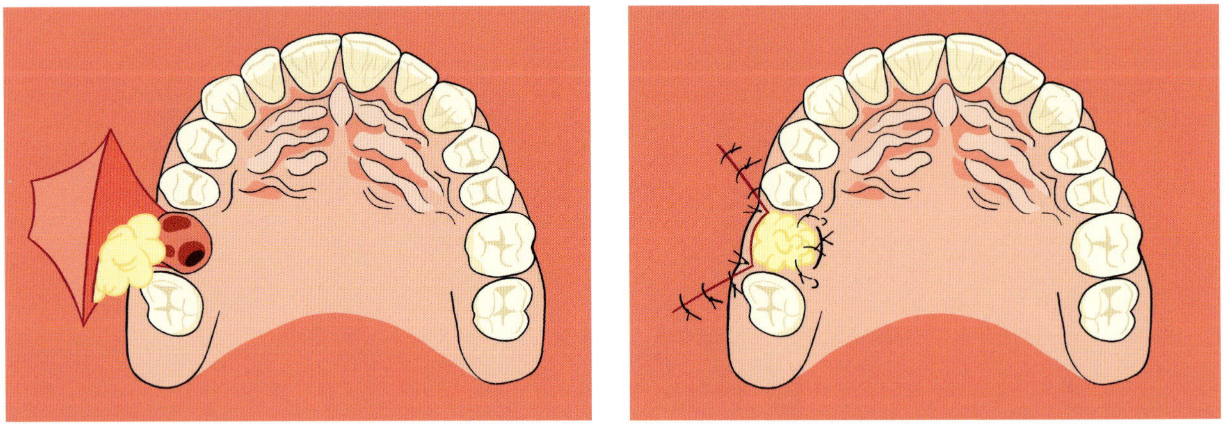

Figs 11-41 and 11-42 Buccal flap with the Bichat fat pad.

Other surgical closure techniques

Buccal flap with the Bichat fat pad

In the case of this technique (Figs 11-41 and 11-42), a trapezoidal flap is initially formed analogous to the Rehrmann buccal flap. However, the incision at the periosteum is made dorsal to the *crista zygomaticoalveolaris* (palpation). After blunt preparation with dissecting scissors as part of the dissection (splitting of the soft tissue), the pedicled Bichat fat pad, usually the intermediate fat flap, or the buccal extension of the posterior fat flap can be mobilized medially to cover the OAC/OAF. The Bichat fat pad can be placed in the OAC/OAF without mucosal coverage and fixed palatally with sutures. In this case, the trapezoidal flap is returned to its original position and fixed with sutures.

Advantages

- High success rate of 93% to 100%, even with a large OAC/OAF[4,5],
- Easy access with minimal dissection,
- The Bichat fat pad can be mobilized well,
- Good vascularization of the Bichat fat pad through branches of the facial, maxillary, and superficial temporal arteries,
- Complete epithelialization of the Bichat fat pad after 2 to 3 weeks[5].

Disadvantages

- Impairment of cheek esthetics due to the prolapse,
- Same success rate as the Rehrmann buccal flap, but associated with more discomfort postoperatively (reduced jaw opening, swelling, and pain)[10],
- Traumatic occlusion occurs in a voluminous Bichat fat pad (hypertrophy),
- It is unclear what happens to the fatty tissue in the alveolar socket over time.

Axhausen buccal flap (dorsally pedunculated)

In this flap technique (Figs 11-43 and 11-44), the incision is made at the mucosa in the vestibule with exposure of the parotid duct. The distally pedicled flap can then be dissected and pivoted palatally over the OAC/OAF (transposition by 90 degrees). Before this, however, the buccal gingiva is completely excised at the OAC/OAF. It is imperative to ensure that the flap is sutured without tension. The Axhausen buccal flap can also be stalked from mesial in its modification.

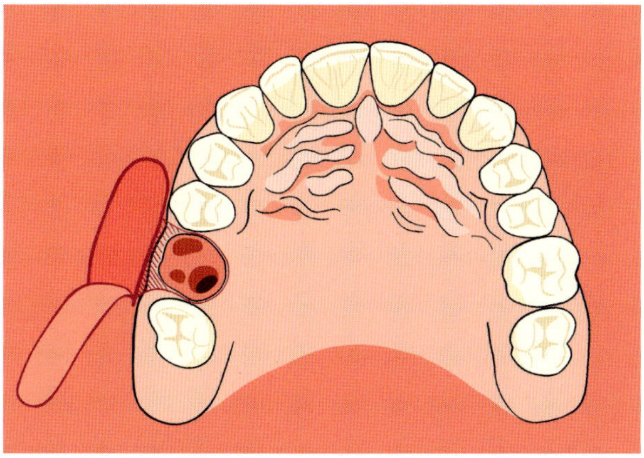
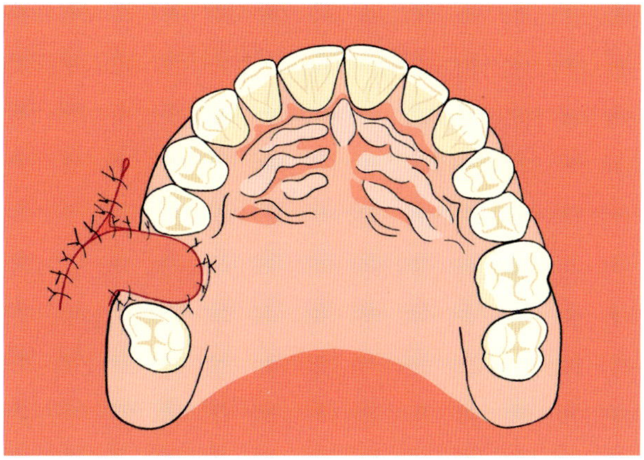

Figs 11-43 and 11-44 Axhausen buccal flap (dorsally pedunculated).

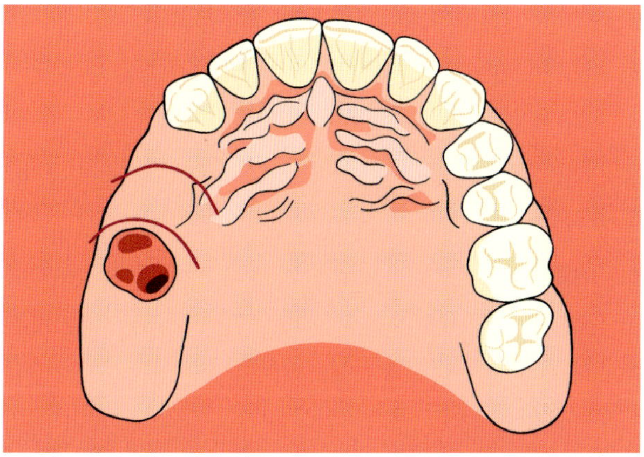
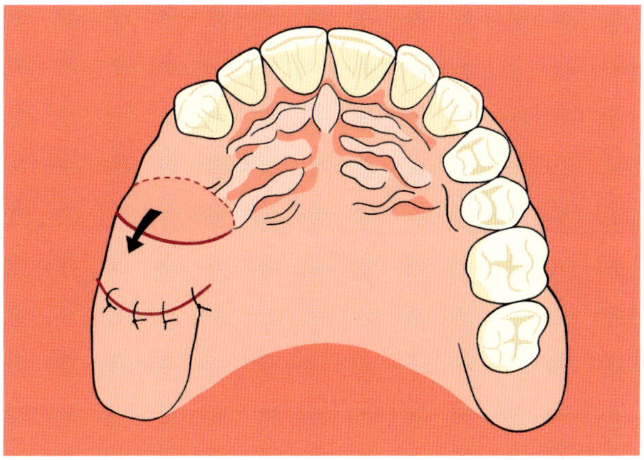

Figs 11-45 and 11-46 Schuchardt bridge flap (from mesial).

Advantages

- Can also be performed on traumatized mucosa/gingiva buccally of the OAC/OAF.

Disadvantages

- Shift of the mucogingival border or loss of the keratinized gingiva,
- Flattening of the vestibule,
- Bone loss due to osteoplasty at the buccal bone lamella.

Schuchardt bridge flap (from mesial)

This flap technique (Figs 11-45 and 11-46) is particularly suitable for a small OAC, provided that the adjacent area is edentulous. The bridge flap consists of two long, curved, and parallel incisions from buccal (within the mobile mucosa) over the alveolar ridge to palatal. The distance between the two incisions should be greater than the mesiodistal width of the alveolus. The bridge flap can either be made from

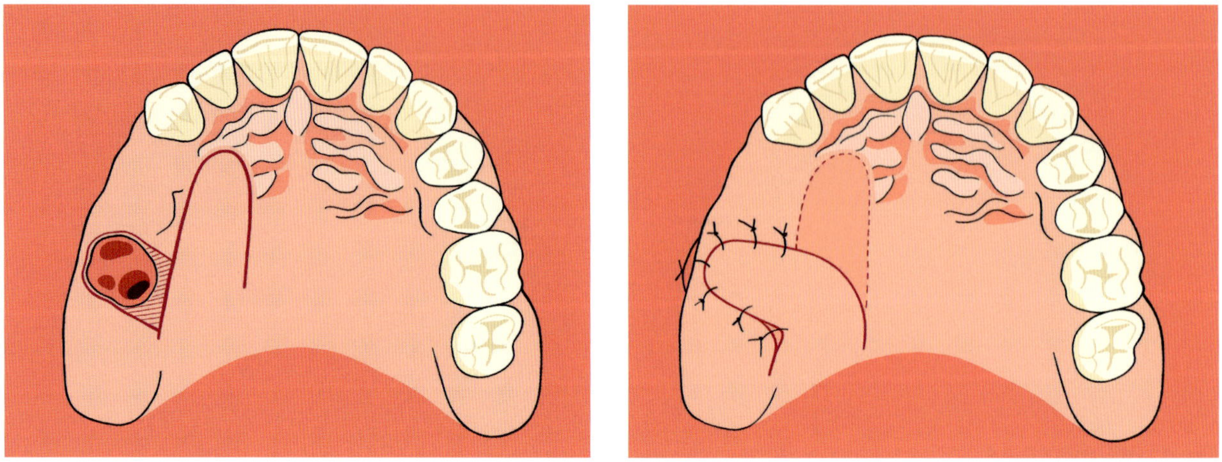

Figs 11-47 and 11-48 Pichler palatal flap.

mesial (according to Schuchardt) or from distal (according to Kazanjia) of an OAC/OAF. The bridge flap is then mobilized by tunneling preparation and moved to the concave side of the incision over the OAC/OAF, then fixed with sutures.

Advantages

- No displacement of the mucogingival border or loss of keratinized gingiva,
- No flattening of the vestibule.

Disadvantages

- Limited indication (adjacent area must be edentulous),
- Difficult technique, often not tension-free (risk of wound dehiscence),
- Postoperatively exposed bone area.

Pichler palatal flap

In this flap technique (Figs 11-47 and 11-48), the cut is made around the palatine artery and the artery is rotated buccally after preparation of the pedicled mucoperiosteal flap. It is imperative to ensure a bony support of the flap, especially in the buccal region of the closure. The bone area in the donor site, which is usually exposed over a large area anteriorly, is covered by an iodoform strip and protective plate and left to heal secondarily.

Advantages

- High success rate of > 95%, even with a large OAC/OAF[1],
- Resistant flap,
- Good vascularization through the palatal artery,
- No displacement of the mucogingival border or loss of keratinized gingiva,
- No flattening of the vestibule.

Disadvantages

- Limited indication (only possible in edentulous posterior region),
- Difficult mobilization and adaptation,
- Palatal bulge due to transposition by 90 degrees,

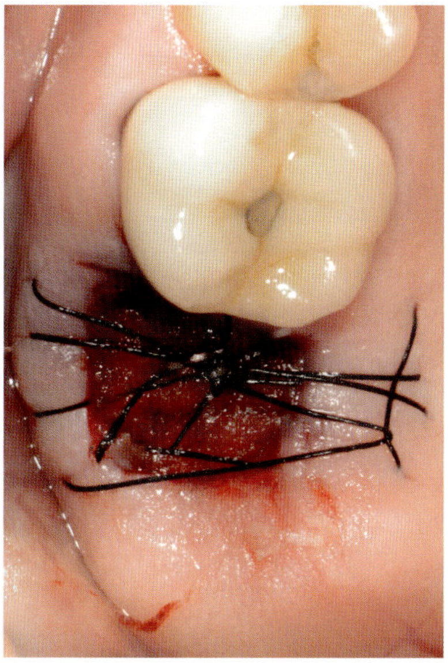

Fig 11-49 Closure of a small OAC (2 mm) with an absorbable collagen cone and sutures.

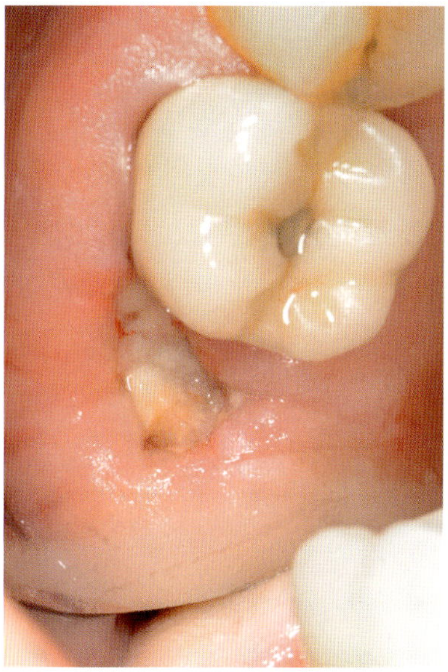

Fig 11-50 Wound situation 10 days postoperatively.

- Postoperatively exposed bone area in the anterior region,
- Pain due to exposed bone palatally,
- Long impairment due to secondary wound healing.

Nonoperative closure techniques

In addition to the various flap techniques, it is repeatedly reported in the literature that a small OAC (< 4 mm) can also heal spontaneously with a stable blood coagulum. However, this should by no means be considered a therapeutic concept because the scientific publications[7,12] that led to this assumption date from the last century and show a low level of evidence.

Nonoperative techniques for closure of a small OAC may include insertion of an absorbable occlusion cone (e.g. a collagen cone) and/or sealing with tissue adhesive (e.g. fibrin glue) (Figs 11-49 and 11-50). However, these variants are controversially discussed despite some evidence[2,3,8,13,15], because even with a small OAC (3 mm), where some authors postulated spontaneous healing with a success rate of 79% to 100%, one cannot really speak of a predictable result due to the wide dispersion.

More decisive for success is the morphology of the alveolus: the deeper the alveolus, the more likely it is that a coagulum will remain stable and successfully close the OAC, even without soft tissue closure.

Furthermore, autogenous bone or bone substitute materials with or without membrane, transplantation of wisdom teeth, and stents for closing the opened maxillary sinus are discussed in the literature. However, higher costs, the existing defect size of an OAC/OAF, an additional harvest site, and the risk of dislocation of the inserted material into the maxillary sinus have to be considered for these variants.

References

1. Anavi Y, Gal G, Silfen R, Calderon S. Palatal rotation-advancement flap for delayed repair of oroantral fistula: a retrospective evaluation of 63 cases. Oral Surg Oral Med Oral Pathol Oral Radiol Endod 2003;96:527–534.
2. Burić N. Use of N-butyl cyanoacrylate with metacryloxisulfolane (glubran 2) surgical glue for flapless closure of oroantral communication. Implant Dent 2013;22:238–243.
3. Burić N, Jovanović G, Krasić D, et al. The use of absorbable polyglactin/polydioxanon implant (Ethisorb®) in non-surgical closure of oro-antral communication. J Craniomaxillofac Surg 2012;40:71–77.
4. Egyedi P. Utilization of the buccal fat pad for closure of oro-antral and/or oro-nasal communications. J Maxillofac Surg 1977;5:241–244.
5. Hanazawa Y, Itoh K, Mabashi T, Sato K. Closure of oroantral communications using a pedicled buccal fat pad graft. J Oral Maxillofac Surg 1995;53:771–775.
6. Ito T, Hara H. A new technique for closure of the oroantral fistula. J Oral Surg 1980;38: 509–512.
7. Keresztesi K. Conservative therapy of oroantral fistula. Z Stomatol 1954;51:317–323.
8. Kniha H, Nentwig GH, Bunnag T. Zum Verschluß oroantraler Verbindungen mit dem Fibrineklebesystem. Dtsch Z Mund Kiefer Gesichts Chir 1985;9:431.
9. Krimmel M. S2k-Leitlinie: Leitlinie odontogene Sinusitis maxillaris – Langfassung. AWMF/ DGMKG 2019;6:1–31.
10. Nezafati S, Vafaii A, Ghojazadeh M. Comparison of pedicled buccal fat pad flap with buccal flap for closure of oro-antral communication. Int J Oral Maxillofac Surg 2012;41:624–628.
11. Punwutikorn J, Waikakul A, Pairuchvej V. Clinically significant oroantral communications – a study of incidence and site. Int J Oral Maxillofac Surg 1994;23:19–21.
12. Schuchardt K. Treatment of oro-antral perforations and fistulae. Int Dent J 1955;5:159–165.
13. Stajcić Z, Todorović LJ, Petrović V. Tissucol in closure of oroantral communication. A pilot study. Int J Oral Surg 1985;14:444–446.
14. Stuck A, Popert U. S2k-Leitlinie: Rhinosinusitis – Langfassung. DGHNO-KHC/DEGAM 2017;4:1–102.
15. Visscher SH, Van Minnen B, Bos RR. Feasibility of conical biodegradable polyurethane foam for closure of oroantral communications. J Oral Maxillofac Surg 2011;69:390–395.

Frena excisions

12

Silvio Valdec, Bernd Stadlinger

Indications

- Reduced tongue mobility,
- Recessions in case of irritating buccal or labial frenulum or lingual of the anterior teeth in the mandible in the case of irritating lingual frenulum,
- Diastema in the case of an interfering labial frenulum,
- Patient suffering from pressure.

Contraindications

- Scleroderma, and caution in collagenosis.

Specific risks

- Adjacent salivary gland excretory ducts,
- Risk of recurrence,
- Recessions on adjacent teeth,
- Caution after radiotherapy in the head and neck region.

Local anesthesia

- Infiltration anesthesia near the ligament.

Step-by-step clinical procedure

There are basically three techniques: V-Y plasty (Figs 12-1 to 12-8), scissor cut (Figs 12-9 to 12-16, Video 12-1), and excision with a CO_2 laser (Figs 12-17 to 12-24).

V-Y plasty

The main steps of the V-Y plasty technique are: clinical inspection of the lingual frenulum (Fig 12-1), incision in a V-shape to the caudal attachment of the lingual frenulum (Fig 12-2), undermining dissection with dissecting scissors to ensure freedom from tension (Fig 12-3), check of mobility after dissection (Fig 12-4), possibly extended lateral undermining dissection for mobilization (Fig 12-5), and primary wound closure with single-button sutures in the

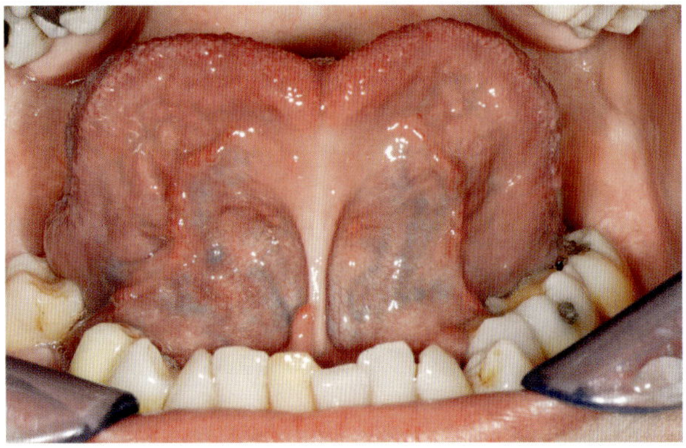

Fig 12-1 Clinical inspection of the lingual frenulum.

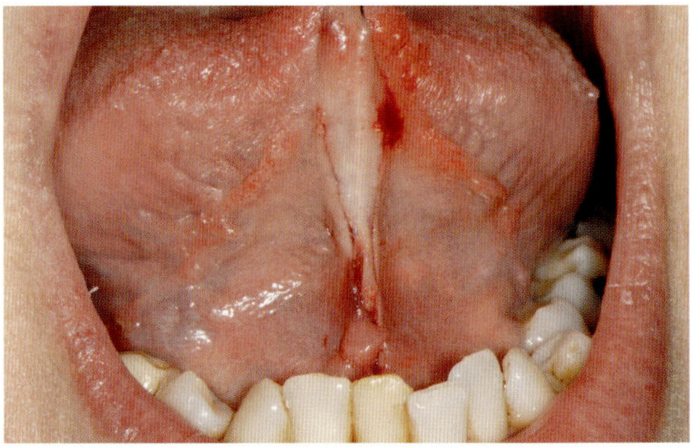

Fig 12-2 V-shaped incision up to the caudal attachment of the lingual frenulum.

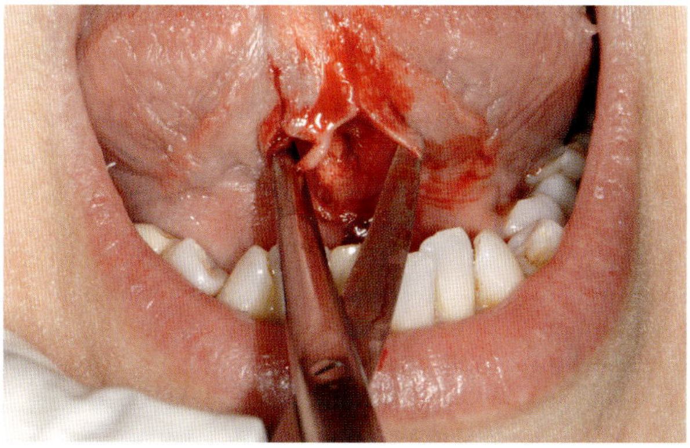

Fig 12-3 Undermining preparation with dissecting scissors to ensure freedom from tension.

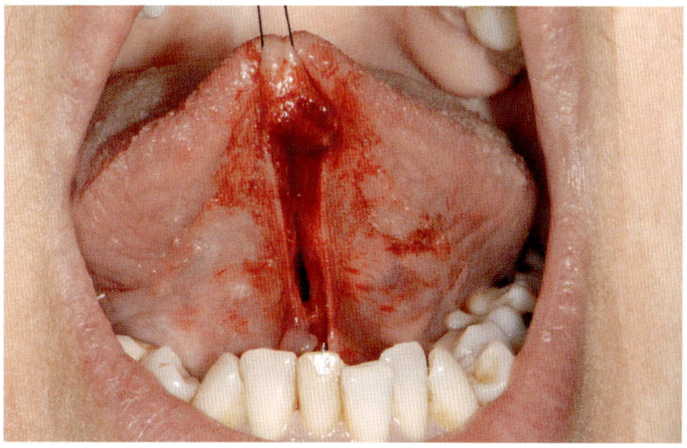

Fig 12-4 Checking the mobility after preparation.

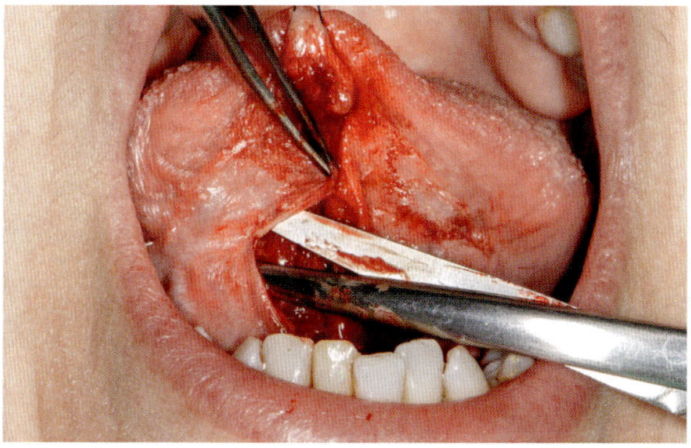

Fig 12-5 Possibly extended lateral undermining preparation for mobilization.

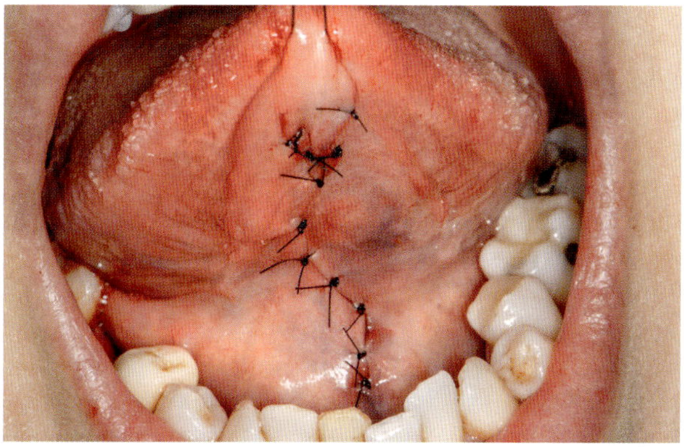

Fig 12-6 Primary wound closure with single-button sutures; Y-shape in the area of the tip of the tongue.

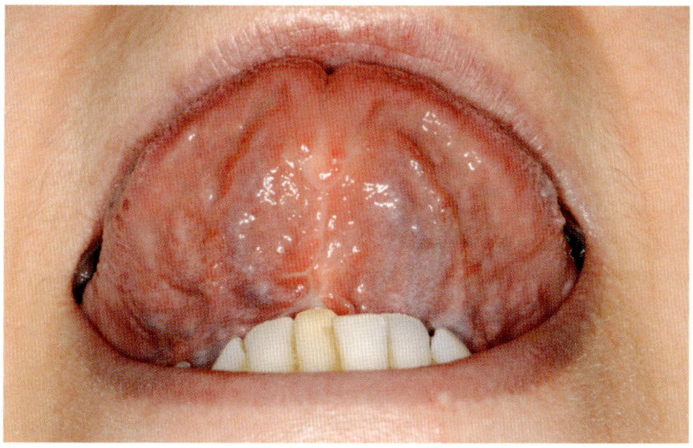

Fig 12-7 Follow-up check after 2 weeks.

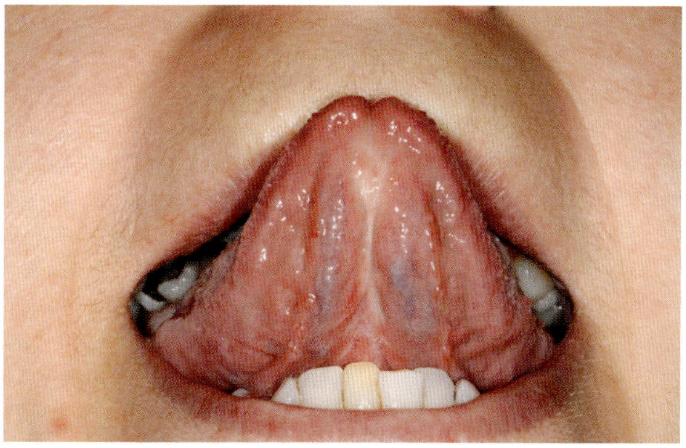

Fig 12-8 Follow-up check after 3 months.

Video 12-1 Tongue frenulum excision using the scissor cut technique.

shape of a Y in the area of the tip of the tongue (Fig 12-6). Suture removal is usually performed after 7 days. The next check should be performed after 2 weeks. Wound healing and mobility are checked at this time (Fig 12-7), and instructions for tongue movement exercises are also given. Further checks are performed after 6 weeks and 3 months (Fig 12-8). Mobility is also checked in each case.

Scissor cut

The main steps of the scissor cut technique (Video 12-1) are: clinical inspection of the lingual frenulum (Fig 12-9), fixation of the lingual frenulum with clamps (Fig 12-10), transection of the lingual frenulum with surgical scissors (Fig 12-11), release of the clamps after the scissor cut (Fig 12-12), inspection of mobility (Fig 12-13), check for residual tension and, if necessary, lateral dissection with dissecting scissors to release residual tension (Fig 12-14), followed by tension-free wound closure with single-button sutures (Figs 12-15 and 12-16). Controls should be performed with suture removal after 7 days, then after 2 weeks, 6 weeks, and 3 months.

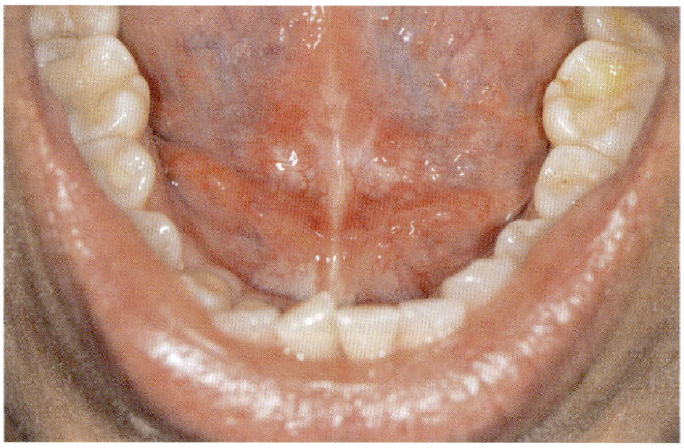

Fig 12-9 Clinical inspection of the lingual frenulum.

Excision with a CO_2 laser

The main steps of the excision with a CO_2 laser technique are: clinical inspection of the buccal or lingual frenulum (Fig 12-17), positioning of the CO_2 laser (Fig 12-18), cutting of the frenulum (Fig 12-19), and check of the tension release at the end (Fig 12-20). The next follow-up is after 2 weeks to check wound healing and mobility, and instructions for tongue movement exercises are also given. The next check is performed 6 weeks after the excision procedure (Fig 12-21). Mobility is also checked at this time. In individual cases, recession coverage with a graft may be necessary in cases of lip or even buccal frenulum (Figs 12-22 and 12-23).

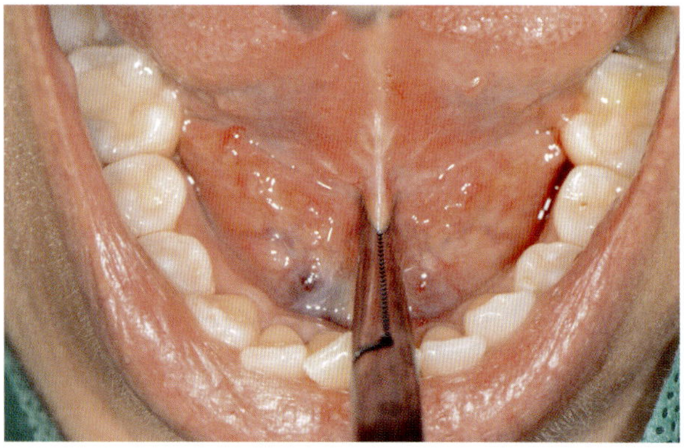

Fig 12-10 Fixation of the lingual frenulum with clamps.

In these cases, suture removal and wound control of the graft is performed 7 days after

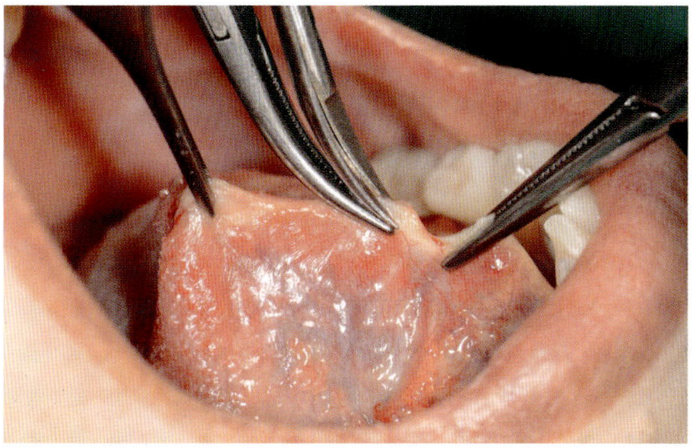

Fig 12-11 Cutting the lingual frenulum with surgical scissors.

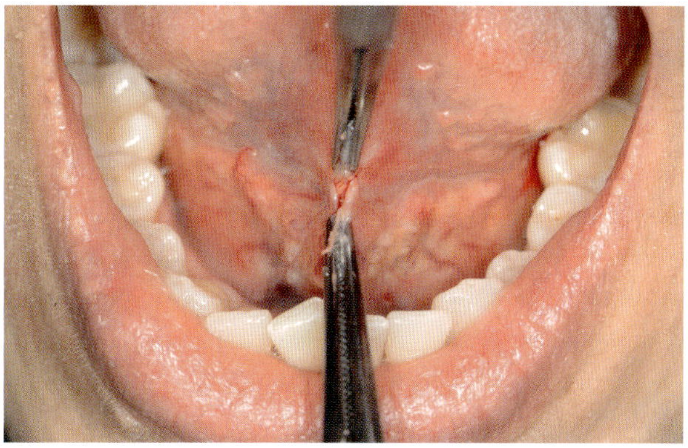

Fig 12-12 Releasing the frenulum after cutting with the scissors.

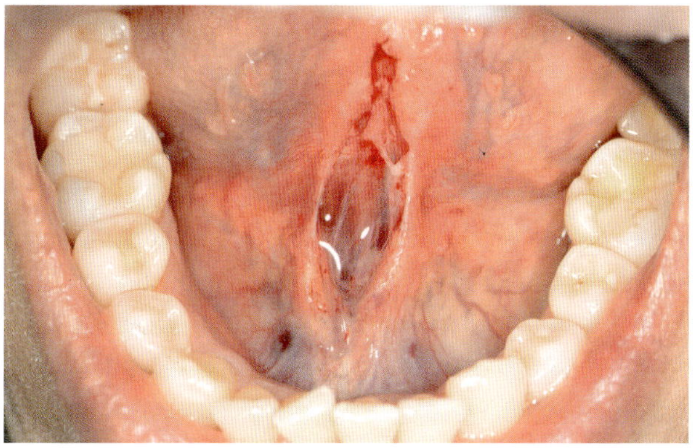

Fig 12-13 Inspection of mobility.

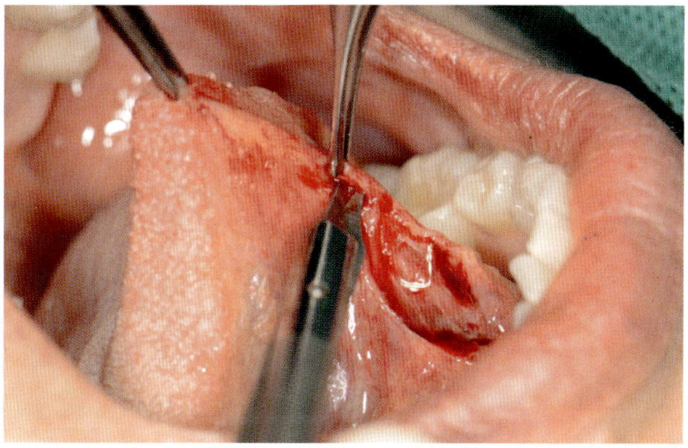

Fig 12-14 Inspection of residual tension: Lateral preparation with dissecting scissors to release residual tension.

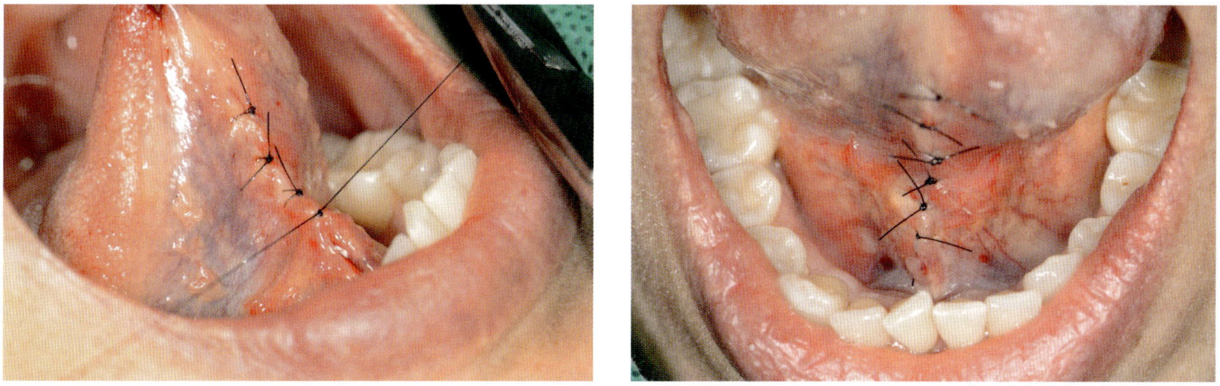

Figs 12-15 and 12-16 Tension-free wound closure with single-button sutures.

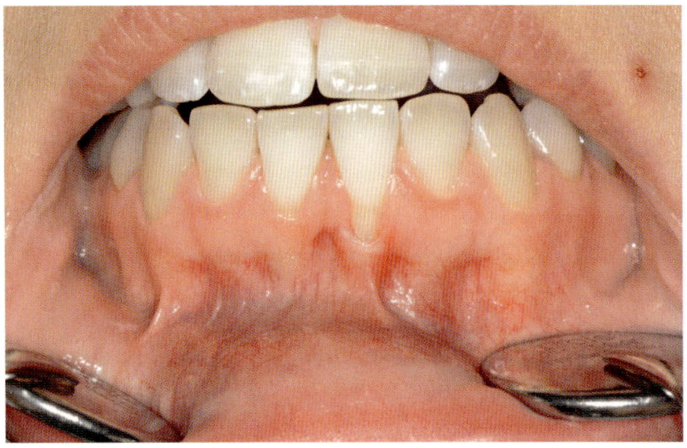

Fig 12-17 Clinical inspection of the ligament.

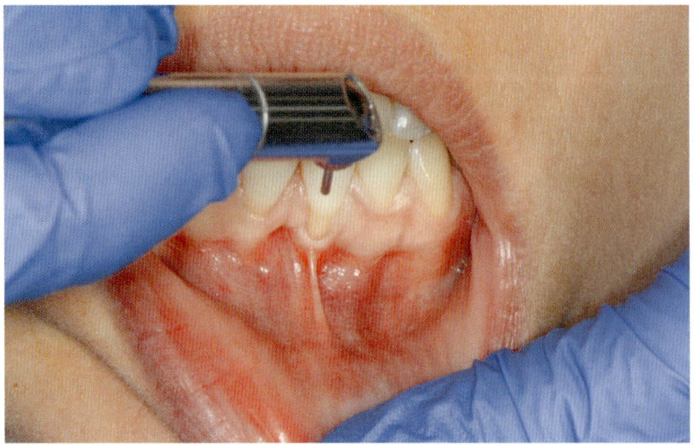

Fig 12-18 Positioning of the CO_2 laser.

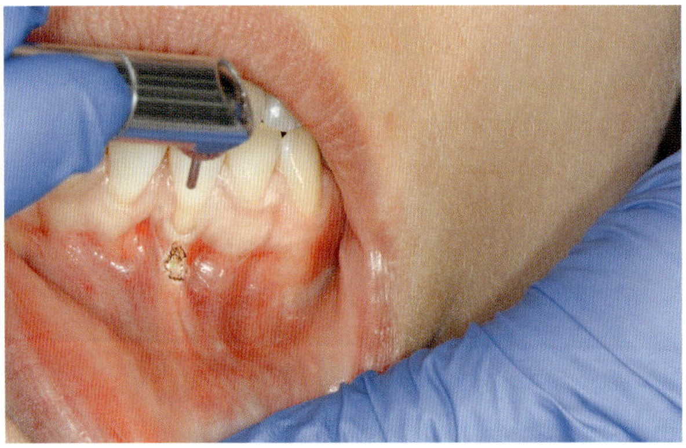

Fig 12-19 Application of the laser at the base of the ligament.

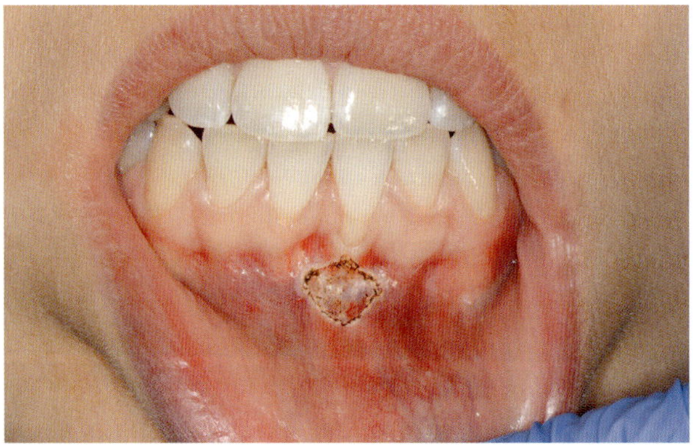

Fig 12-20 Checking the tension release.

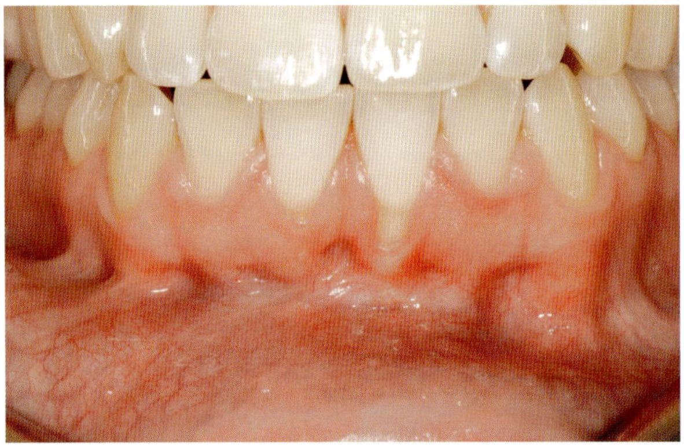

Fig 12-21 Check after 6 weeks, including mobility check.

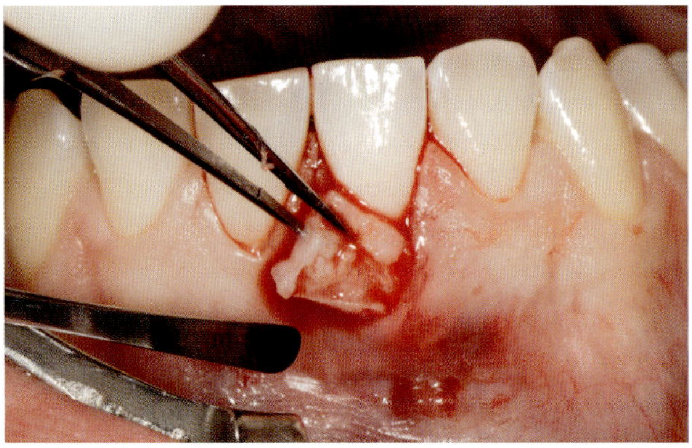

Fig 12-22 In labial frenulum, recession coverage...

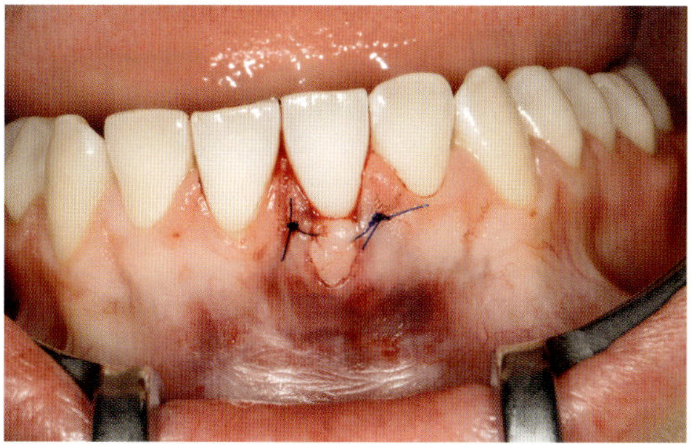

Fig 12-23 ... could be performed with a graft, if necessary.

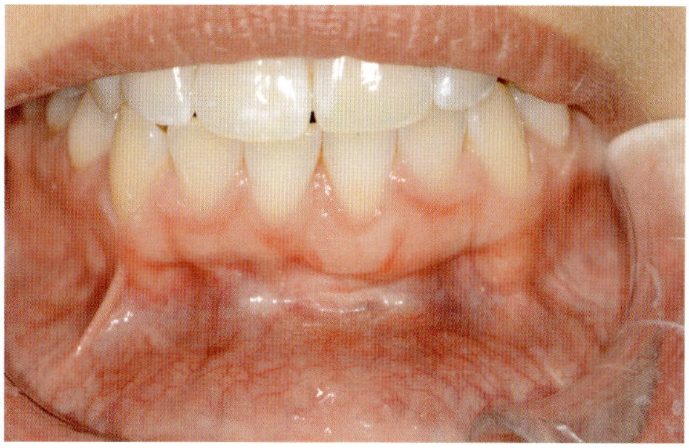

Fig 12-24 Follow-up check after 1 year.

grafting. Further checks are indicated after 3 months to verify mobility, then again after 1 year (Fig 12-24).

Wound care and closure

- Single-button sutures after V-Y plasty and scissor cut,
- Polidocanol-containing dental adhesive paste after excision with a CO_2 laser.

Postoperative controls and course

After V-Y plasty and scissor cut, suture removal is performed after approximately 7 days; further follow-up checks are advisable after 2 weeks, 6 weeks, and 3 months. After excision with a CO_2 laser, epithelialization of the wound is complete after about 2 weeks. Suture removal is not necessary in this case. Throughout the postoperative period, the patient should perform tongue mobility exercises.

Recommended literature

1. Dunsche A, Lambrecht JT. Chirurgie der intraoralen Weichgewebe. In: Lambrecht JT (Hrsg). Zahnärztliche Operationen. Berlin: Quintessenz, 2008.
2. Suter V, Bornstein M, Steffen R, Hitz Lindenmüller I. Ankyloglossie. In: Filippi A, Hitz Lindenmüller I (Hrsgs). Die Zunge. Berlin: Quintessenz, 2016.

13 Excisional and incisional biopsies of the soft tissue

Zeynab Ahmed, Irène Hitz Lindenmüller

Changes in the oral mucosa recur in dental practice and require a thorough systematic examination that includes inspection of the inside of the cheeks, the floor of the mouth, the tongue, the palate, and the gingiva. Corresponding changes should always be assessed through lateral comparison.

Together with the anamnestic data, the findings can thus be assigned to a common main symptom. Differential diagnoses can be made on the basis of age, gender, possible risk factors, and statistical frequencies. To arrive at a definitive diagnosis, histopathologic examination of the tissue is required in most cases, which is the gold standard for clarifying an oral mucosal lesion.

Indications

Biopsy is recommended as soon as there are suspicious findings in the oral cavity. These may be white or red changes with suspicion of precancerous lesions, but also persistent ulcerations and swellings that do not reveal a cause.

Oral mucosal changes that do not show improvement 7 to 10 days after cause elimination or drug therapy should be biopsied immediately for clarification as to whether they are benign or malignant in order to avoid unnecessarily delaying therapy that may be needed. Often, a biopsy is also taken in order to make a (histopathologically verified) diagnosis in the first place.

Contraindications

In the case of changes that are indurated and sunken into the epithelium or show cauliflower-like exophytic growth, which may be painless (with or without lymph node findings), the dentist should not perform a biopsy, as these may be symptoms of a malignant finding. In this case, the patient must be referred to a specialized clinic with appropriate treatment options for further diagnosis.

Specific risks

As with any oral surgery procedure, the presence of an updated medical history and a complete medication list is essential. In the case of anticoagulation or other high-risk factors in patients, it is recommended to consult with the general practitioner.

Local anesthesia

Tissue removal should be performed under local anesthesia. However, direct injection into the tissue to be biopsied should be avoided, as otherwise correct histopathologic findings may be compromised by the production of edematous swelling. A conduction anesthesia is therefore preferred. If infiltration anesthesia is nevertheless necessary, it is important to place several small deposits circularly around the biopsy site. Especially in areas with a high blood supply such as the tongue, it is recommended to use a local anesthetic with a vasoconstrictor to improve intraoperative visibility and minimize the intraoperative risk of bleeding.

Biopsy techniques

Different options are available for obtaining a tissue sample, depending on the location and size as well as general medical factors (e.g. anticoagulants). Generally, the sample is taken from a representative site of the change. For this purpose, the biopsy specimen must be taken at a sufficient depth. For an evaluation, the sampling of the entire epithelium as well as portions of subepithelial connective tissue is essential.

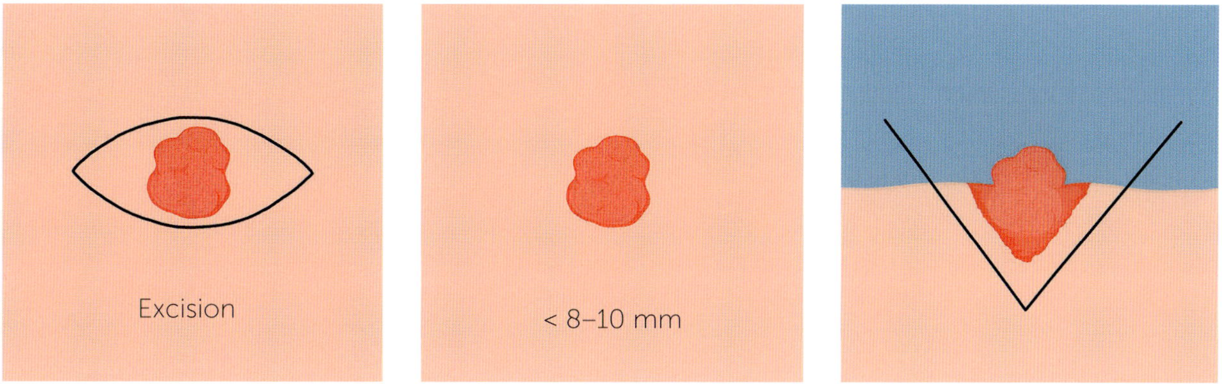

Figs 13-1 to 13-3 Excisional biopsy.

Excisional biopsy

At best, the main goal of a biopsy is the complete removal of the oral mucosal lesion through an excisional biopsy. This can be performed for lesions that appear suspicious of < 1 cm (e.g. fibroma, leukoplakia, salivary gland cysts). The advantage of excisional biopsy is that the findings can be sent and evaluated in toto for histopathologic clarification. The excision should be performed in healthy tissue (*in sano*) and should have a safety margin of 1 to 2 mm. Consequently, there is a larger postoperative wound area than with incisional biopsy, which must be subsequently treated (Figs 13-1 to 13-3).

Incisional biopsy

Incisional biopsy is indicated for suspicious findings that do not allow complete excision because of their extension of > 1 cm or unclear limitation (e.g. oral lichen planus, lichenoid reaction, blistering disease). In these cases, it may be appropriate to biopsy at different sites. To obtain a biopsy that is as representative as possible, portions should be taken from the altered as well as the healthy oral mucosa. Note that the incision is made in the marginal area and not in the center of the change since, especially in the case of ulcers, the central portion contains only necrotic and non-evaluable tissue (Figs 13-4 to 13-6).

Clinical procedure

Biopsies can be performed with a scalpel, punch, or CO_2 laser. The choice of appropriate instrumentation depends on the extent, risk factors, medical history, surrounding anatomical structures of the sampling site, and operator preference or experience.

Scalpel biopsy

Biopsy with straight and angled scalpels (Fig 13-7) is a common method that can be used relatively easily in everyday practice. In the vicinity of anatomically critical structures, such as the palatine artery on the palate, or in esthetically challenging areas, an angled scalpel may be helpful. Surgical or diamond-tipped forceps are used to hold the tissue at the sampling site until detachment without pressure, and then the tissue is placed in the pathology transport tube (with 4% buffered formalin solution). Bruising of the biopsy specimen should be avoided to ensure histopathologic evaluation of the architecture of the epithelium and thus the degree of dysplasia. Depending on the type and size of excision, primary wound closure or wound care with dental adhesive paste is recommended.

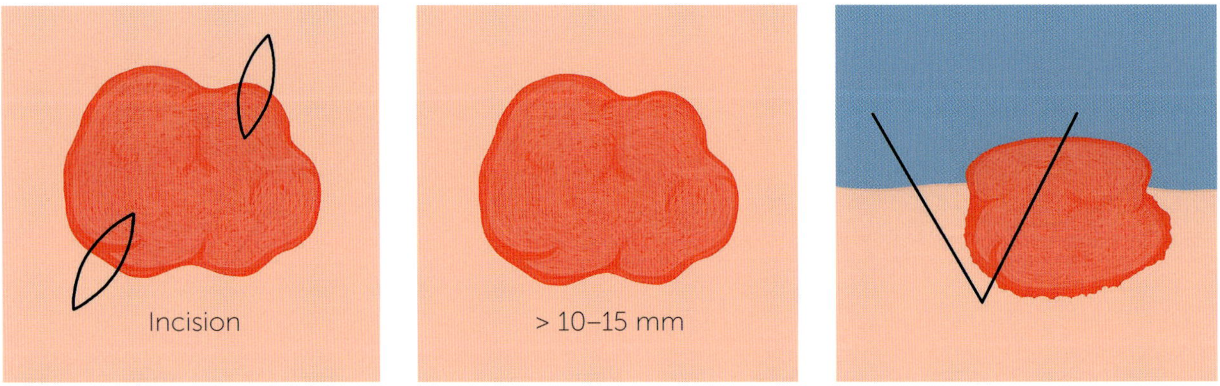

Figs 13-4 to 13-6 Incisional biopsy.

Punch biopsy

Punches of different diameters (usually 3 to 6 mm) (Fig 13-8) can be used to remove a biopsy specimen with a defined diameter by applying pressure and simultaneously rotating the specimen. Also in this case, postoperative care with sutures is recommended because of the bleeding that occurs, although it is not always possible. Punch biopsies are performed especially in cases of blistering diseases. If a vascular malformation is suspected, the use of a punch should be avoided.

CO_2 laser

Biopsies can also be taken with the aid of a CO_2 laser. Here, the photothermal effect is used to cut or ablate the tissue. At the same time, the laser beam can be used to occlude smaller blood vessels up to 0.5 mm in diameter. Therefore, in most cases, covering the wound surface with dental adhesive paste is sufficient and suturing can be omitted. The biopsy specimen subsequently shows a zone of carbonization, necrosis, and edema, which cannot be evaluated histopathologically. For this reason, a safety margin of 1 mm should be maintained. On the submission form for histopathologic examination, it is therefore essential to specify the type of removal by a CO_2 laser. Due to the ease of handling as well as the simpler postoperative management, the CO_2 laser technique is used more frequently in the case studies shown than removal with a scalpel.

Wound care and closure

Wound closure depends on the biopsy method chosen and the general condition of the patient. In the case of biopsy by scalpel or punch, suturing may be recommended due to the bleeding that is induced. However, primary wound closure often results in an uncomfortable feeling of tightness due to the loss of substance. A biopsy wound caused by a CO_2 laser, on the other hand, can be covered with dental adhesive paste and left to heal secondarily. In addition to the dental adhesive paste, which is applied at home until superficial epithelialization, an analgesic can be prescribed. If the risk of bleeding is increased, local compression with swabs (soaked in tranexamic acid, if necessary) is recommended.

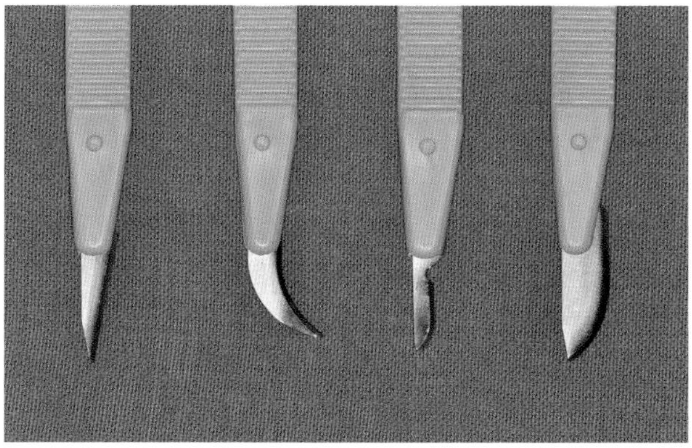

Fig 13-7 Straight and angled scalpels.

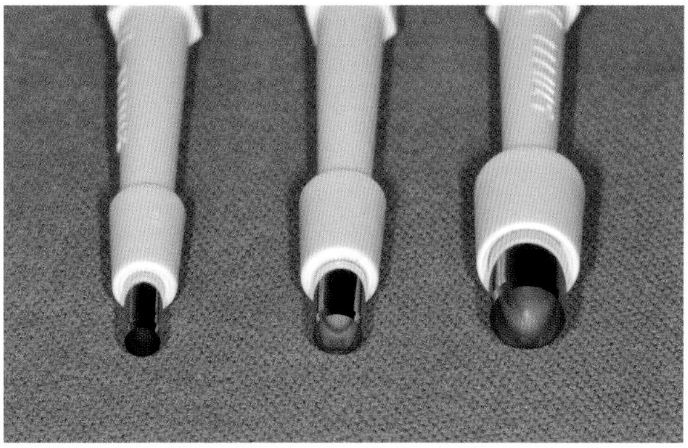

Fig 13-8 Punches of different diameters.

Postoperative controls and course

Postoperative oral hygiene with a soft toothbrush is recommended. Although acidic and spicy foods and drinks should be avoided during the wound healing phase, food can be taken as usual immediately after the local anesthetic has worn off. A wound check and, if necessary, suture removal can take place after 1 week. The histopathologic report should also be available at this time for discussion with the patient and to determine any further procedure. The course of wound healing also depends on the patient's general medical situation. In smokers and high-risk patients, further follow-up examinations may be indicated due to delayed wound healing.

Excision biopsies

Epulis/pyogenic granuloma

Clinic and etiology

- Soft to coarse, rather spherical structure that grows rapidly and appears on the gingiva or alveolar mucosa,
- May bleed easily when touched,
- Traumatic in origin,
- Often hormonally co-caused and associated with plaque.

Indications

- Removal indicated for increasing growth, discomfort, restriction in eating or brushing teeth; for diagnosis; for clarification to check for malignancy.

Contraindications

- None; in pregnant women, wait until the end of pregnancy and lactation due to the risk of recurrence due to pregnancy hormones.

Specific risks

- Risk of recurrence high unless completely excised surgically and subgingival cleaning of the adjacent tooth is performed,
- Local bleeding in certain forms of epulis reduces optimal view of the surgical field, thus insufficient excision or curettage and thus possible recurrence.

Local anesthesia

- Infiltration anesthesia useful to reduce local bleeding and thus obtain a better view of the surgical field.

Step-by-step clinical procedure

- See Figures 13-9 to 13-16.

Wound care and closure

- Primary wound closure is not always possible if the finding occurs on the gingiva,
- Hemostasis by local compression,
- Wound covering with dental adhesive paste,
- Instructions on oral hygiene are very important: soft manual toothbrush; domestic tooth cleaning under visual control to ensure absolute absence of plaque; gingiva must not be traumatized by toothbrush bristles, otherwise there is a risk of recurrence; additional local antiseptic (e.g. chlorhexidine gel).

Postoperative controls and course

- Wound check after 1 to 2 weeks is useful to check oral hygiene and possible recurrence,
- Further checks after 4 weeks and 6 months,
- If necessary, repeat excision/vaporization using a CO_2 laser.

Recommended literature

1. Filippi A, Hitz Lindenmüller I (Hrsg). Die Zunge. Berlin: Quintessenz, 2016.
2. Kumar A, Cascarini L, McCaul JA, et al. How should we manage oral leukoplakie? Br J Oral Maxillofac Surg 2013;51:377–383.
3. Tambuwala A, Sangle A, Khan A, Sayed A. Excision of oral leukoplakia by CO_2 lasers versus traditional scalpel: a comparative study. J Maxillofac Oral Surg 2014;13:320–327.

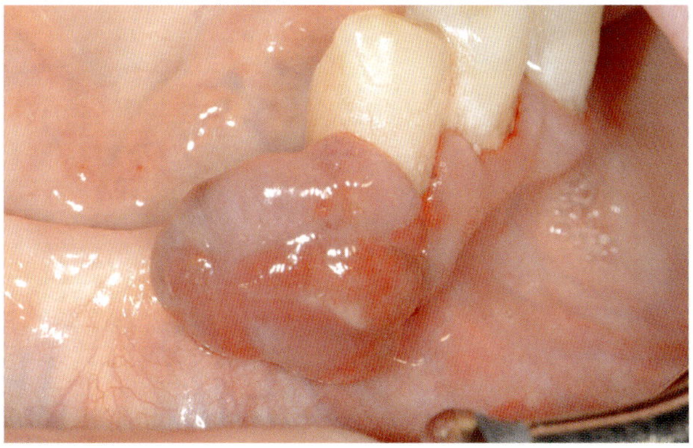

Fig 13-9 Initial clinical situation: Prominent, red-purple, inflammatory, ball-like tissue proliferation close to tooth 33. All visible teeth also show significant plaque accumulation.

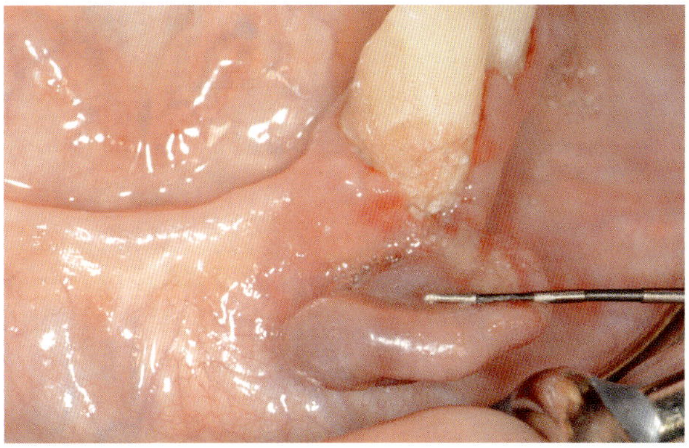

Fig 13-10 Each finding should be inspected prior to removal to determine how and whether the structure appears on the mucosa (here the gingiva). In this case, the finding appears pedunculated marginal to tooth 33, which simplifies the removal. The wound area is correspondingly small.

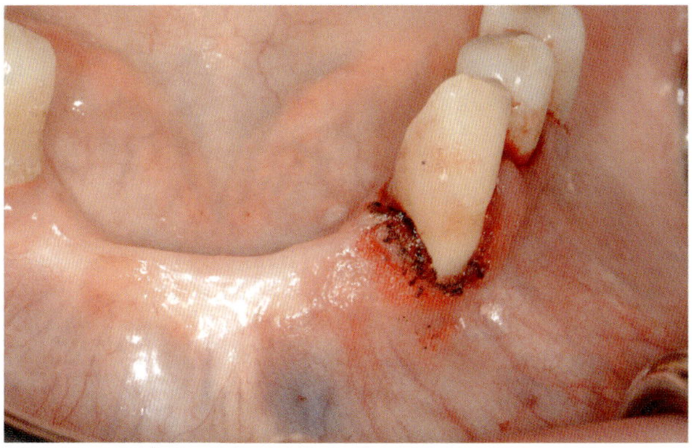

Fig 13-11 After infiltration anesthesia, a scalpel/CO_2 laser is used to separate the findings on the pedicle. Depending on the degree of inflammation, diffuse hemorrhage may occur locally, impairing further procedures due to clouding of the surgical field. Since it is still unclear at this point whether the wound is actually an epulis/pyogenic granuloma, the wound area must be curetted down to the periosteum or vaporized with a CO_2 laser. In the case of an epulis, the (co-)involved tooth must also be thoroughly curetted to minimize the risk of recurrence.

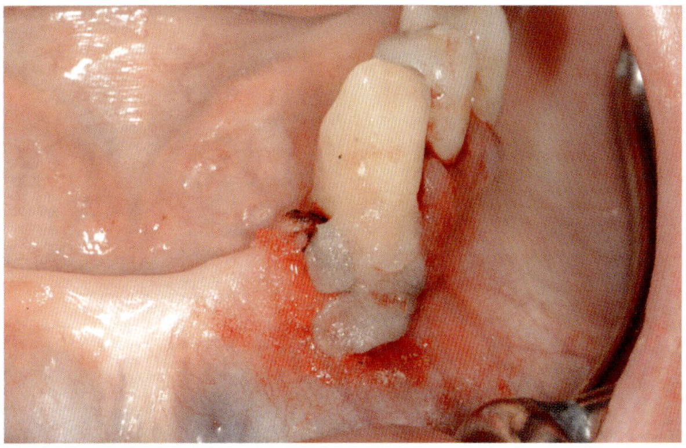

Fig 13-12 The wound area cannot be primarily closed and is therefore covered with dental adhesive paste. This procedure must be performed regularly at home for pain relief and to protect the wound area. The use of a local antiseptic (e.g. chlorhexidine gel) is also recommended.

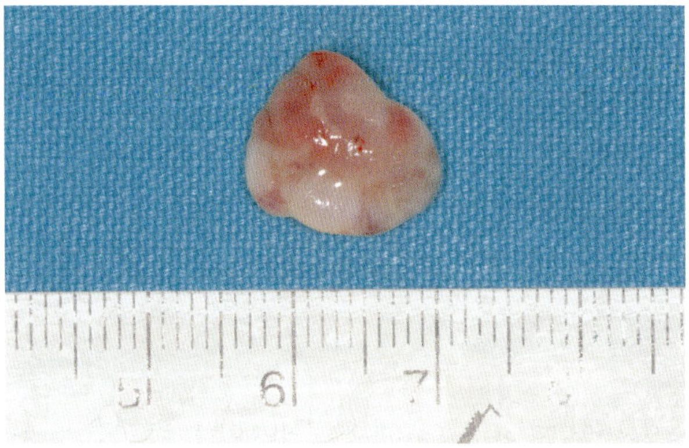

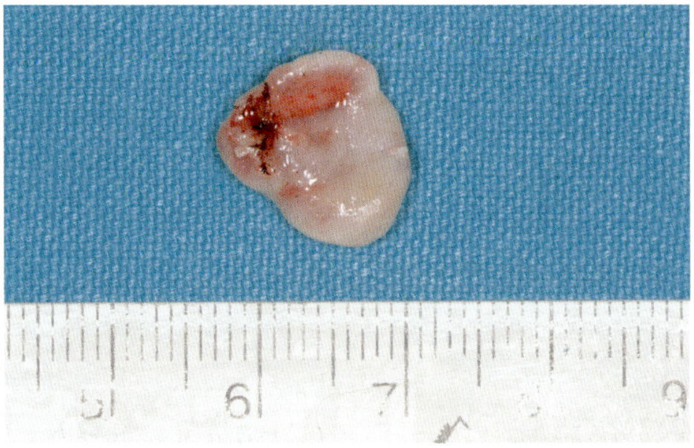

Figs 13-13 and 13-14 All removed findings must be examined histopathologically. Shown here are the findings (external and internal view) after removal. In the internal view, the ulcerated area is clearly visible.

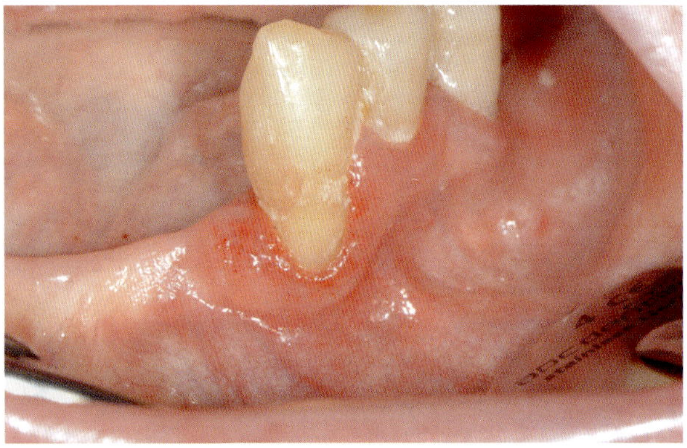

Fig 13-15 Wound control should be performed 1 week postoperatively, especially to check oral hygiene and thus prevent recurrence. In the present case, the inflammation marginal to tooth 33 and the clear plaque accumulation are striking.

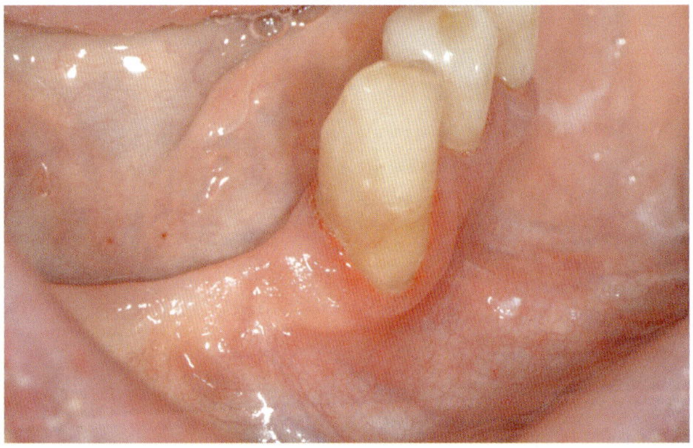

Fig 13-16 Check at 4 weeks postoperatively: The marginal gingiva is still slightly reddened, but oral hygiene is clearly better.

Fibroma

Clinic and etiology

- Round, oval, elongated, pedunculated or broad-based pink polyp,
- Initially soft, hardening after prolonged persistence,
- Traumatic in origin.

Indications

- Removal indicated for increasing growth, discomfort, restrictions in eating, speaking, and oral hygiene; for diagnosis; for clarification to check for malignancy.

Contraindications

- None.

Specific risks

- Fibromas on the gingiva carry the risk of possible recession; therefore, detailed patient education is required.

Local anesthesia

- Conduction anesthesia or infiltration anesthesia.

Step-by-step clinical procedure

- See Figures 13-17 to 13-24.

Wound care and wound closure

- In the case of CO_2 laser, open wound healing; if necessary, wound covering with dental adhesive paste,
- In the case of scalp excision, primary wound closure by means of (resorbable) sutures is not always possible, depending on the localization.

Postoperative controls and course

- Depending on the suture material selected (resorbable/non-resorbable) or whether a CO_2 laser is used: 1 to 2 weeks,
- Elimination of possible irritating factors, otherwise there is a risk of recurrence.

Recommended literature

1. Filippi A, Hitz Lindenmüller I (Hrsg). Die Zunge. Berlin: Quintessenz, 2016.
2. Suter VJ, Reichart PA, Warnakulasuriya S, Altermatt HJ, Bornstein MM. Fibrome und fibröse Hyperplasien: Diagnostik, Therapie und klinische Relevanz einer häufigen oralen Veränderung. Quintessenz 2014;65:711–721.
3. Valério RA, de Queiroz AM, Romualdo PC, Brentegani LG, de Paula-Silva FW. Mucocele and fibroma: treatment and clinical features for differential diagnosis. Braz Dent J 2013;24: 537–541.

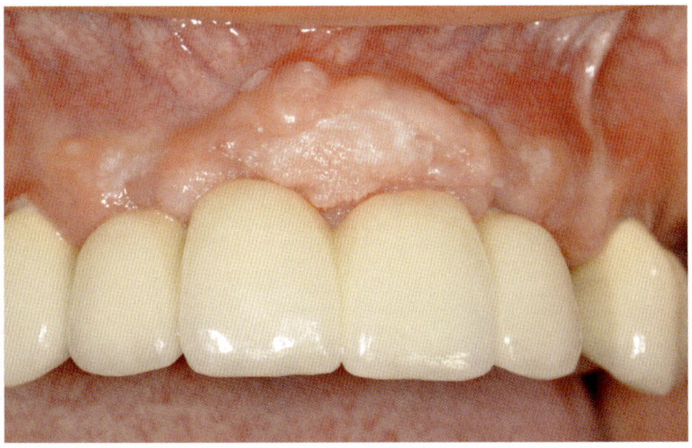

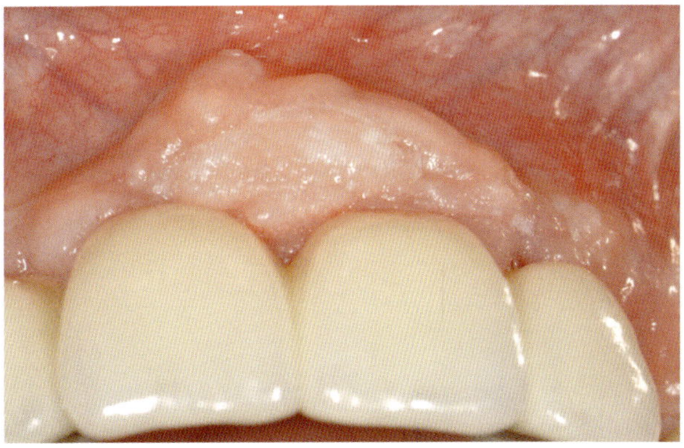

Figs 13-17 and 13-18 Baseline clinical situation: Prominent pinkish, coarse, broad-based, seated finding in the maxillary anterior region. The surface shows white and papillomatous areas.

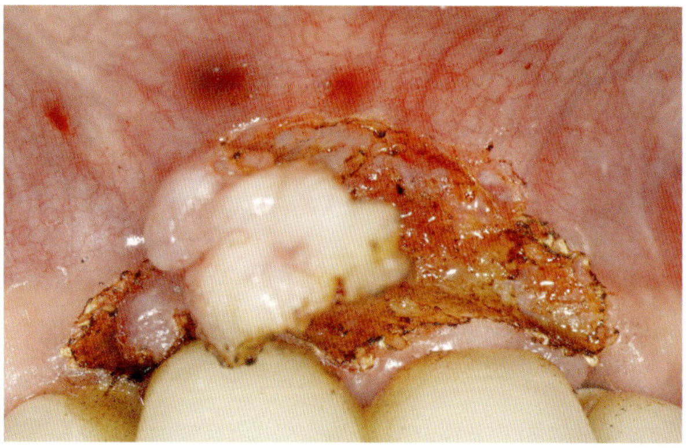

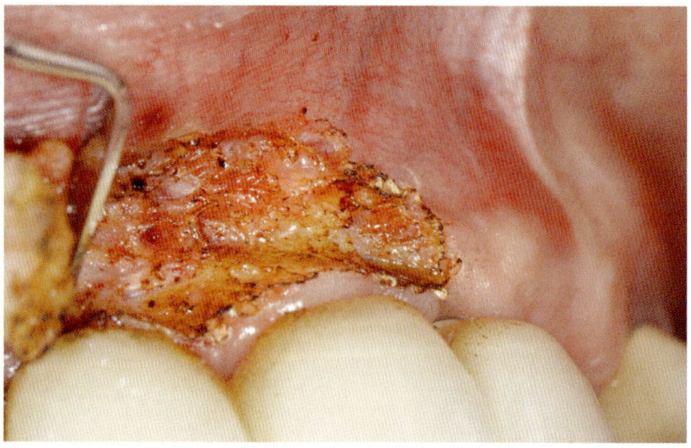

Figs 13-19 and 13-20 Each finding should be inspected before removal to see how it appears on the mucosa (here the gingiva). This gives a better estimate of the size of the expected wound area. In this case, the finding appears broad-based, resulting in a larger wound area during excision. After local anesthesia has been administered (in this case, infiltration anesthesia), the fibroma is separated from the base with a scalpel/CO_2 laser. Bleeding is usually kept within limits in the case of a fibroma.

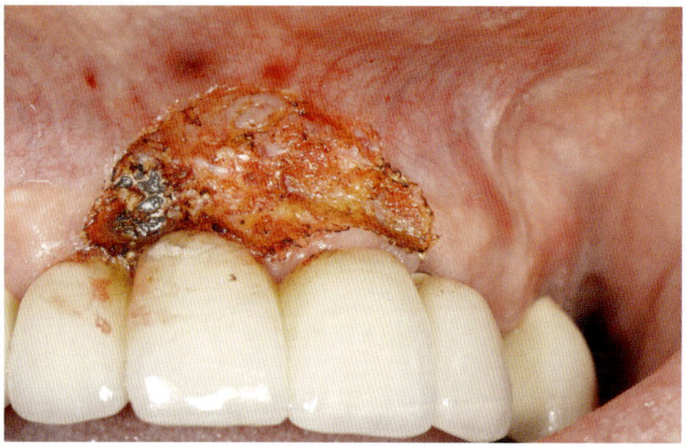

Fig 13-21 If bleeding does occur, compression is applied with a swab, or the vessel/bleeding area is obliterated with a CO_2 laser or electrotome (black area). The wound area cannot be closed primarily and is therefore covered with dental adhesive paste. This procedure must be repeated regularly at home for pain relief and protection of the wound area.

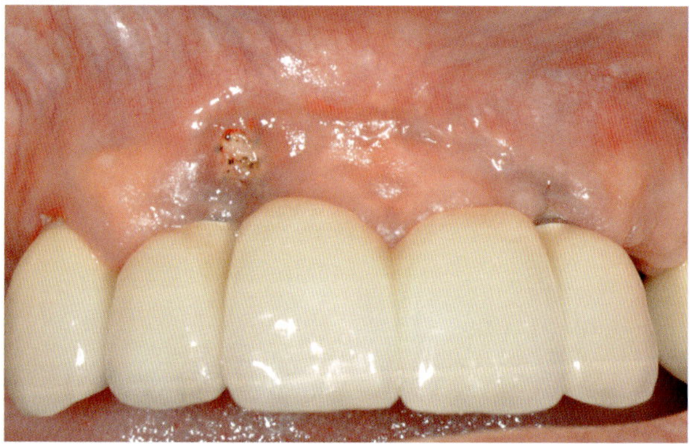

Fig 13-22 Clinical situation 3 weeks after excision: wound healing of region 11/12 (in the area of vaporization) is somewhat delayed. A wound check is usually performed 1 to 2 weeks after excision, among other things to check oral hygiene and inform the patient about the histopathologic findings. Here, the suspected diagnosis of fibroma was confirmed.

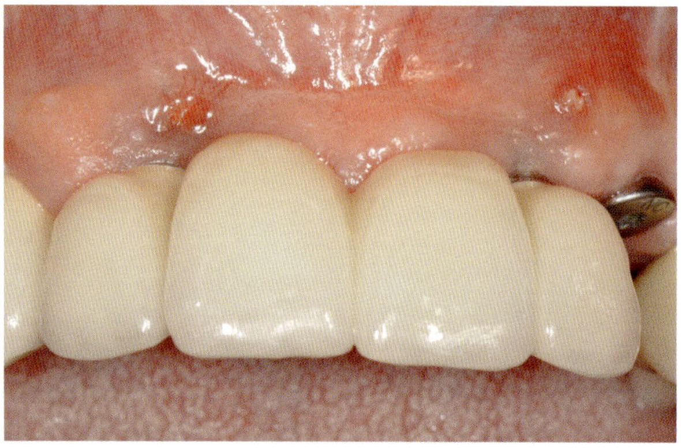

Fig 13-23 Clinical situation 6 weeks after excision: Wound healing is probably delayed due to the patient's smoking habits.

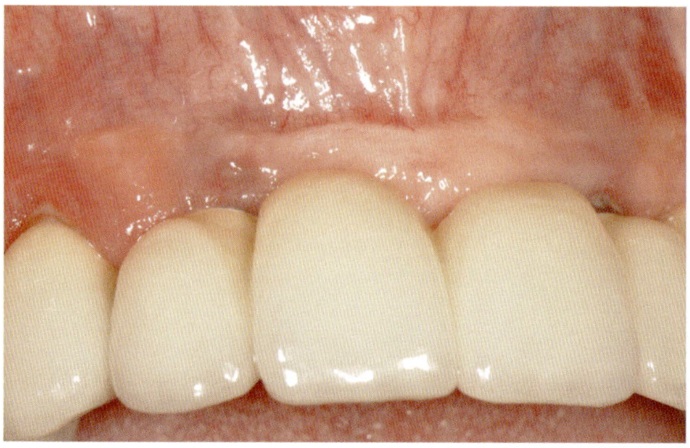

Fig 13-24 Clinical situation 1 year postoperatively.

Hemangioma/vascular malformation

Clinic and etiology

- Light to dark red or purplish, slightly raised, bulging, depressible lesion with increasing size,
- Increasing in older age,
- May be traumatic in origin.

Indications

- Removal indicated for esthetic reasons, rapidly increasing growth, discomfort, restriction in eating; for diagnosis; for clarification of malignancy.

Contraindications

- None, possibly unfavorable anatomical location.

Specific risks

- Hemangiomas often extend deeply ("tip of the iceberg"); often the size is unclear; especially deep and osseous hemangiomas must be referred to a specialist clinic,
- Risk of bleeding, especially in regions with a good blood supply such as the tongue, and with blood-thinning medication,
- Recurrence possible with incomplete removal.

Local anesthesia

- Line anesthesia and infiltration anesthesia useful for local hemostasis.

Step-by-step clinical procedure

- See Figures 13-25 to 13-36.

Wound care and closure

- This depends on the size of the wound area, the anatomical location, and the bleeding tendency: In the case of open wound healing (CO_2 laser), wound covering using dental adhesive paste or primary wound closure using (resorbable) sutures (in the case of scalp excision).

Postoperative controls and course

- Depending on the suture material chosen (resorbable/non-resorbable) or whether a CO_2 laser is used: 1 to 2 weeks. To check for a possible recurrence, further control is advisable 6 months postoperatively.

Recommended literature

1. Filippi A, Hitz Lindenmüller I (Hrsg). Die Zunge. Berlin: Quintessenz, 2016.
2. Schneider AC, Altermatt HJ, Reichart PA, Bornstein MM. Gutartige Tumoren der Mundhöhlenschleimhaut. Teil 2: Mesenchymale Neoplasien. Quintessenz 2010;61:1193–1200.

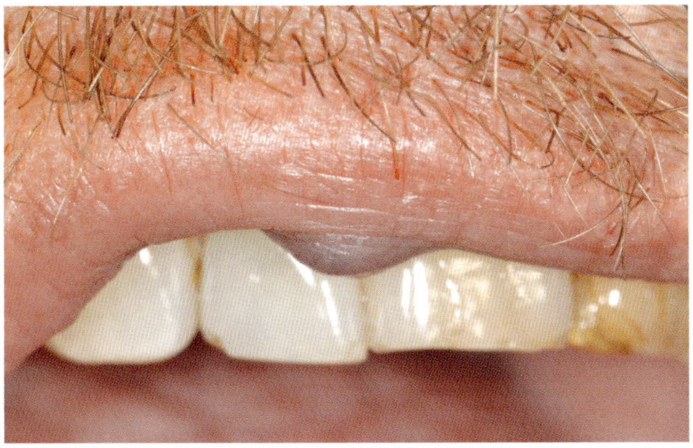

Fig 13-25 The patient is disturbed by the lip appearance. A drooping, purplish-bluish finding in the middle of the upper lip is striking.

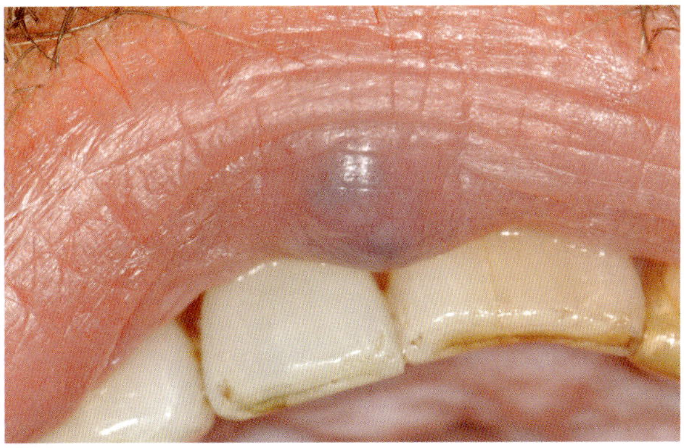

Fig 13-26 The palpable and clinically visible vascular tangles are indicative of a vascular malformation.

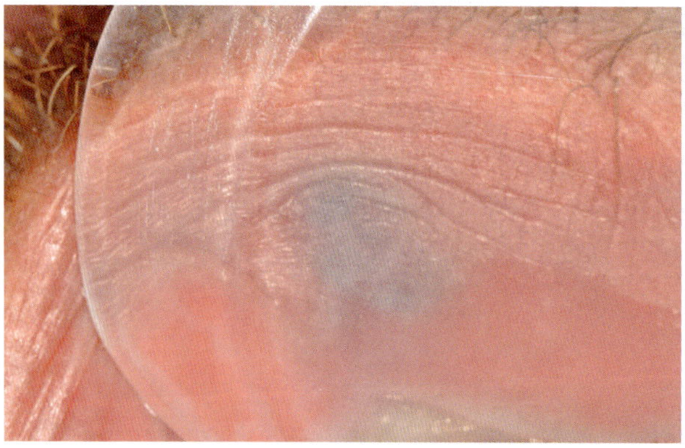

Fig 13-27 Using a glass spatula, it is easier to ascertain whether the suspected diagnosis of a hemangioma/vascular malformation is plausible: When pressure is applied with the glass spatula, the findings lose color as the blood is pushed away from the vessels.

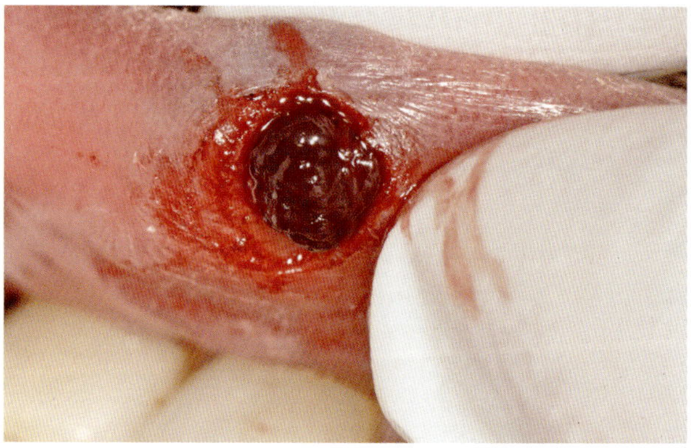

Fig 13-28 A superficial incision is made at the *punctum maximum* and perpendicular to the dentition with a scalpel/CO_2 laser. Finger pressure from the outside allows the blood vessel clusters to be pressed out and be optimally visualized.

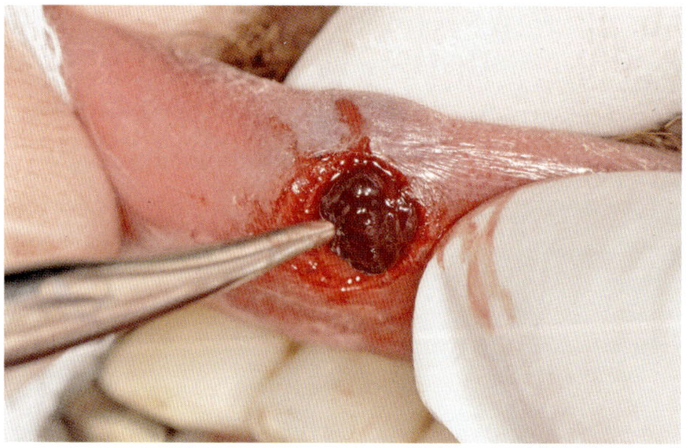

Fig 13-29 Using blunt scissors or forceps, the findings are carefully detached from the surrounding soft tissue to avoid opening the vessels and causing bleeding.

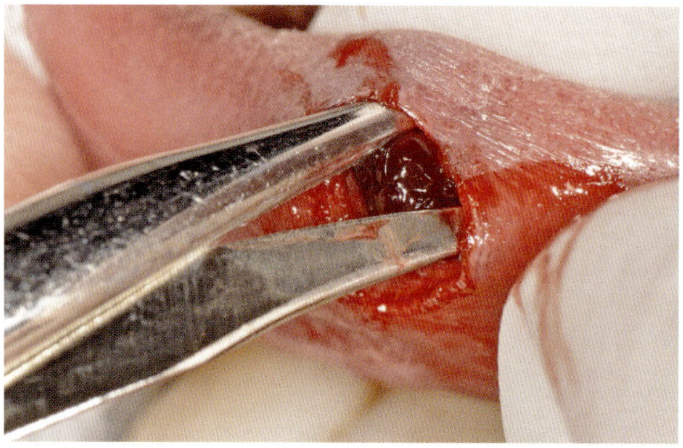

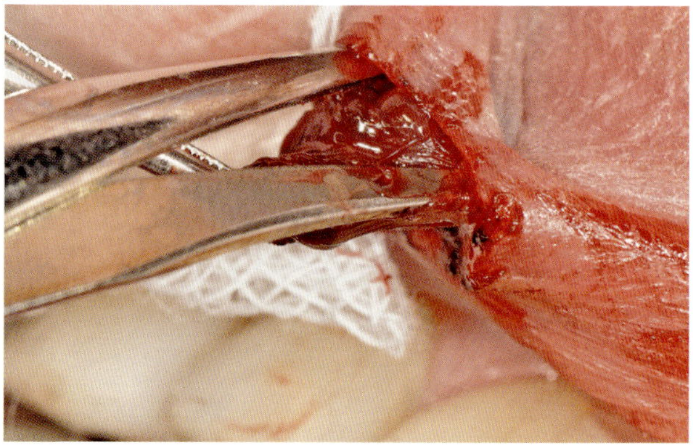

Figs 13-30 and 13-31 If necessary, the access must be opened further using blunt scissors, and the hemangioma pushed through the opening by applying pressure from the outside of the lip. The process can be accelerated by gently pulling on the finding with dental forceps.

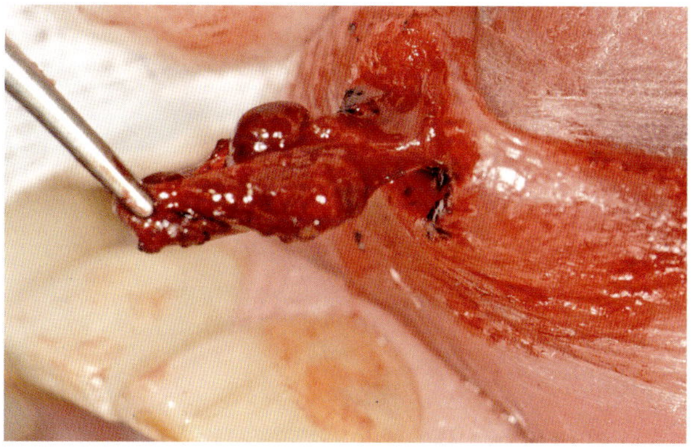

Fig 13-32 The vascular tangle is completely detached from the surrounding soft tissue by gentle traction, separated, and then examined histopathologically.

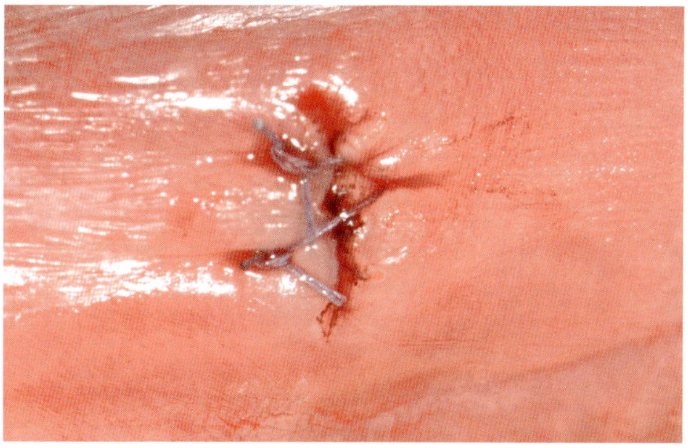

Fig 13-33 Wound closure is performed here using resorbable sutures. Wound healing is hardly disturbed by the teeth, since the incision was made at a 90-degree angle to the row of teeth, thus providing a minimal surface of attack.

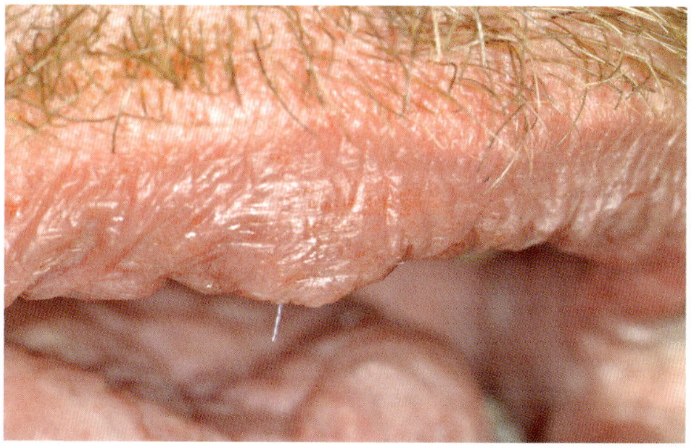

Fig 13-34 Lip image immediately postoperatively. Since the hemangioma has stretched the mucosa like an expander, the lip line is not yet harmonious.

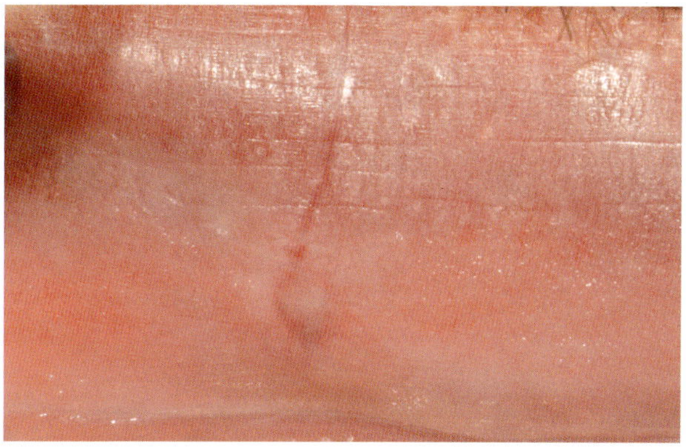

Fig 13-35 Clinical situation 6 weeks postoperatively. Wound healing has long since been completed and only a minimal scar is visible but not noticeable.

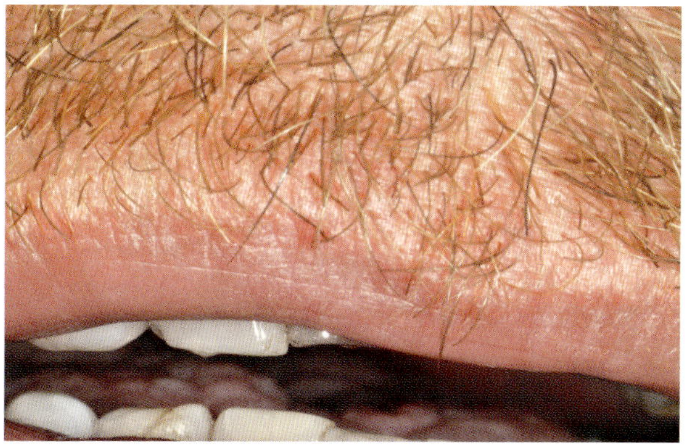

Fig 13-36 The lip now appears harmonious.

Leukoplakia

Clinic and etiology

- Sharply demarcated white spot, not wipeable, homogeneously smooth, white-red speckled or verrucous,
- Mechanical-irritative causes, tobacco, alcohol, human papillomavirus (HPV).

Indications

- Removal indicated for increasing size, verrucous or inhomogeneous appearance,
- For risk factors such as smoking, alcohol, other drugs; for diagnosis; for clarification of malignancy.

Contraindications

- None, but consider anatomy.

Specific risks

- None.

Local anesthesia

- Conduction or infiltration anesthesia.

Step-by-step clinical procedure

- See Figures 13-37 to 13-49.

Wound care and wound closure

- In case of CO_2 laser, open wound healing; if necessary, wound covering with dental adhesive paste,
- In case of scalp excision, primary wound closure by means of (resorbable) sutures is not always possible (depending on localization).

Postoperative controls and course

- Depending on the suture material selected (resorbable/non-resorbable) or whether a CO_2 laser was used: 1 to 2 weeks,
- Exclude possible irritation factors and other noxae, otherwise there is a risk of recurrence,
- Progress checks, depending on noxae, usually every 3 to 6 months.

Recommended literature

1. Filippi A, Hitz Lindenmüller I (Hrsg). Die Zunge. Berlin: Quintessenz, 2016.
2. Kumar A, Cascarini L, McCaul JA, et al. How should we manage oral leukoplakie? Br J Oral Maxillofac Surg 2013;51:377–383.
3. Tambuwala A, Sangle A, Khan A, Sayed A. Excision of oral leukoplakia by CO_2 lasers versus traditional scalpel: a comparative study. J Maxillofac Oral Surg 2014;13:320–327.

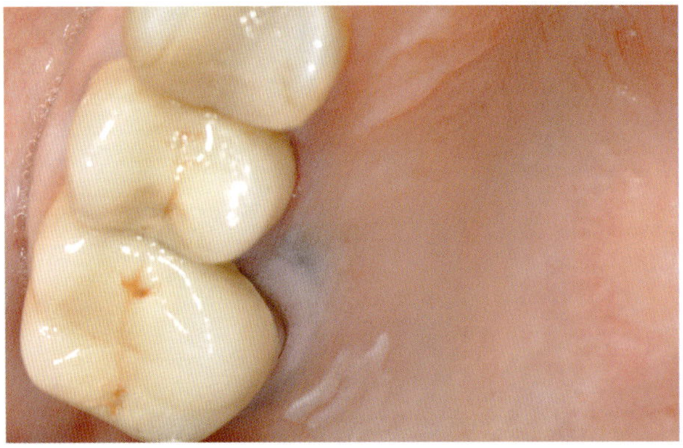

Fig 13-37 Clinical situation: Clearly defined leukoplakia palatal to tooth 16.

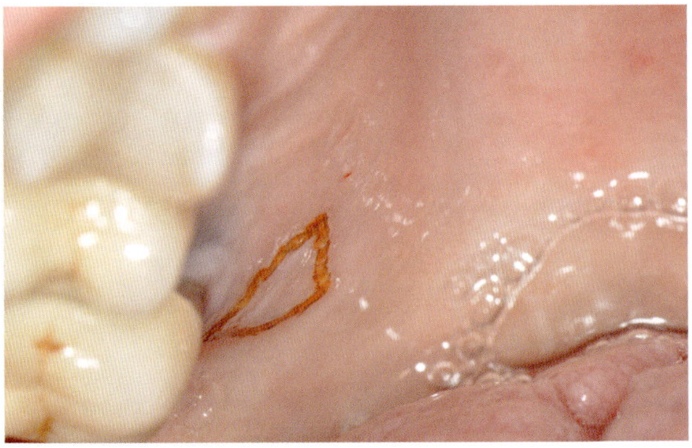

Fig 13-38 After local anesthesia has been administered (in this case, infiltration anesthesia for local hemostasis), the entire finding is circularly marked with a scalpel/CO_2 laser.

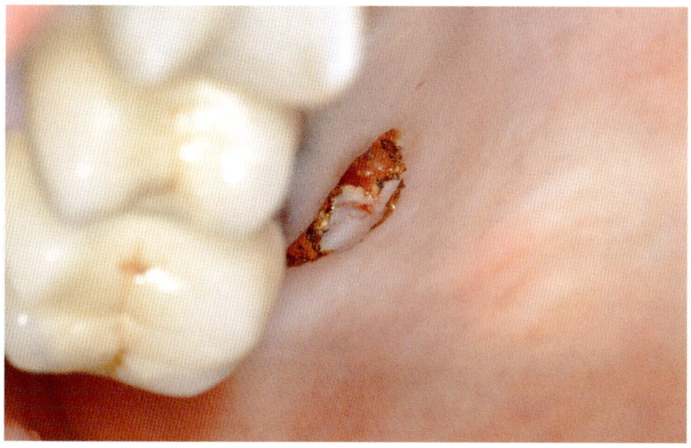

Fig 13-39 The finding is detached from the surrounding soft tissue with a scalpel/CO_2 laser. Any bleeding can be stopped with a CO_2 laser or an electrotome, otherwise compression with a cotton swab helps.

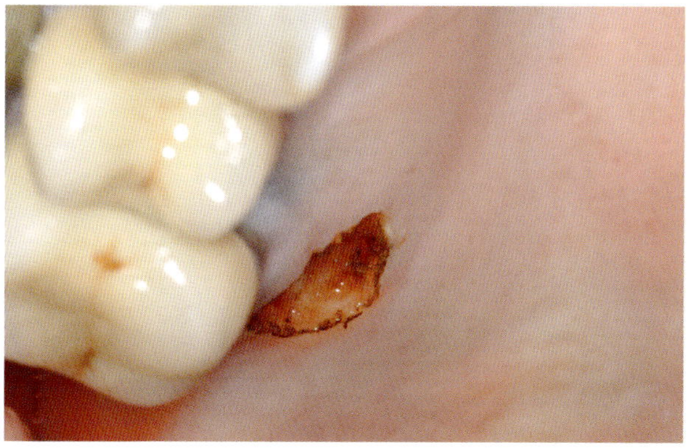

Fig 13-40 The wound area cannot be closed primarily and is therefore covered with dental adhesive paste. This procedure must be continued regularly at home for pain relief and protection of the wound area.

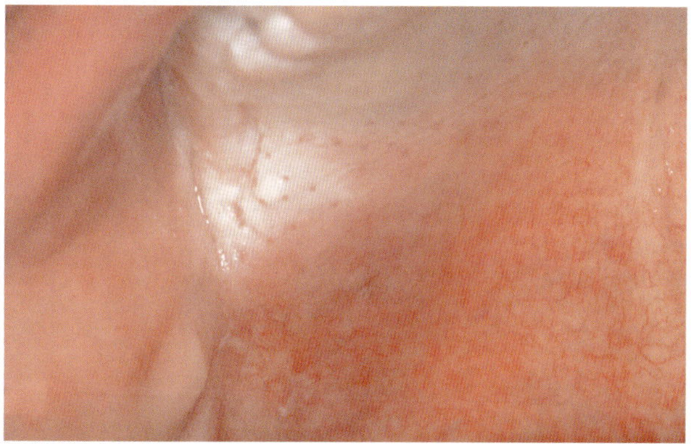

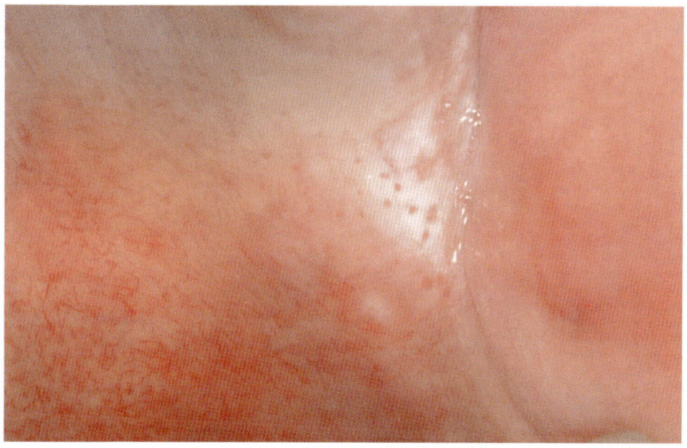

Figs 13-41 and 13-42 Initial clinical situation: Leukoplakic change palatally at the transition to the soft palate, more conspicuous on the right than on the left. For this reason, the decision was made to biopsy on the right side. The patient is a heavy smoker (two packs per day).

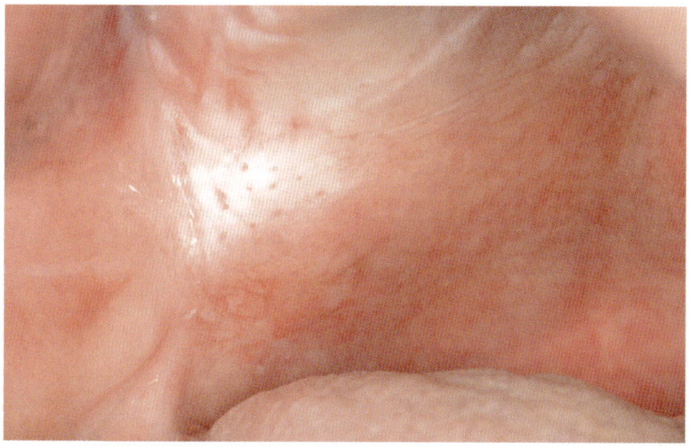

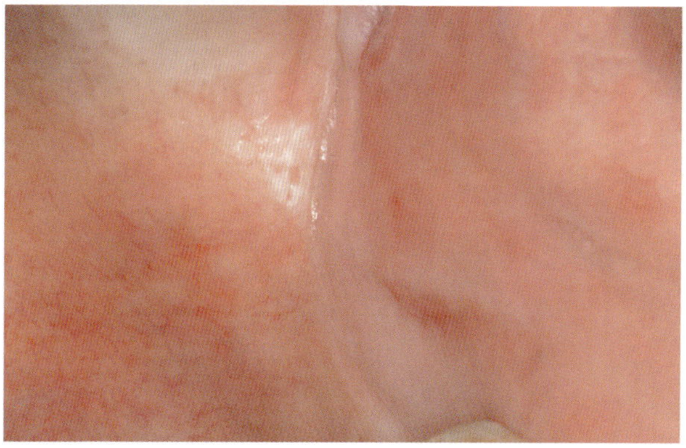

Figs 13-43 and 13-44 Clinical situation after reduction of smoking to one pack per day: The leukoplakic changes have decreased somewhat as a result.

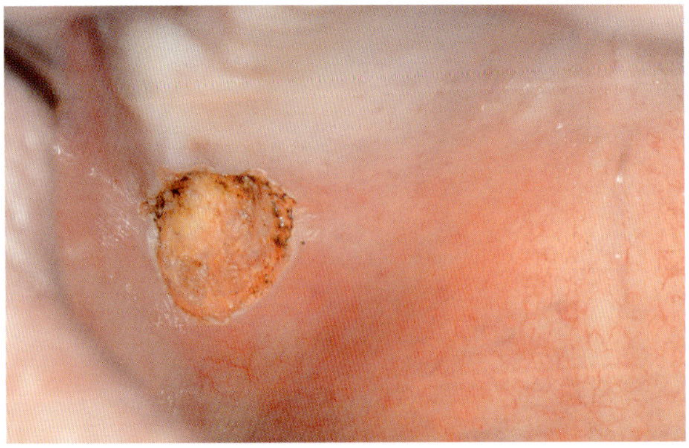

Fig 13-45 After local anesthesia has been administered (in this case, infiltration anesthesia for local hemostasis), the entire finding is circumscribed with a scalpel/CO_2 laser and detached from the surrounding soft tissue. Any bleeding can be stopped with a CO_2 laser or an electrotome, otherwise compression with a cotton swab helps. The wound area cannot be closed primarily and is therefore covered with dental adhesive paste. This procedure must be repeated regularly at home for pain relief and protection of the wound area.

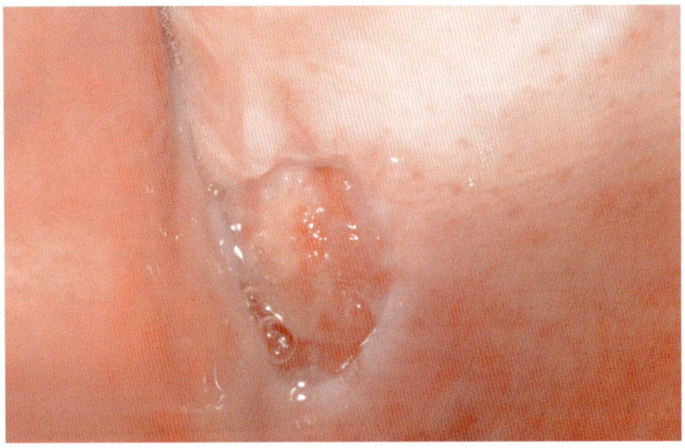

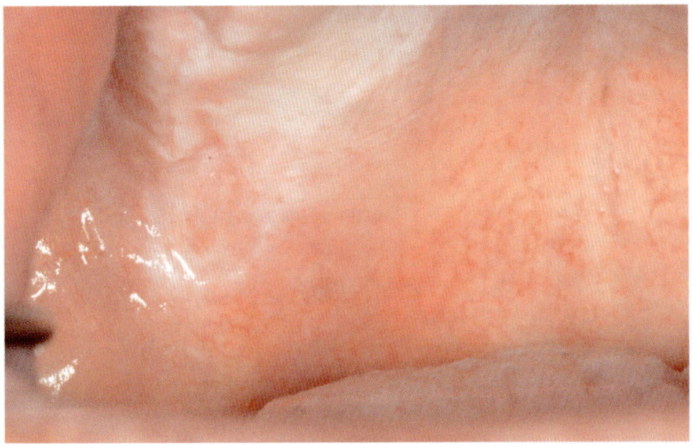

Figs 13-46 and 13-47 Clinical situation 2 and 5 weeks after excision: Wound healing is somewhat delayed because the patient still smokes, despite being informed. Heat development causes disruption of wound healing.

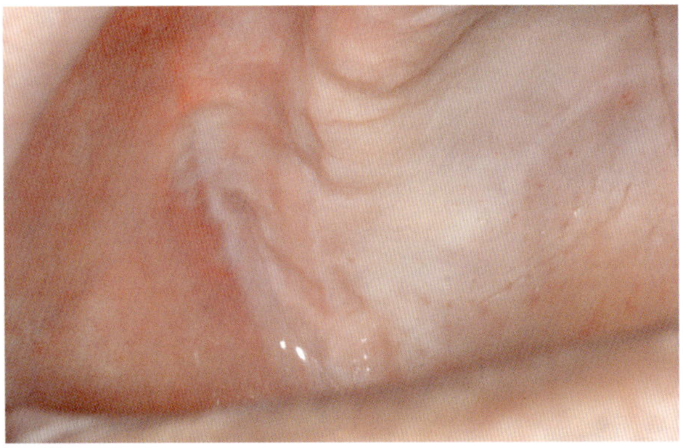

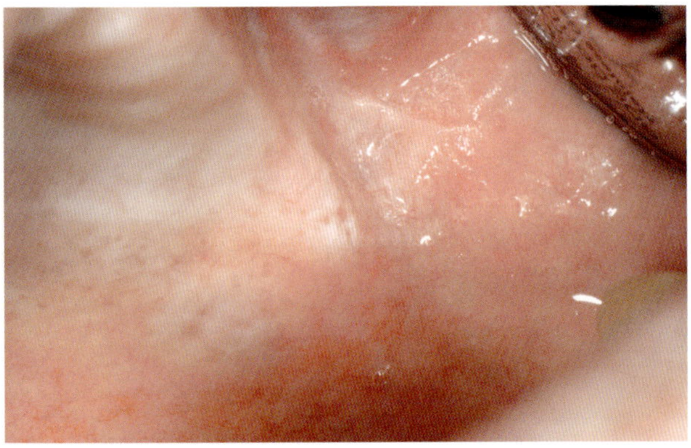

Figs 13-48 and 13-49 Histopathologic examination with subsequent in situ hybridization revealed an oncogenic human papillomavirus (HPV-18 – high risk) as a possible (co-)causative agent of the leukoplakia. For this reason, regular clinical controls must be performed.

Lipoma

Clinic and etiology

- Bulging, spherical structure with a smooth surface and a yellow color shining through,
- Slow growing,
- Benign mesenchymal tumor.

Indications

- Removal indicated for increasing size, discomfort, limitation in eating or speaking; for diagnosis; for clarification of malignancy.

Contraindications

- None, possibly in case of difficult anatomical location.

Specific risks

- High risk of recurrence if surrounding capsule is not also completely removed.

Local anesthesia

- Conduction anesthesia more useful than infiltration anesthesia because the outline of the finding can be better assessed this way.

Step-by-step clinical procedure

- See Figures 13-50 to 13-60.

Wound care and wound closure

- In the case of CO_2 laser, open wound healing; if necessary, wound coverage with dental adhesive paste,
- In the case of scalpel excision, primary wound closure with (resorbable) sutures.

Postoperative controls and course

- Depending on the suture material selected (resorbable/non-resorbable) or whether a CO_2 laser was used: 1 to 2 weeks,
- To check for a possible recurrence, a further 6-month postoperative check is advisable.

Recommended literature

1. Egido-Moreno S, Lozano-Porras AB, Mishra S, Allegue-Allegue M, Marí-Roig A, López-López J. Intraoral lipomas: Review of literature and report of two clinical cases. J Clin Exp Dent 2016;8:e597–e603.
2. Filippi A, Hitz Lindenmüller I (Hrsg). Die Zunge. Berlin: Quintessenz, 2016.
3. Harnisch H, Altermatt HJ, Bornstein M. Intraorales Lipom im Bereich des Nervus mentalis. Schweiz Monatsschr Zahnmed 2007;117: 373–381.

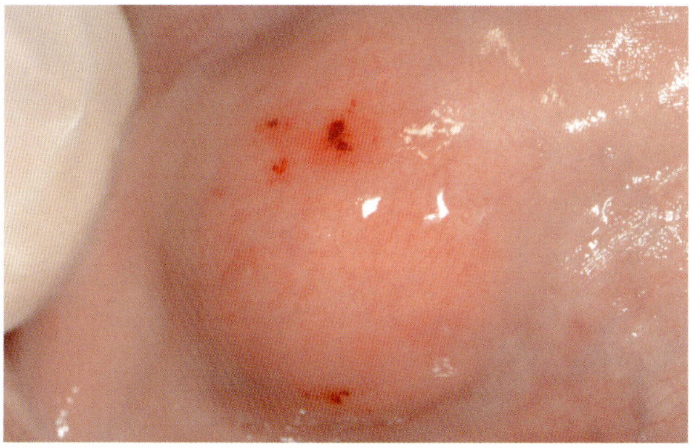

Fig 13-50 Initial clinical situation: Raised, rather coarse finding on the lower lip with hemorrhages (probably bite injury due to the disturbing elevation) and distinct vascular markings (indicative of a lipoma).

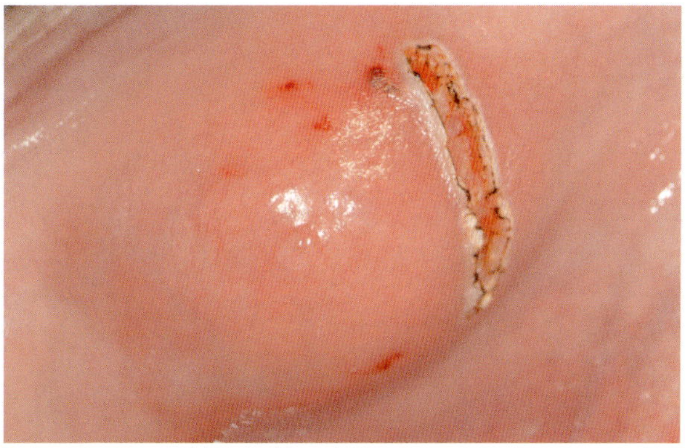

Fig 13-51 Incision (here by a CO_2 laser) at the *punctum maximum* of the elevation and transverse/perpendicular to the dentition (in order not to disturb wound healing by mechanical irritation by the dentition).

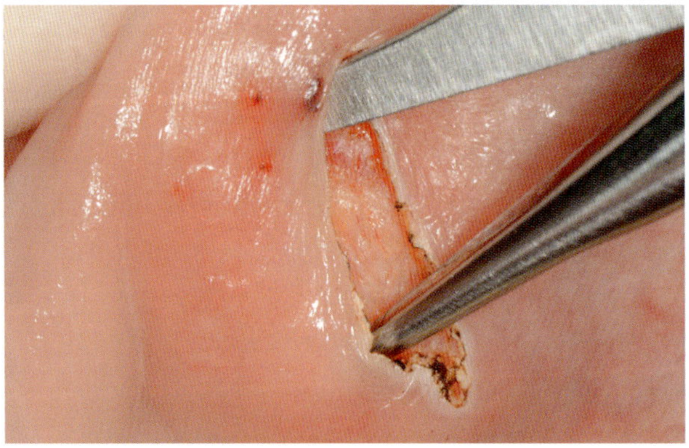

Fig 13-52 Using blunt scissors, the mucosa is carefully detached from the capsular surface in a circular manner.

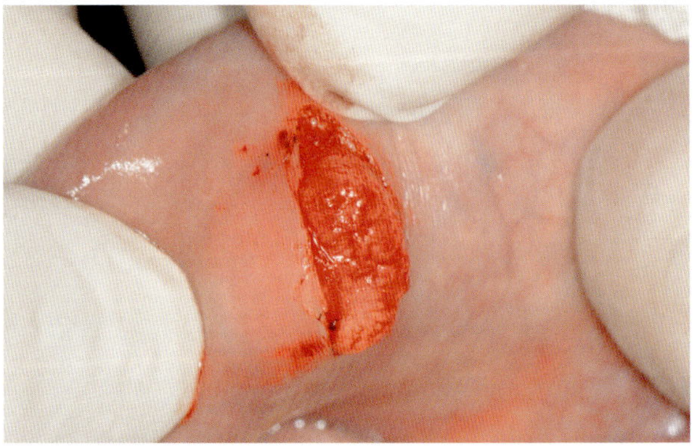

Fig 13-53 Finger pressure from the outside pushes the finding through the slit to the surface. The lobulation of the tissue mass and the yellowish color suggest a lipoma.

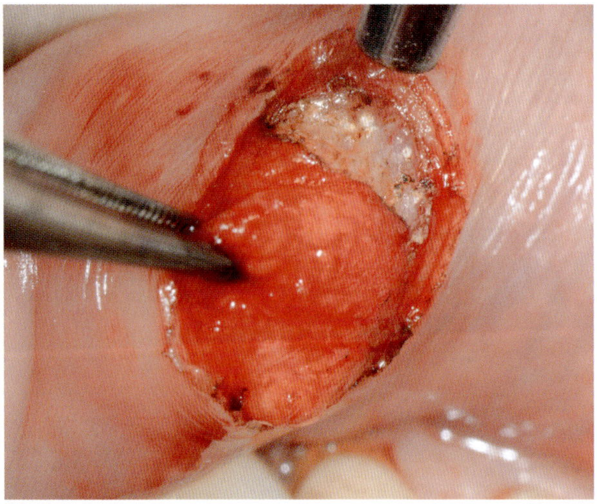

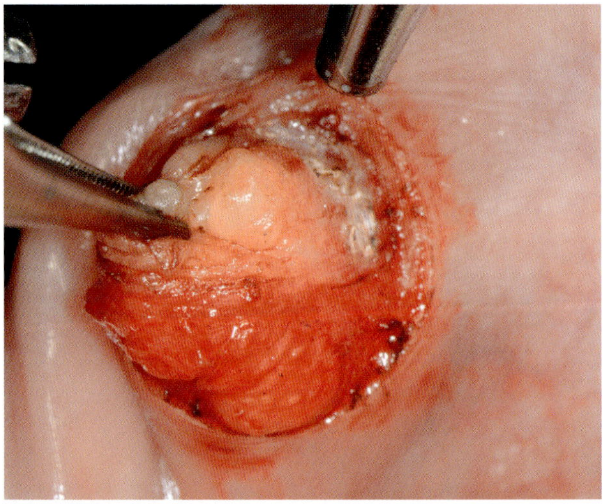

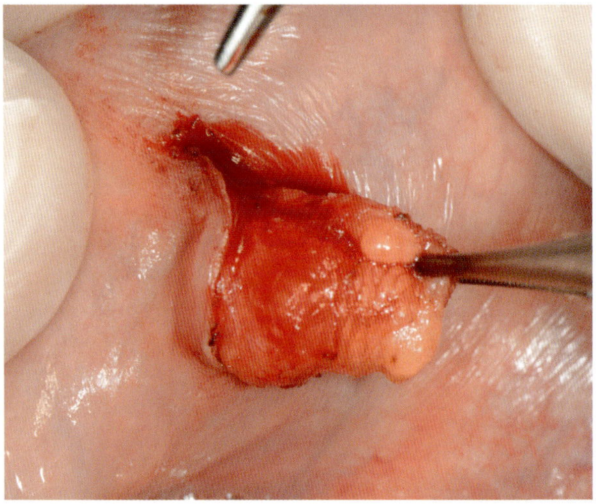

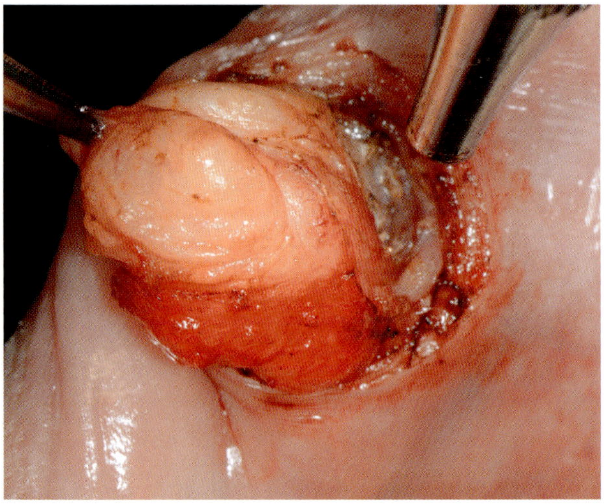

Figs 13-54 to 13-57 Using surgical forceps, the encapsulated finding is carefully lifted off the underlying musculature and completely detached from it, together with the capsule, using a scalpel/CO_2 laser.

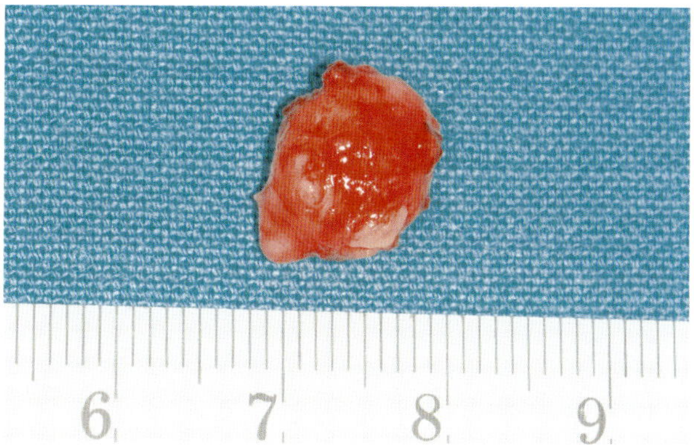

Fig 13-58 Excisate for subsequent histopathologic examination. The capsule surrounding the finding appears to be complete. Residual capsule in the lip would inevitably lead to recurrence.

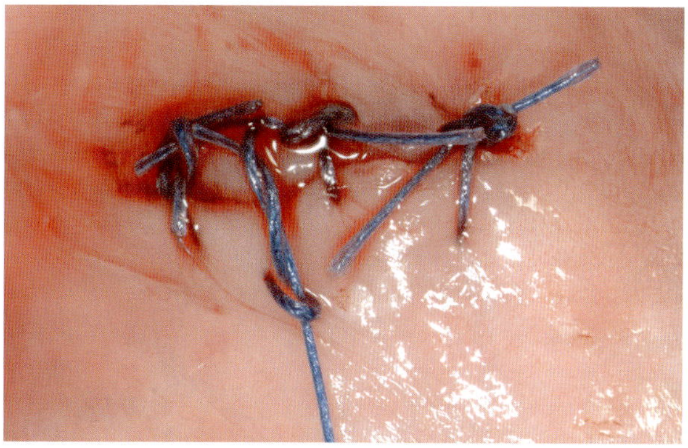

Fig 13-59 Wound closure using resorbable sutures.

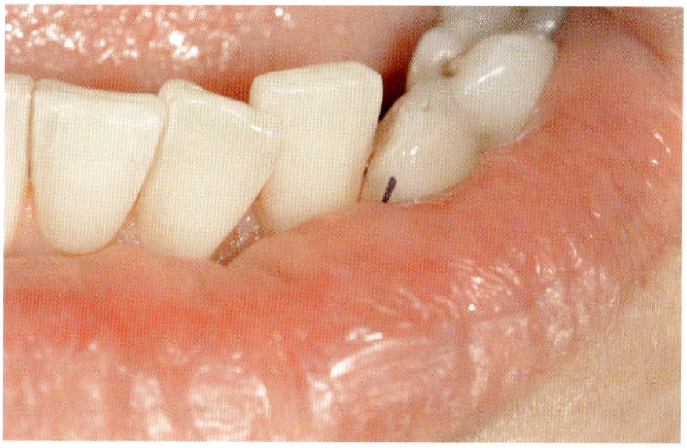

Fig 13-60 The tooth row hardly interferes with wound healing because the incision was performed at a 90-degree angle to the tooth row.

Papilloma

Clinic and etiology

- Exophytic, cone-like mucosa, sometimes cauliflower-like, usually pedunculated; pink or white,
- Most commonly caused by HPV.

Indications

- Removal indicated for increasing size, irritation; for diagnosis; for clarification of malignancy and genesis (HPV).

Contraindications

- None.

Specific risks

- Risk of recurrence in case of incomplete excision,
- In case of viral genesis (HPV), oncogenic high-risk types are also possible (HPV-16, -18, -33; in situ hybridization for HPV),
- Transmission via smear infection possible.

Local anesthesia

- Conduction anesthesia or infiltration anesthesia.

Step-by-step clinical procedure

- See Figures 13-61 to 13-66.

Wound care and wound closure

- In the case of CO_2 laser, open wound healing; if necessary, wound covering with dental adhesive paste,
- In the case of scalpel excision, primary wound closure by means of (resorbable) sutures.

Postoperative controls and course

- Depending on the suture material selected (resorbable/non-resorbable) or whether a CO_2 laser was used: 1 week, also possible irritation factors must be ruled out,
- To check for a possible recurrence, a further 6-month postoperative control is recommended,
- If an oncogenic HPV is detected, the controls must be more closely monitored.

Recommended literature

1. Araújo Andrade S, Pratavieira S, Fracalossi Paes S, Ribeiro MM, Salvador Bagnato V, de Pilla Varotti F. Oral squamous papilloma: a view under clinical, fluorescence and histopathological aspects. Einstein (Sao Paolo) 2019;17(2):eRC4624. doi: 10.31744/einstein_journal/2019RC4624.
2. Chaitanya NC, Allam NS, Gandhi Babu DB, Waghray S, Badam RK, Lavanya R. Systematic meta-analysis on association of human papilloma virus and oral cancer. J Can Res Ther 2016;12:969–974.
3. Filippi A, Hitz Lindenmüller I (Hrsg). Die Zunge. Berlin: Quintessenz, 2016.
4. Toledano-Serrabona J, López-Ramírez M, Sánchez-Torres A, España-Tost A, Gay-Escoda C. Recurrence rate of oral squamous cell papilloma after excision with surgical scalpel or laser therapy: A retrospective cohort study. Med Oral Patol Oral Cir Bucal 2019;24:e433–e437. 10.4317/medoral.22943

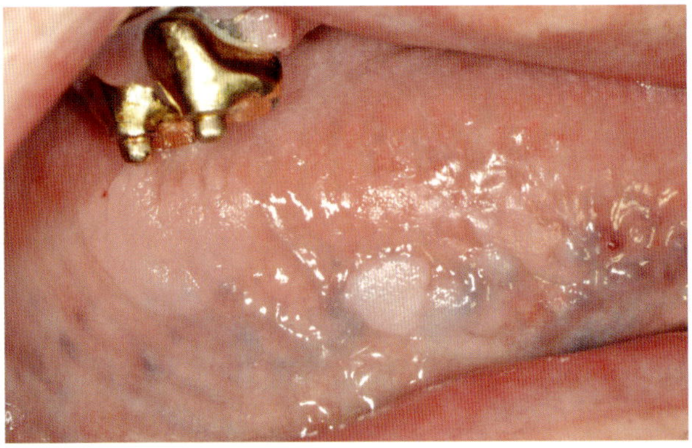

Fig 13-61 Initial clinical situation: White, flat findings with a slightly verrucous surface.

Fig 13-62 After local anesthesia (infiltration anesthesia is advisable on the well-perfused tongue), the entire finding is circumnavigated with a scalpel/CO_2 laser. Since a blood vessel was clearly visible mesially of the finding, a CO_2 laser was used to make it easier to stop any bleeding. If excision with a scalpel is planned, a vascular clamp should be provided to quickly stop any bleeding. In the event of severe bleeding, the wound is closed primarily by suturing.

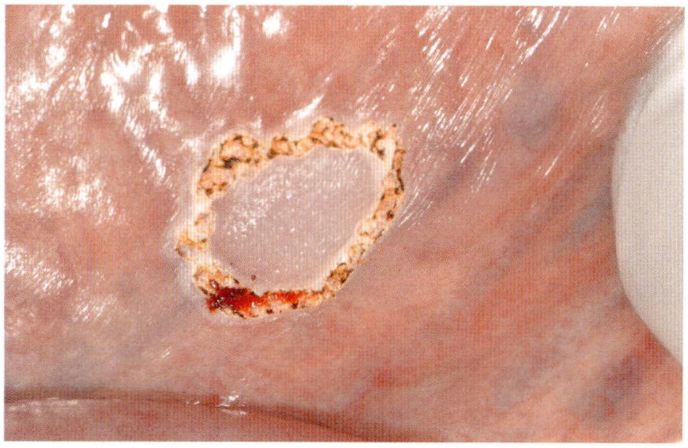

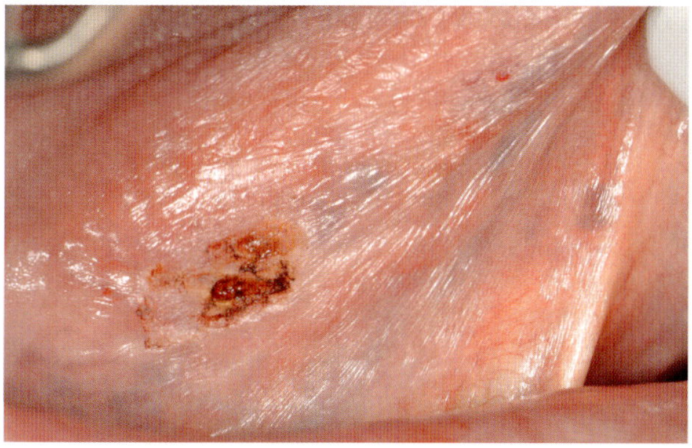

Fig 13-63 The wound is separated from the underlying musculature.

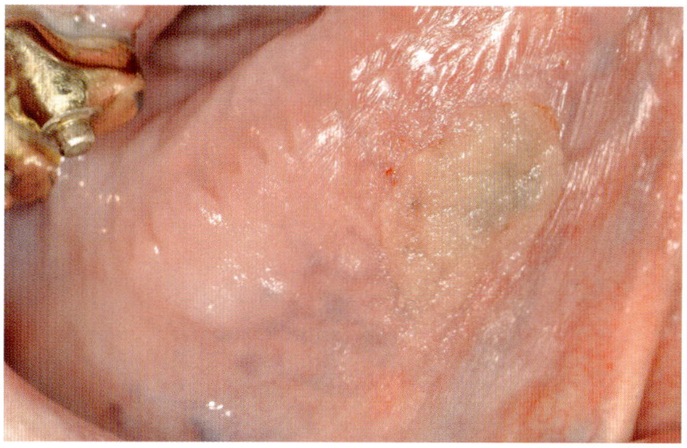

Fig 13-64 The wound area can be closed primarily or left to heal secondarily. In open wound healing, the wound is covered with dental adhesive paste. This procedure must be repeated regularly at home for pain relief and protection of the wound area.

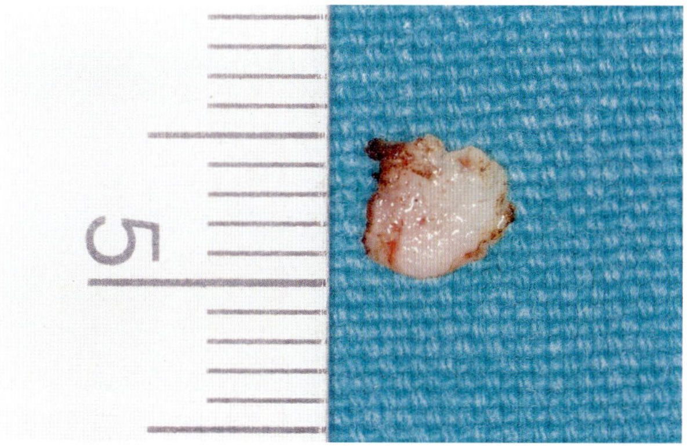

Fig 13-65 The excisate is sent for histopathologic examination for further clarification.

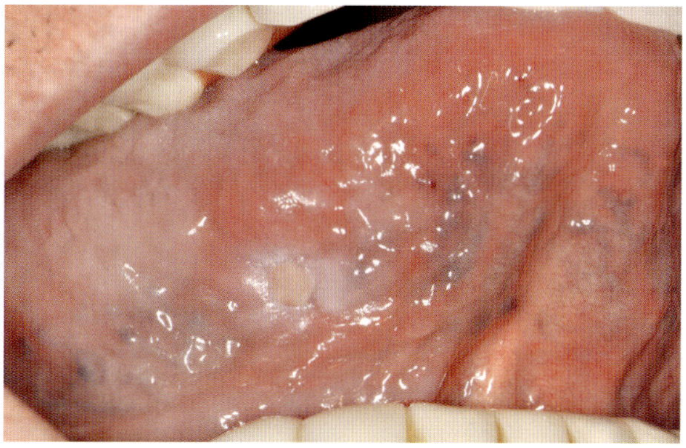

Fig 13-66 Clinical situation 1 week after excision: Wound healing was somewhat delayed in this case, possibly because the (open) wound area was regularly disturbed by the dentition due to the localization during eating, drinking, and swallowing. The histopathologic report showed no evidence of a viral genesis, so in situ hybridization to clarify an oncogenic HPV was not necessary.

Salivary gland cyst/mucocele

Clinic and etiology

- Recurrent swelling, vesicular, soft and fluctuant, usually containing clear fluid, with a bluish color shining through,
- Often traumatic in origin or caused by a small salivary stone.

Indications

- Removal indicated for increasing size, discomfort, limitation in eating or speaking; for diagnosis; for clarification of malignancy.

Contraindications

- None.

Specific risks

- Risk of recurrence is high, especially if one of the minor salivary glands is injured during excision of the lesion.

Local anesthesia

- Conduction anesthesia is more useful because infiltration anesthesia leads to an increase in volume and thus the outline of the finding cannot be optimally assessed.

Step-by-step clinical procedure

- See Figures 13-67 to 13-82.

Wound care and wound closure

- In the case of CO_2 laser, open wound healing; if necessary, wound covering with dental adhesive paste and covering of orthodontic appliances with wax,
- In the case of scalp excision, primary wound closure with (resorbable) sutures is not always necessary and advisable due to possible injury to minor salivary glands and thus increased risk of recurrence (depending on the localization).

Postoperative controls and course

- Depending on the suture material selected (resorbable/non-resorbable) or whether a CO_2 laser was used: 1 to 2 weeks,
- Check possible irritation factors, otherwise recurrence is possible.

Recommended literature

1. Bahadure RN, Fulzele P, Thosar N, Badole G, Baliga S. Conventional surgical treatment of oral mucocele: a series of 23 cases. Eur J Paediatr 2012;13:143–146.
2. Filippi A, Hitz Lindenmüller I (Hrsg). Die Zunge. Berlin: Quintessenz, 2016.
3. Hitz Lindenmüller I. Gewebeschonende Technik zur Entfernung von Speicheldrüsenzysten an der Lippe. Quintessenz 2010;61:1185–1190.
4. Valério RA, de Queiroz AM, Romualdo PC, Brentegani LG, de Paula-Silva FW. Mucocele and fibroma: treatment and clinical features for differential diagnosis. Braz Dent J 2013;24: 537–541.

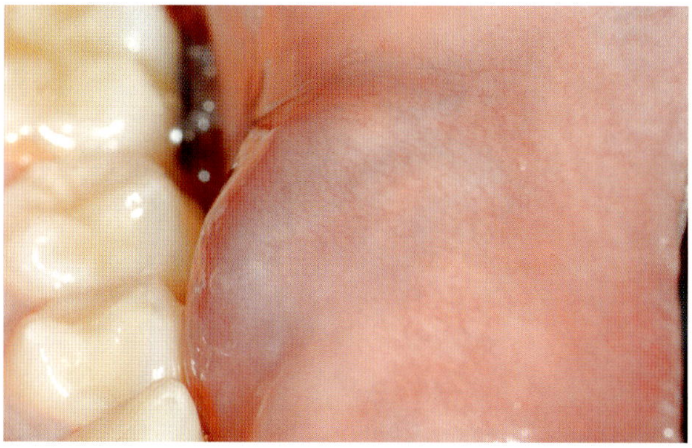

Fig 13-67 Initial clinical situation with prominent, bluish translucent and depressible findings on the lower lip/inner cheek on the left. The orthodontic brackets are clearly visible and may have caused trauma to the mucosa, resulting in a salivary gland cyst.

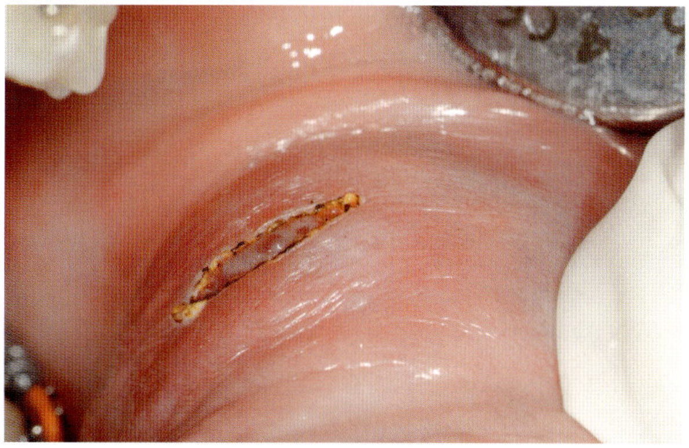

Fig 13-68 Careful opening of the swelling at the *punctum maximum* in a vertical direction (so as not to disturb wound healing by the dentition/brackets) under local anesthesia (conduction anesthesia). The epithelium is only lightly scratched with a scalpel or opened with a CO_2 laser.

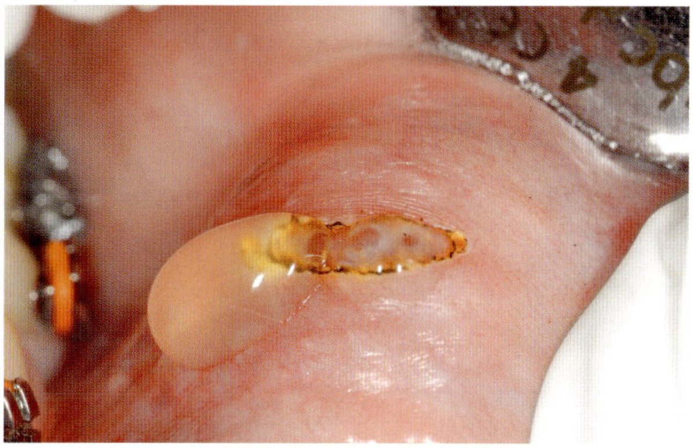

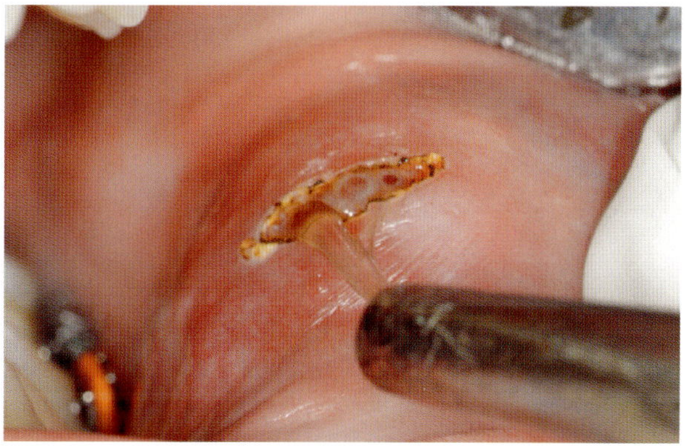

Figs 13-69 and 13-70 The emerging mucous saliva confirms the suspected diagnosis of a salivary gland (extravasation) cyst. Even though extremely careful preparation was performed here, the cyst lumen was nevertheless opened because, strictly speaking, it is not a true cyst but a pseudocyst.

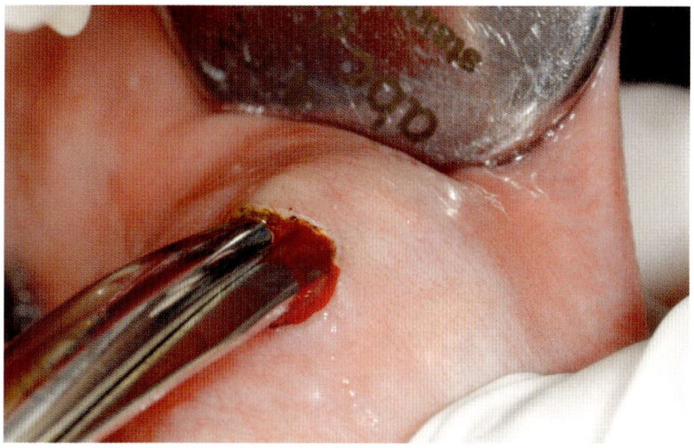

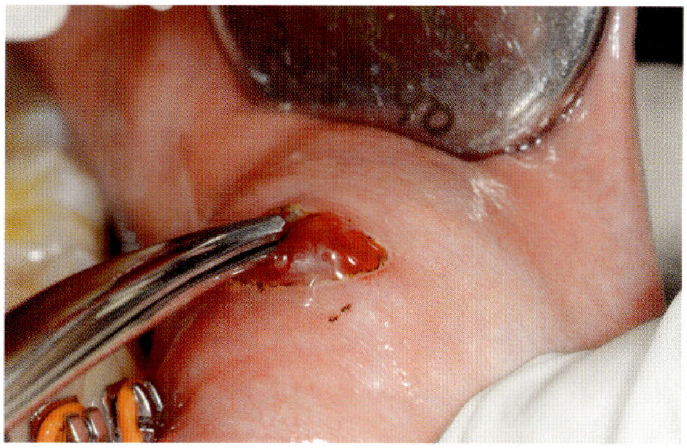

Figs 13-71 and 13-72 Dissecting the involved minor salivary glands circularly from the epithelium and underlying musculature with blunt dissecting scissors.

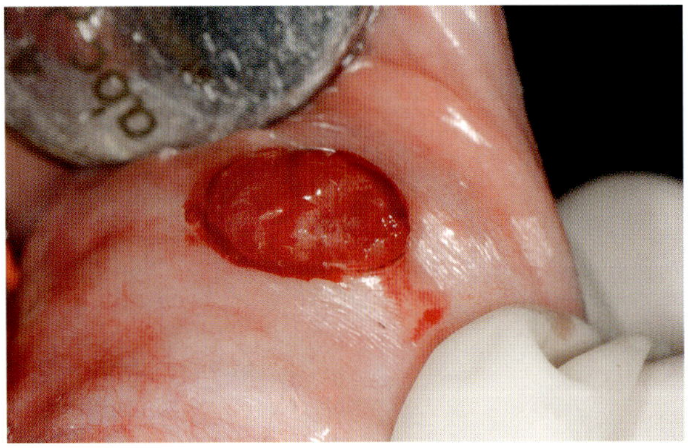

Fig 13-73 Finger pressure from the outside of the lip/cheek presents an adjacent minor salivary gland conglomerate.

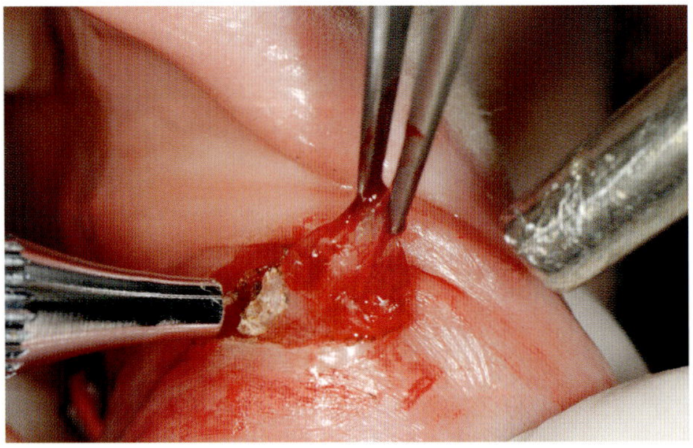

Fig 13-74 The salivary gland conglomerate is carefully pulled out with forceps.

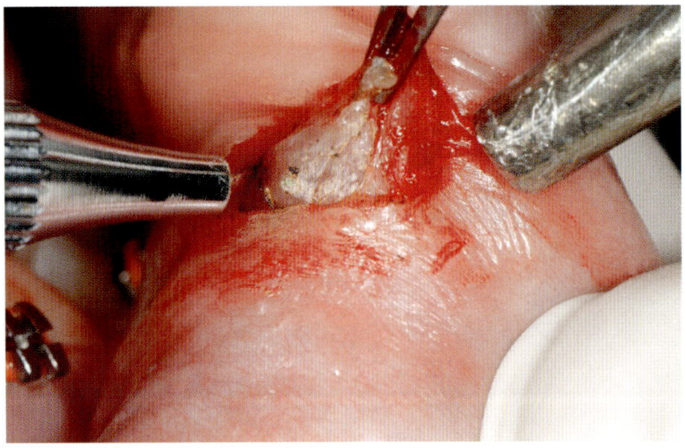

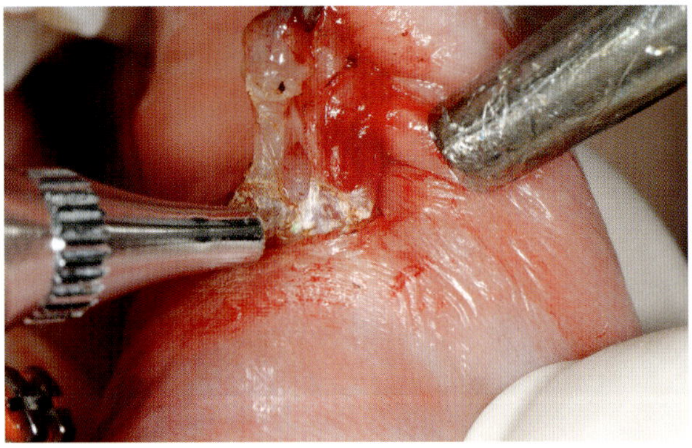

Figs 13-75 and 13-76 Subsequently, separation below the circumference of the salivary gland conglomerate is performed from all directions.

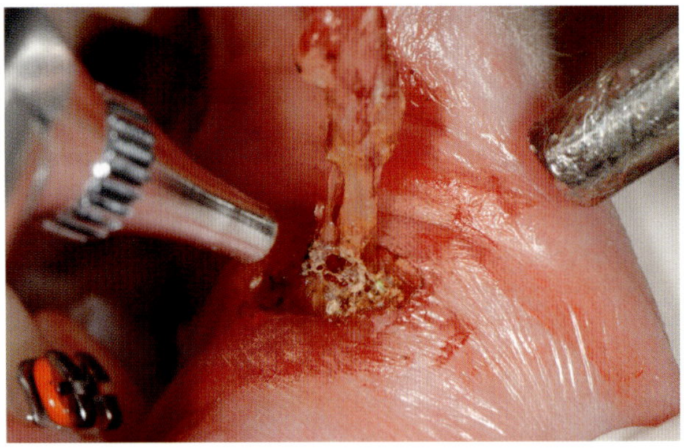

Fig 13-77 Finally, the salivary gland conglomerate is separated from the underlying musculature at the base with a scalpel/CO_2 laser.

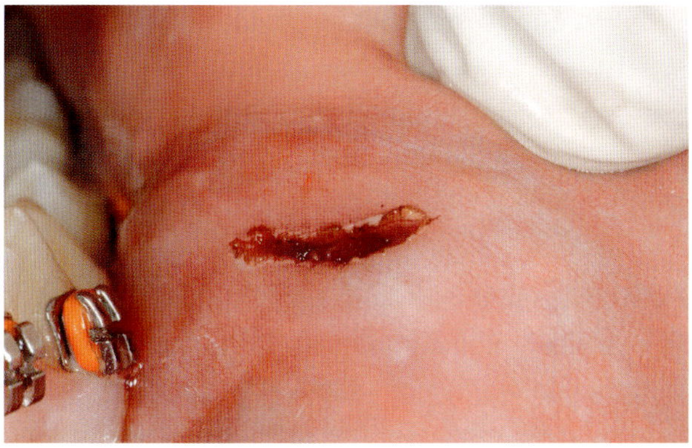

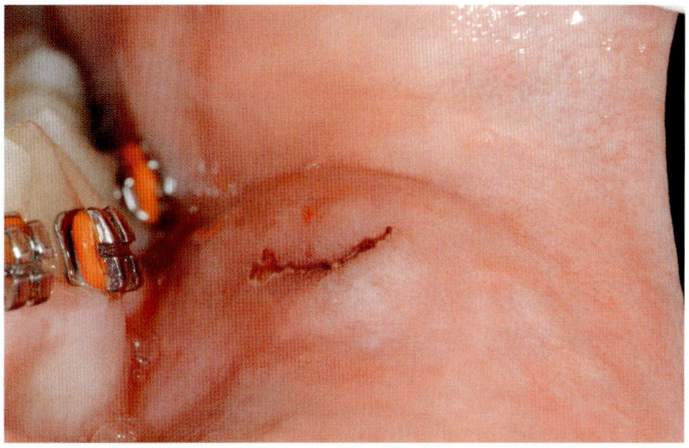

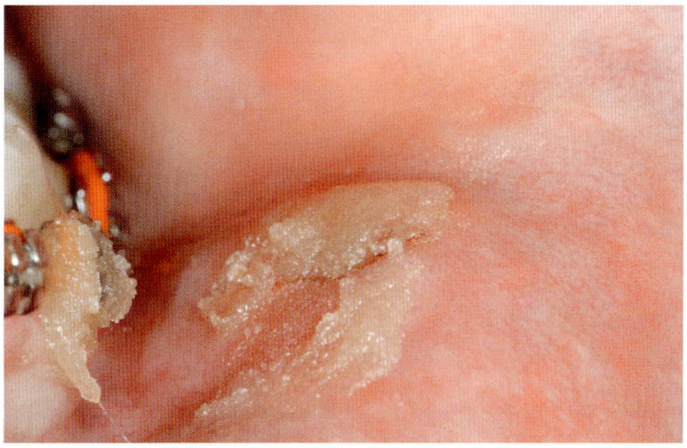

Figs 13-78 to 13-80 The wound edges do not yet close immediately after excision due to the surgical procedure with traction. Only after a few minutes is the tissue relaxed and, in the best case, the wound edges lie against each other. If this is the case, suturing can be omitted and the minimal wound area can be covered with dental adhesive paste, if necessary.

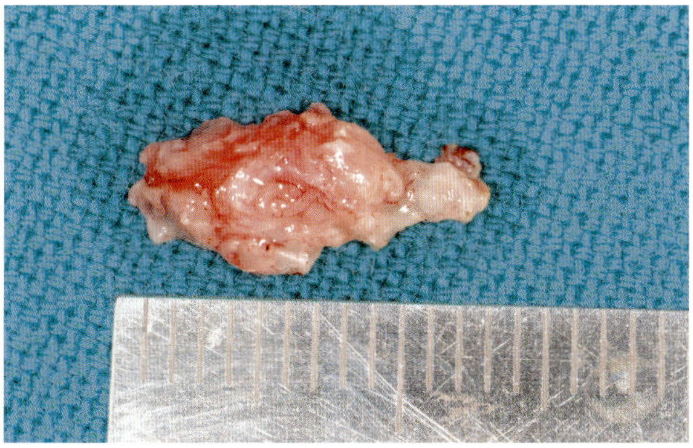

Fig 13-81 The salivary gland conglomerate is subsequently examined histopathologically.

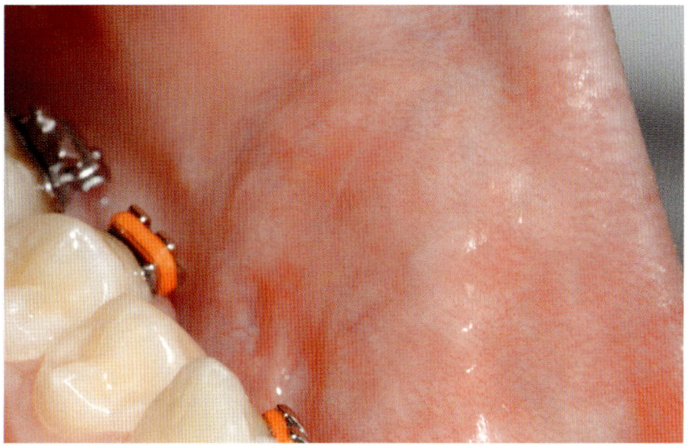

Fig 13-82 Clinical situation 1 month postoperatively: Thanks to the minimally invasive incision chosen perpendicular to the dentition as well as the postoperative covering of the orthodontic brackets with wax, wound healing was hardly affected.

Incisional biopsies

Blistering diseases

Clinic and etiology

- Clear or blood-filled blisters and ulcerations (burst blister) on reddened mucosa,
- Caused by genetic autoimmune disease or medication (antibiotics, antihypertensives, nonsteroidal anti-inflammatory drugs, etc).

Indications

- For diagnosis of blistering diseases/findings; for clarification of malignancy.

Contraindications

- None.

Specific risks

- Since there is a cross-linking disorder of the epithelium, a biopsy/mechanical trauma can lead to a large-scale detachment of the epithelium and thus to severe bleeding.

Local anesthesia

- Conduction anesthesia or infiltration anesthesia.

Step-by-step clinical procedure

- See Figures 13-83 to 13-102.

Wound care and wound closure

- Wound closure often difficult due to cross-linking disorder of the epithelium,
- Wound covering with dental adhesive paste.

Postoperative controls and course

- Usually 1 to 2 weeks after biopsy to discuss pathology report and further procedures (usually drug therapy with corticosteroids or other immunosuppressants),
- Close clinical controls usually every 3 to 6 months, depending on the severity of the disease.

Recommended literature

1. Filippi A, Hitz Lindenmüller I (Hrsg). Die Zunge. Berlin: Quintessenz, 2016.
2. Kamaguchi M, Iwata H. The diagnosis and blistering mechanisms of mucous membrane pemphigoid. Front Immunol 2019;10:34.
3. Levitt J, Bernardo S, Whang T. Videos in clinical medicine. How to perform a punch biopsy of the skin. N Engl J Med 2013;369:e13.
4. Schmidt E, Zillikens D. Pemphigoid diseases. Lancet 2013;381:320–332.

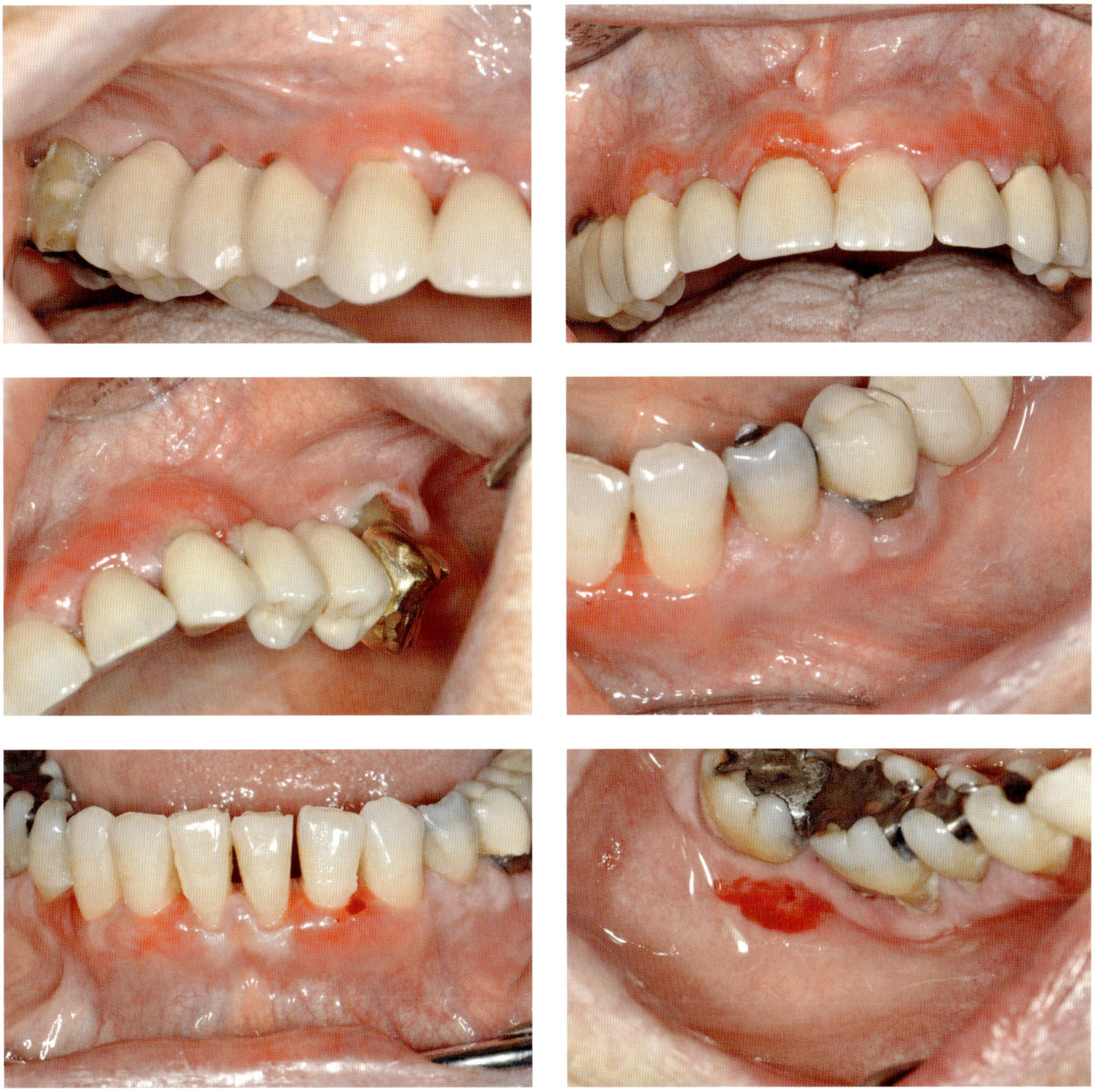

Figs 13-83 to 13-88 Areas of erosion, desquamation, and ulceration can be seen on the attached gingiva, primarily along the *margo gingivae* vestibularly, in all four quadrants. Vestibularly at region 13, an ulceration (probably an already torn blister) is well recognizable. A blood-filled blister is visible at region 46/47.

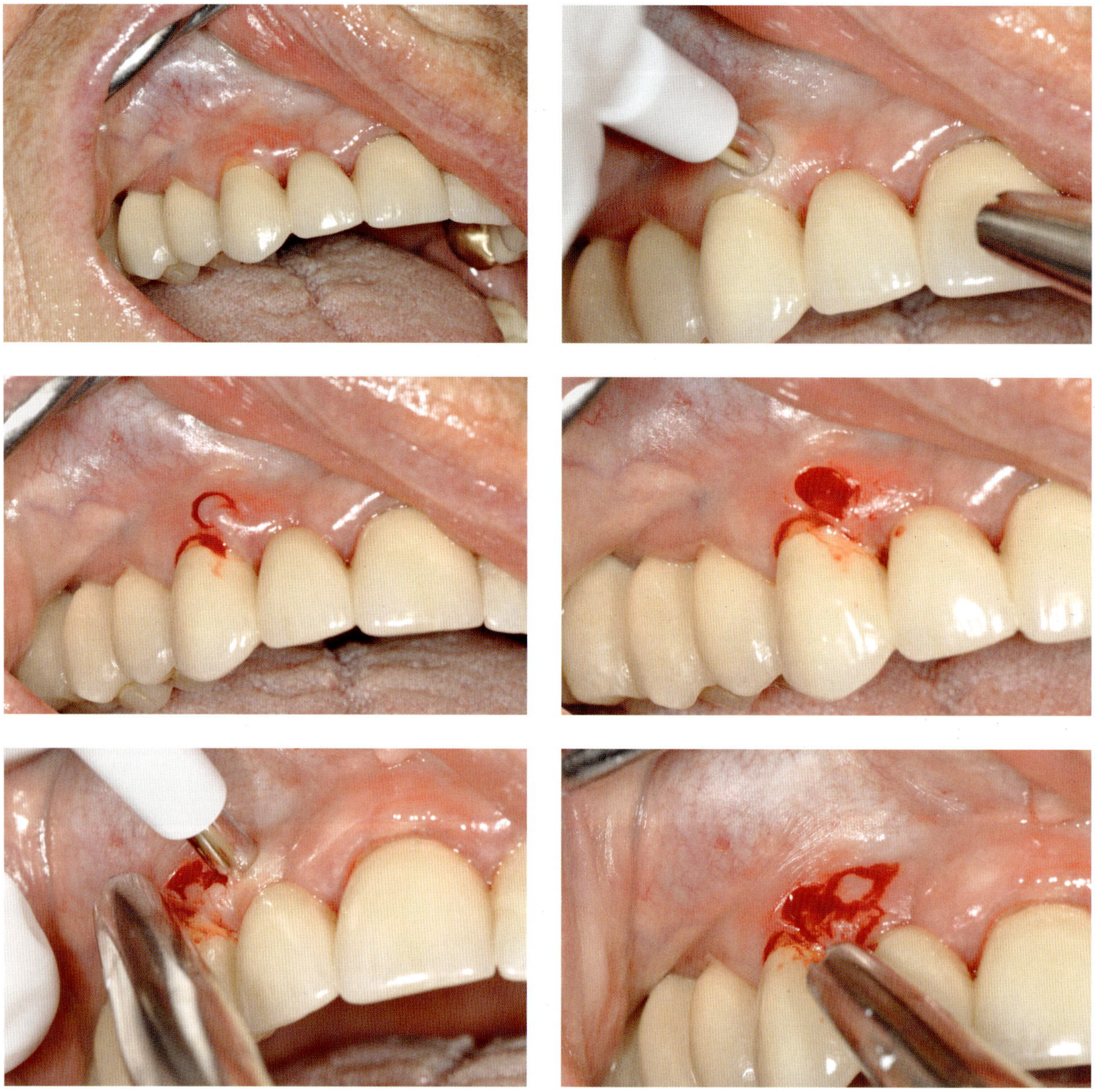

Figs 13-89 to 13-94 Based on the clinical situation alone, a blistering disease can be assumed; however, two biopsies are needed to differentiate between a *pemphigus vulgaris* and a bullous mucous membrane pemphigoid. After local anesthesia (for local hemostasis, it is better to use infiltration anesthesia) in region 12/13, a punch biopsy (biopsy punch boot, 4-mm diameter) is therefore taken approximately 1 mm away from the gingival margin of tooth 13 (in order not to provoke recession). The biopsy must be taken in the marginal area here, since the center of the blister has no valuable histopathologic information due to the necrosis. The biopsy specimen is placed in formalin solution. A second punch biopsy is taken in the perilesional tissue (further away from the blister margin). This is used to determine the site of blister formation (intraepithelial or subepithelial) by direct immunofluorescence (DIF). For this reason, the biopsy specimen is placed in Michels solution. The blister should now be aspirated extremely carefully because the epithelium is particularly fragile due to the cross-linking disorder.

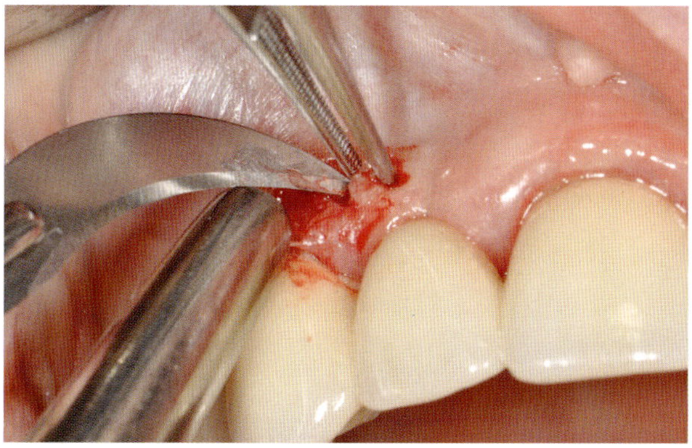
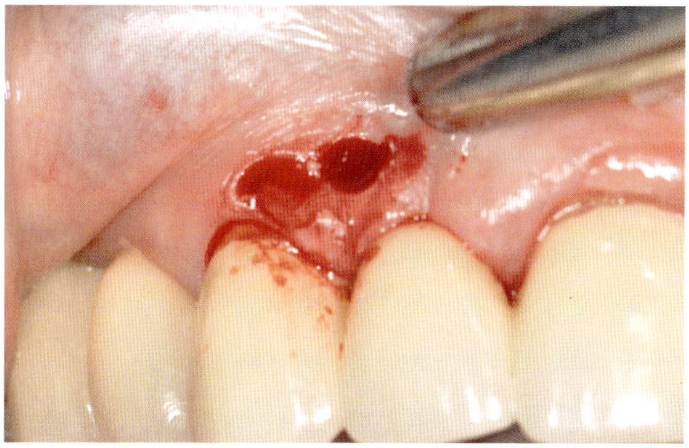

Figs 13-95 and 13-96 The two tissue samples, each of which have been circularly transected by punching, are both carefully dissected from the lower surface with a scalpel. This procedure requires the highest precision.

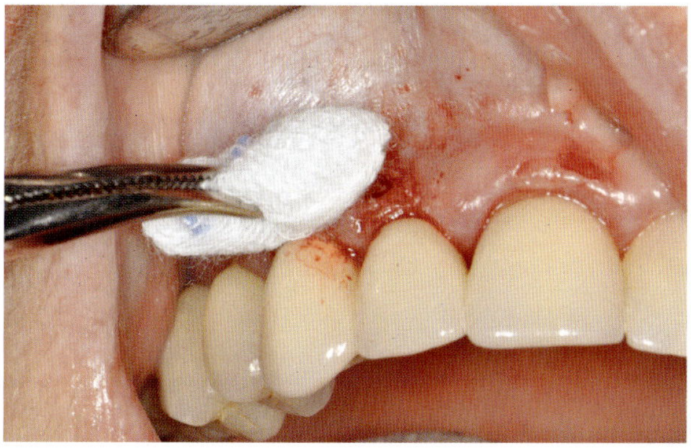
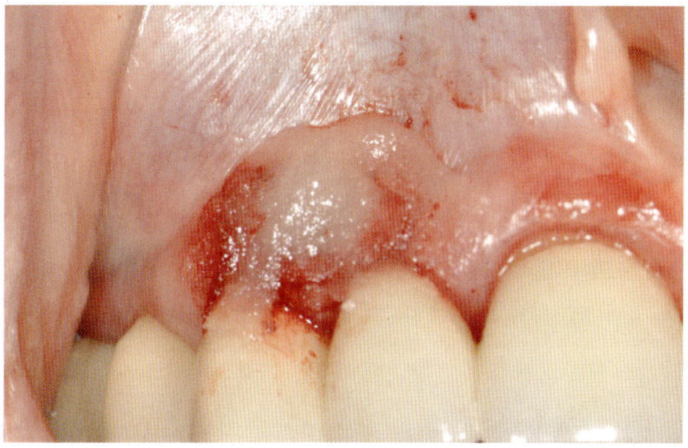

Figs 13-97 and 13-98 Typically, the tissue bleeds profusely during this procedure. The bleeding can be contained somewhat by compression with a swab. Suture restoration is virtually impossible because the epithelium is not properly anchored on the lower surface, so wound coverage with dental adhesive paste is an option.

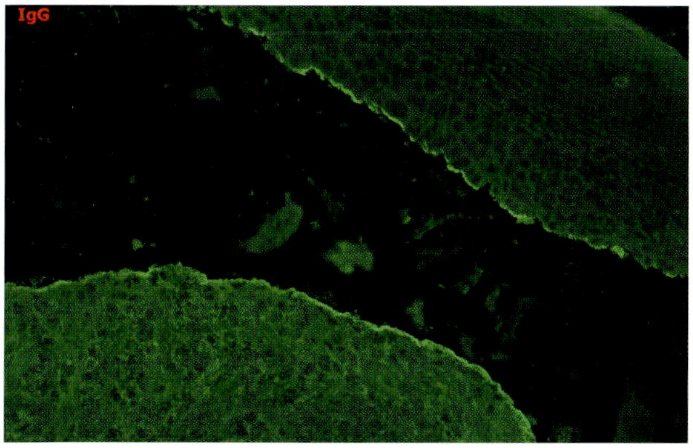

Fig 13-99 The two tissue samples are now examined histopathologically. The first biopsy specimen is used for conventional histopathologic examination, and the second for immunohistologic examination (DIF; green). The image shows subepithelial detachment of the epithelium, which is indicative of a bullous pemphigoid.

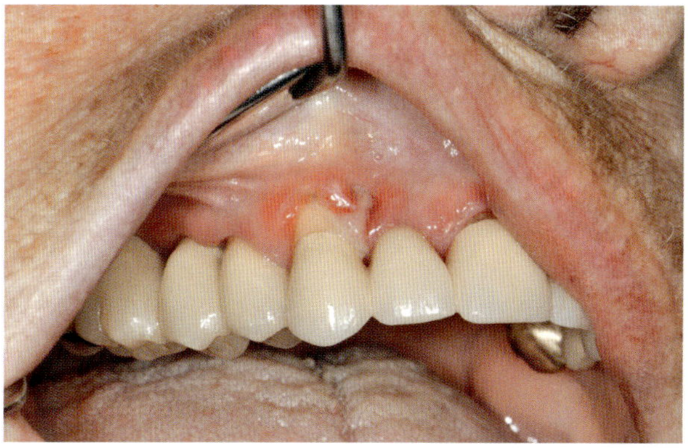

Fig 13-100 Clinical situation 10 days after biopsy: The two biopsy sites are still covered with fibrin in places.

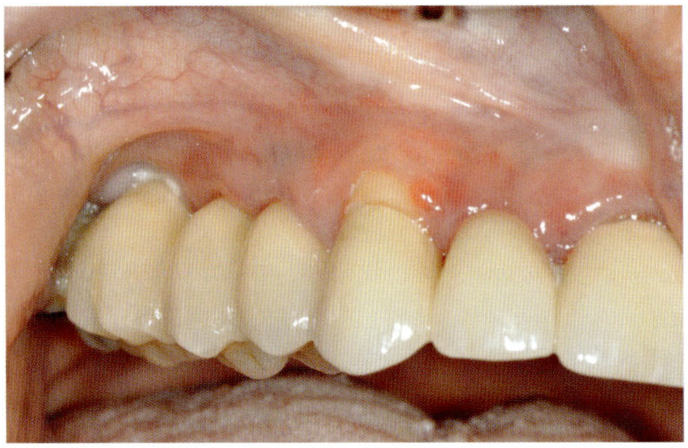

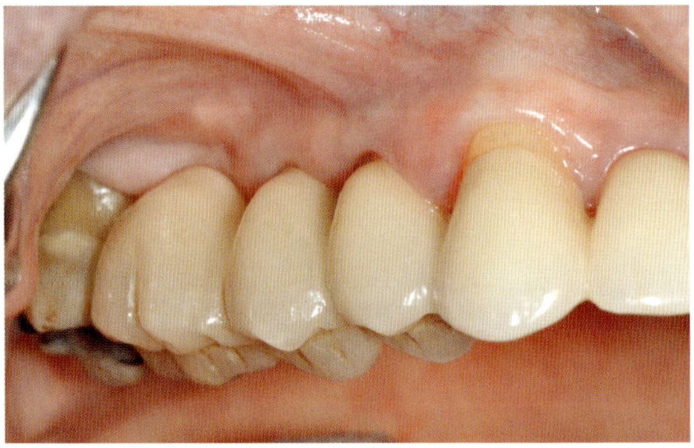

Figs 13-101 and 13-102 Clinical control 3 weeks and 1 year postoperatively shows irritation-free mucosal conditions.

Leukoplakia

Clinic and etiology

- Sharply demarcated white spot, not wipeable, homogeneously smooth, white-red speckled or verrucous,
- Induced by mechanical irritant, tobacco, alcohol, HPV.

Indications

- Removal indicated in case of increasing size, verrucous or inhomogeneous appearance,
- In case of risk factors such as smoking, alcohol, other drug use; for diagnosis; for clarification of malignancy.

Contraindications

- None, but consider anatomy.

Specific risks

- None.

Local anesthesia

- Conduction anesthesia or infiltration anesthesia.

Step-by-step clinical procedure

- See Figures 13-103 to 13-112.

Wound care and wound closure

- In the case of CO_2 laser, open wound healing; if necessary, wound covering with dental adhesive paste,
- In the case of scalp excision, primary wound closure by means of resorbable sutures is not always possible (depending on localization).

Postoperative controls and course

- Depending on the suture material selected (resorbable/non-resorbable) or whether a CO_2 laser was used: 1 to 2 weeks,
- Exclude possible irritation factors and other noxae, otherwise there is a risk of recurrence,
- Progress checks depending on noxae, usually every 3 to 6 months.

Recommended literature

1. Filippi A, Hitz Lindenmüller I (Hrsg). Die Zunge. Berlin: Quintessenz, 2016.
2. Kumar A, Cascarini L, McCaul JA, et al. How should we manage oral leukoplakie? Br J Oral Maxillofac Surg 2013;51:377–383.
3. Tambuwala A, Sangle A, Khan A, Sayed A. Excision of oral leukoplakia by CO_2 lasers versus traditional scalpel: a comparative study. J Maxillofac Oral Surg 2014;13:320–327.

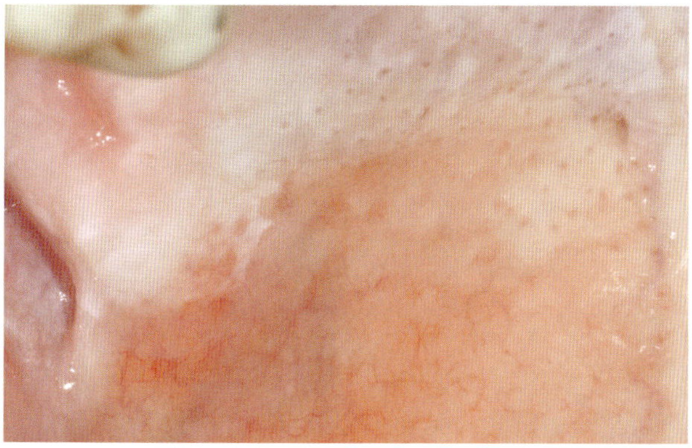

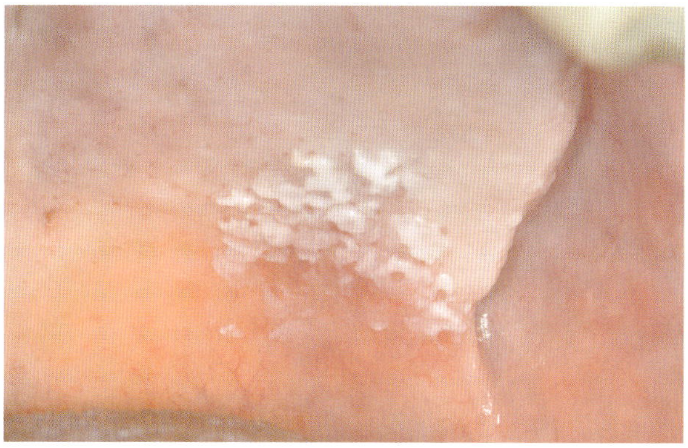

Figs 13-103 and 13-104 Initial clinical situation: Leukoplakic change palatally at the transition to the soft palate. A biopsy was performed on the left side because the findings were more conspicuous on that side.

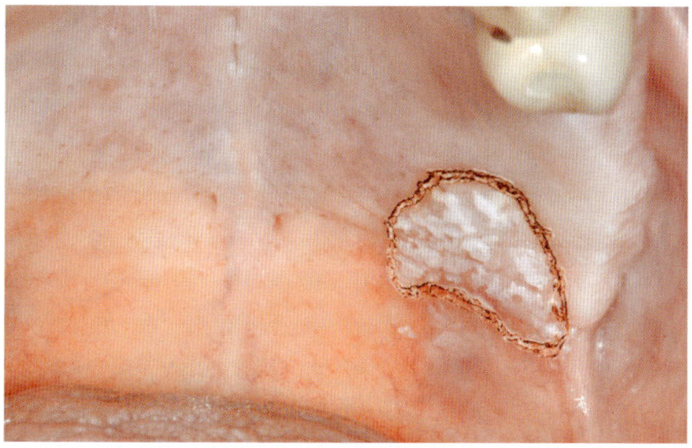

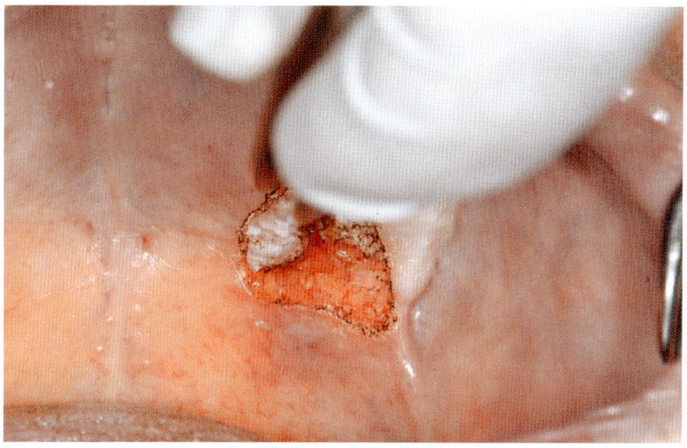

Figs 13-105 and 13-106 After local anesthesia (in this case, infiltration anesthesia for local hemostasis), the entire finding is circularly incised with a scalpel/CO_2 laser and detached from the base. Any bleeding can be stopped with a CO_2 laser or with an electrotome, otherwise compression with a swab helps.

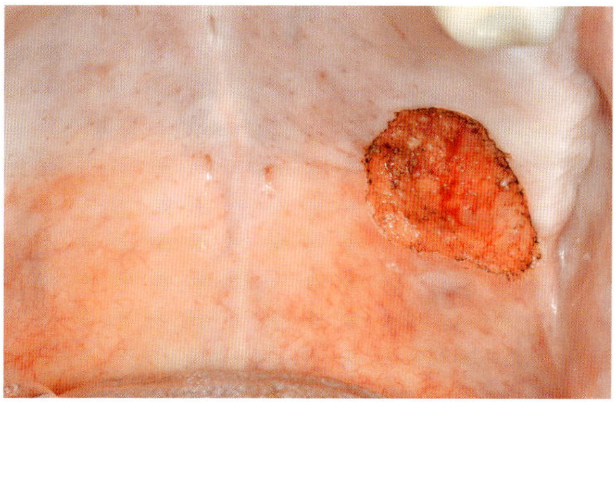

Fig 13-107 The wound area cannot be closed primarily and is therefore covered with dental adhesive paste. This procedure must be repeated regularly at home for pain relief and protection of the wound area.

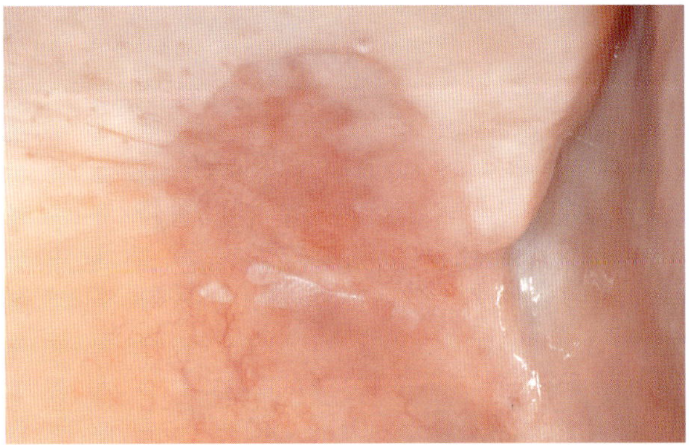

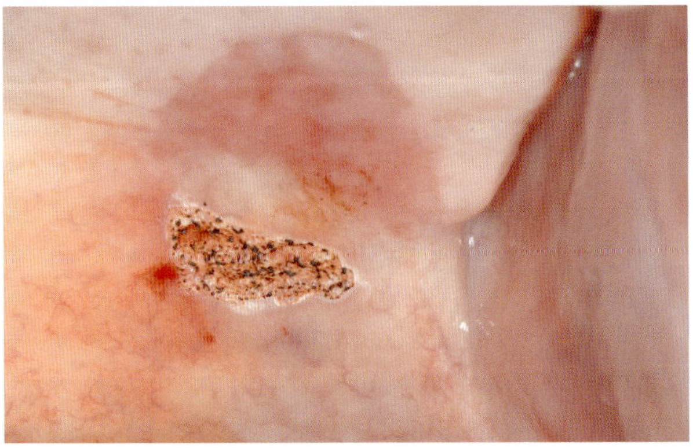

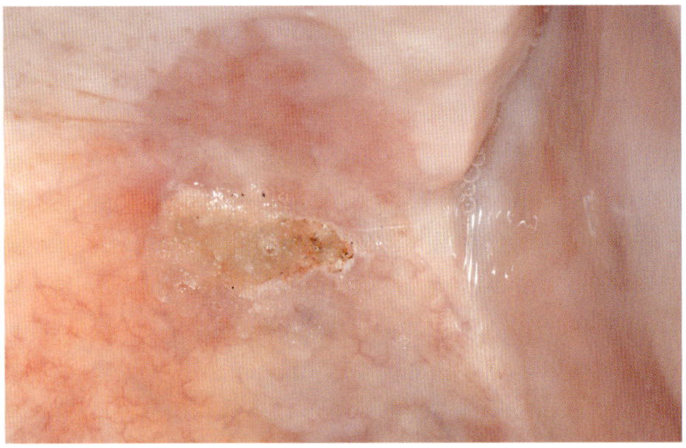

Figs 13-108 to 13-110 Clinical situation 3 weeks after excision: wound healing is complete. At this time, it is also possible to assess whether recurrence may have occurred. Histopathologic examination revealed focal epithelial dysplasia. Distally, a small residual area of leukoplakia is visible. The finding is immediately removed, and the wound area is covered with dental adhesive paste.

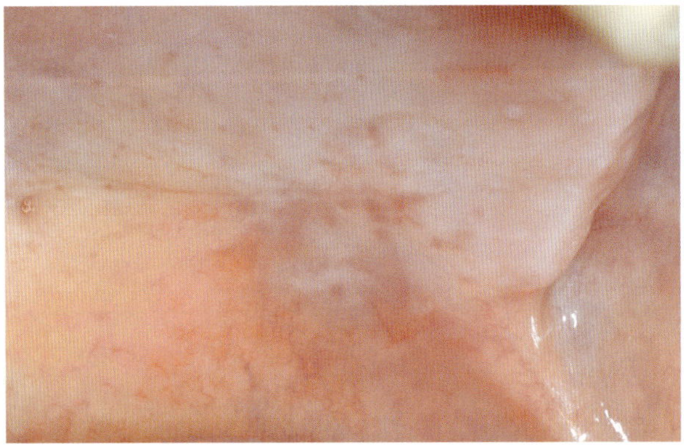

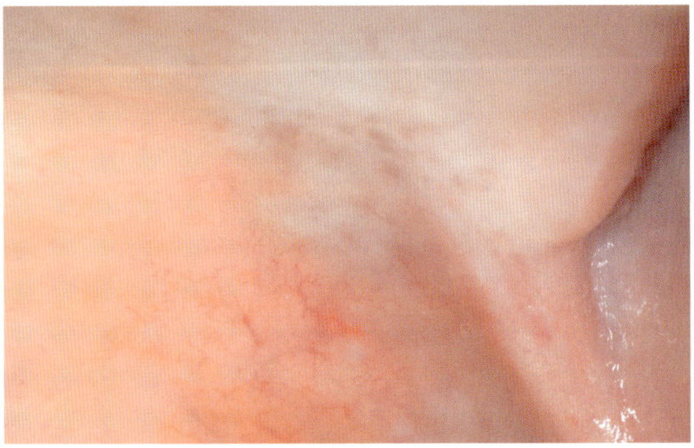

Figs 13-111 and 13-112 Clinical situation at 6 months, then 1 year after the 6-month check-up. The patient has stopped smoking, so recurrence is no longer expected.

Lichenoid reactions

Clinic and etiology

- Oral mucosal reaction triggered by dental materials, causing contact hypersensitivity,
- May also be caused by medications such as specific antihypertensives or oral antidiabetics,
- Additional symptoms are possible such as dry mouth, burning of the mucosa, impaired taste,
- Removal of the cause may result in symptom relief or regression of the findings.

Indications

- Incision indicated for no improvement of symptoms or regression of findings despite elimination of irritation.

Contraindications

- None.

Specific risks

- Consider anatomy and general anamnesis.

Local anesthesia

- Conduction anesthesia or infiltration anesthesia.

Step-by-step clinical procedure

- See Figures 13-113 to 13-118.

Wound care and wound closure

- In the case of CO_2 laser, open wound healing; if necessary, wound covering with dental adhesive paste,
- In the case of scalpel excision, primary wound closure.

Postoperative controls and course

- Depending on the patient's general medical condition: 1 to 2 weeks,
- Recall depending on degree of dysplasia, noxious agents, and success of therapy.

Recommended literature

1. Filippi A, Hitz Lindenmüller I (Hrsg). Die Zunge. Berlin: Quintessenz, 2016.
2. Höller S, Hitz Lindenmüller I. Oraler Lichen Planus. MKG-Chirurg 2018;11:4–11.
3. Marell L, Tillberg A, Widman L, Bergdahl J, Berglund A. Regression of oral lichenoid lesions after replacement of dental restorations. J Oral Rehabil 2014;41:381–391.

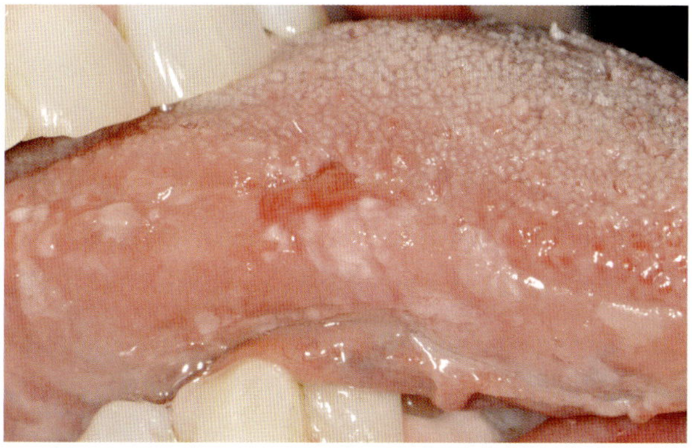

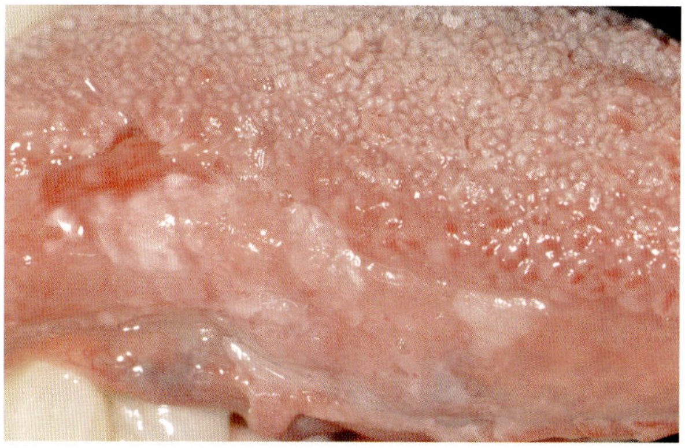

Figs 13-113 and 13-114 Initial clinical situation with pronounced white changes and reddened ulcer on the right tongue margin. Despite pretreatment with a deep-drawn splint, the lichenoid findings had not regressed and should therefore be clarified with further diagnostics.

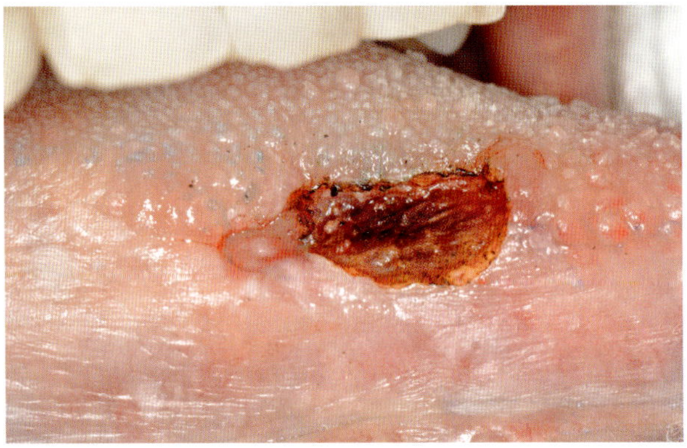

Fig 13-115 After local anesthesia (in this case, infiltration anesthesia for local hemostasis), part of the lesion is circularly incised at a representative site with a scalpel/CO_2 laser and detached from the base. Any bleeding can be stopped with a CO_2 laser or with an electrotome, otherwise compression with a swab helps.

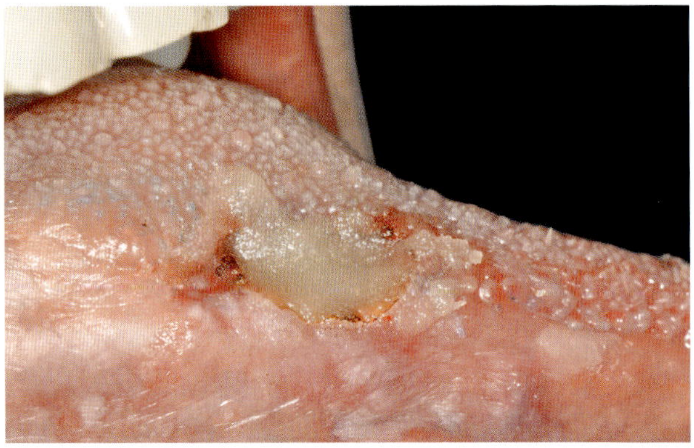

Fig 13-116 The wound area cannot be primarily closed after the biopsy with a CO_2 laser, so covering with dental adhesive paste is performed. This procedure must be repeated regularly at home for pain relief and protection of the wound area.

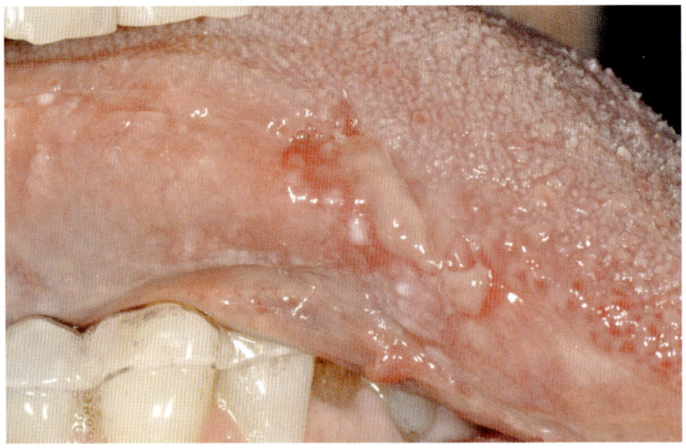

Fig 13-117 Delayed wound healing at the incision site can be seen 3 weeks after biopsy removal. This delay in wound healing may be an indication of possible malignancy. In the case report described, the histopathologic findings revealed a microinvasive carcinoma. In such cases, the patient should be referred to a specialized clinic for further diagnosis and treatment.

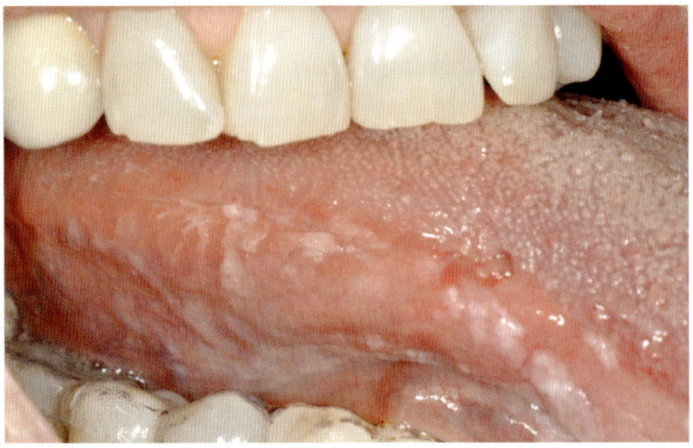

Fig 13-118 The clinical situation 2 months after biopsy removal still shows insufficient wound healing and a clear persistent clinical change at the entire tongue margin.

Oral lichen planus

Clinic and etiology

- Mucocutaneous, noninfectious inflammation with autoimmune component; complete etiology is still unclear,
- Different forms (reticular, papular, plaque-like, erosive-atrophic, bullous, ulcerative) that may occur simultaneously; often a symmetrical affection of the oral mucosa,
- "Wickham's streak" represents a pathognomonic symptom; since the clinical picture is almost identical to oral lichenoid reaction, both clinically and histopathologically, an accurate history and clinical findings are essential for making the diagnosis.

Indications

- Incision indicated when irritant elimination (mechanical and chemical) or drug therapy does not result in symptom relief.

Contraindications

- None, but consider anatomy.

Specific risks

- None.

Local anesthesia

- Conduction anesthesia or infiltration anesthesia.

Step-by-step clinical procedure

- See Figures 13-119 to 13-124.

Wound care and wound closure

- In the case of CO_2 laser, open wound healing; if necessary, wound covering with dental adhesive paste,
- In the case of scalpel excision, primary wound closure.

Postoperative controls and course

- Depending on the patient's general medical condition: 1 to 2 weeks,
- Recall depending on degree of dysplasia, noxious agents, and symptoms.

Recommended literature

1. Filippi A, Hitz Lindenmüller I (Hrsg). Die Zunge. Berlin: Quintessenz, 2016.
2. Gupta S, Jawanda MK. Oral lichen planus: an update on etiology, pathogenesis, clinical presentation, diagnosis and management. Indian J Dermatol 2015;60:222–229.
3. Höller S, Hitz Lindenmüller I. Oraler Lichen Planus. MKG-Chirurg 2018;11:4–11.

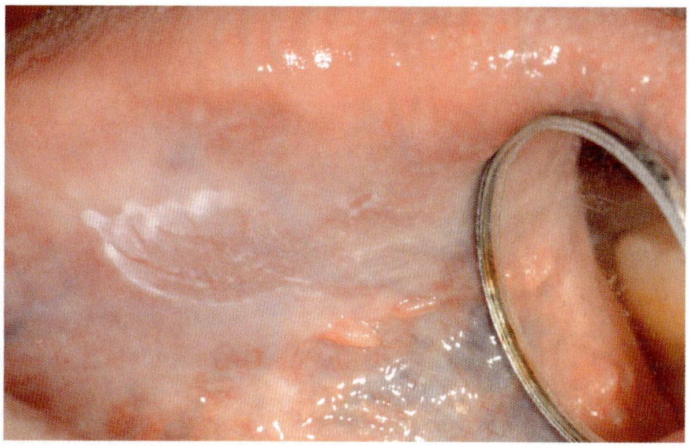

Fig 13-119 Initial clinical situation: Whitish-reticular change on the right tongue margin with extension toward the floor of the mouth.

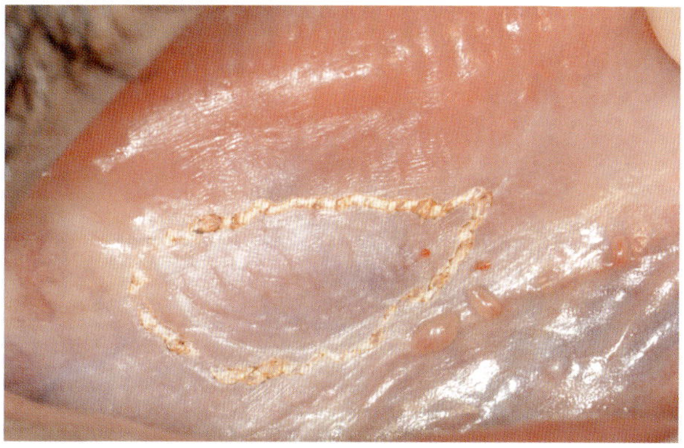

Fig 13-120 After local anesthesia (in this case, infiltration anesthesia for local hemostasis) has been administered, the entire finding is circumcised with a scalpel/CO_2 laser.

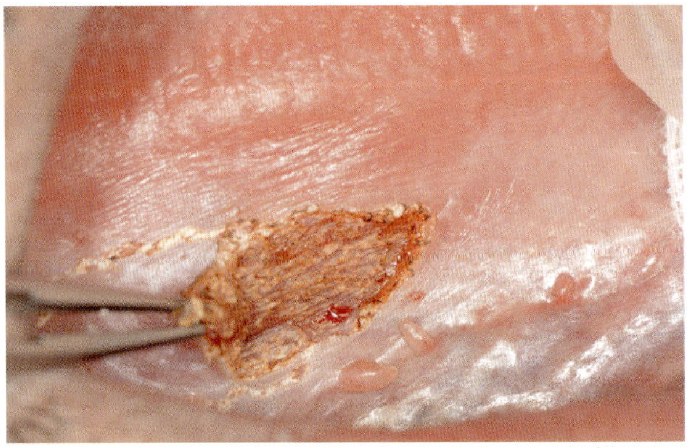

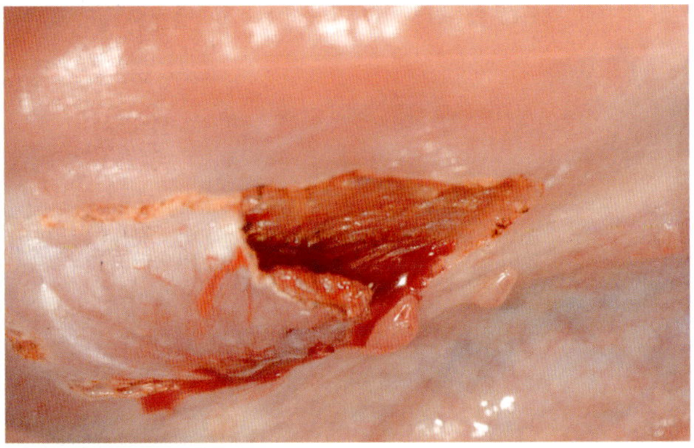

Figs 13-121 and 13-122 Detachment of the altered oral mucosa from the muscular support.

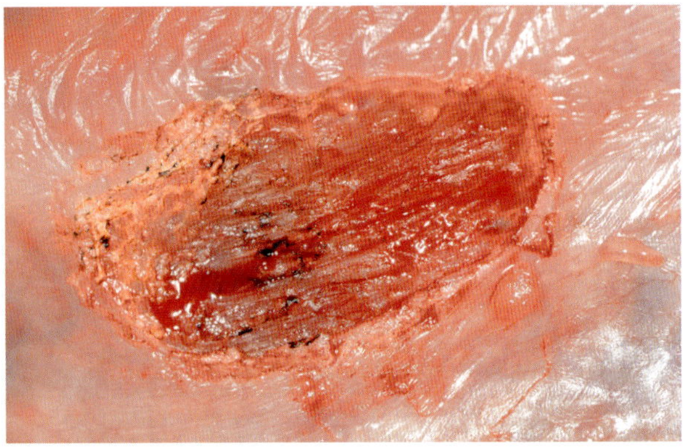

Fig 13-123 The wound area cannot be primarily closed due to the CO_2 laser excision and is therefore covered with dental adhesive paste. This procedure must be continued regularly at home for local analgesia and protection of the wound area.

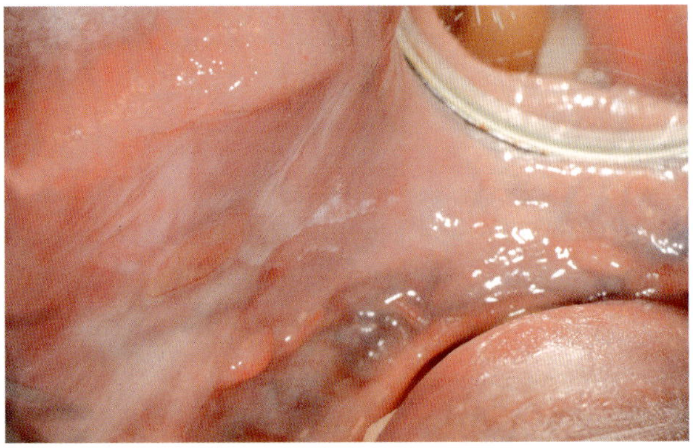

Fig 13-124 Clinical situation 2 weeks after incisional biopsy: Wound healing is complete.

Pre- and posttreatment with medication

14

Petra Rugani, Stephan Acham, Norbert Jakse

The risk and extent of postoperative complaints and infection-related complications are influenced by factors on two levels: firstly, by the specific procedure, localization, clinical findings, invasiveness, extent, and duration of the procedure; secondly, by the individual patient's general condition, previous illnesses, medication history, and immune status.

Prevention and therapy or alleviation of postoperative complaints are an obligatory and intrinsic part of medical assistance. In addition, patients judge the quality of a surgical procedure primarily on the basis of the resulting pain and complications that occur.

Accordingly, clear recommendations for pain prevention that consider procedure-specific and patient-individual factors are of great importance in surgical therapy planning.

Perioperative pain prophylaxis

Perioperative pain medication aims to reduce the patient's distress to such an extent that normal daily activities are not (or only slightly) impaired. Accordingly, values of ≤ 3 on the 10-item numerical rating scale (NRS) for pain should be aimed for.

Most oral surgical procedures are performed on an outpatient basis. Therefore, pain therapy should be as standardized as possible, have few side effects, and be easy to administer, i.e. usually peroral. Especially on the first two postoperative days, pain that is > 3 on the NRS can be expected without analgesia. Accordingly, analgesia should be initiated perioperatively and then be routinely continued for 2 postoperative days as basic pain prophylaxis.

If more severe pain is expected, additional on-demand medication should be offered as sufficient prevention. The patient must be precisely informed about the maximum dose and duration of the therapy.

In most cases, pain occurs as a symptom of a postoperative inflammatory reaction. Therefore, nonsteroidal anti-inflammatory drugs (NSAIDs) are considered the drug of choice for basic pain prophylaxis (e.g. diclofenac or dexibuprofen).

Only in the presence of a proven contraindication to classic COX-1- and COX-2-acting NSAIDs (e.g. kidney disease, ongoing cortisone therapy, 3rd trimester pregnancy) must a substitute medication be used. The first-choice substitute medication is paracetamol, which, however, lacks the postoperative desired antiphlogistic effect.

If severe swelling and pain are to be expected, the adjuvant use of a glucocorticoid with a medium to longer half-life has proven effective in addition to the basic medication. In outpatient oral surgery, for example, 40 mg of methylprednisolone, administered orally as a single dose immediately preoperatively, can significantly reduce swelling and pain.

Metamizole, which has been used since the 1920s and has only a small anti-inflammatory component, is very well suited as an additive medication for severe pain or as a reserve medication when the maximum daily dose of NSAIDs has been reached. However, the drug has been repeatedly discredited for decades because of the feared side effect of blood count changes (agranulocytosis). In some countries, metamizole was even temporarily withdrawn from the market. From today's perspective, metamizole can certainly be recommended as a short-term, very potent additive demand medication. Nevertheless, patients should in any case be informed about the risk of life-threatening agranulocytosis, which is usually accompanied by the typical symptom triad of fever, sore throat, and inflammatory mucosal lesions.

If more severe pain is expected or the basic analgesic medication is not sufficient, a low-potency opioid (e.g. dihydrocodeine 60 mg ret. 0-0-1 p.o.) can be offered as an alternative additional medication on an outpatient basis after appropriate patient education about possible side effects and interactions. It is also recommended in stage II of the WHO staging scheme for analgesia.

In case of long-term NSAID administration or corresponding risk situations (especially gastroduodenal ulcers), the administration of a proton pump inhibitor is indicated to prevent gastrointestinal complications.

For many years, the University Clinic for Dentistry and Oral Health in Graz has routinely used medication for perioperative pain prophylaxis that considers the extent of the procedure and the individual patient situation (Tables 14-1 and 14-2).

Table 14-1 Intervention groups.

Level 1	No/minor pain expected	Minor procedures, e.g. removal of loosened teeth, biopsies
Level 2	Moderate pain expected	Oral/implant surgery, e.g. wisdom tooth removal, simple implant placement
Level 3	Severe pain expected	Oral/implant surgery, e.g. extensive osteotomies, augmentative surgery

Table 14-2 Scheme for outpatient perioperative pain medication in relation to the intervention group (modified according to Acham and Jakse[1]).

Indication	Active substances	Intervention groups and order recommendation	
Basic medication	Dexibuprofen 400 mg, 3x1 Diclofenac 50 mg, 3x1	1 2 3	If required Obligatory Obligatory
Alternative to basic medication	Paracetamol 500 mg, 3x1 Metamizole 500 mg, (max) 4x1	1 2 3	If required Obligatory Obligatory
Extension	Methylprednisolone 40 mg, 1x1 Dexamethasone 8 mg, 1x1	1 2 3	– If required Obligatory
Extension	Dihydrocodeine 60 mg, 0-0-1	1 2 3	– – If required
Supplementary	Pantoprazole or esomeprazole 20 mg 1-0-0 for prophylaxis or 40 mg 1-0-0 for therapy	1–3	In case of previous gastrointestinal disease

Perioperative antibiotic prophylaxis

The natural colonization of the oral cavity by microorganisms, collectively known as the oral microbiome, means that the oral cavity is not an aseptic area per se. Oral surgical procedures are therefore usually described as clean contaminated or as contaminated.

It is not uncommon for perioperative antibiotic prescriptions to be habitual, based on patient expectation, without proper indication, for forensic corroboration. Overall, these prescriptions are offered rather generously. Dentists are among the top prescribers of antibiotics, accounting for approximately 10% of antibiotic prescriptions worldwide.

In contrast, there is a general consensus in favor of a restrictive use of antibiotics, not least because antibiotic resistance is becoming a relevant threat, and possible side effects such as allergic reactions or serious intestinal complications must be considered.

Taking into account that oral bacteremia is not only triggered by dental procedures but also occurs during daily living activities such as eating or brushing the teeth, the indications for perioperative antibiotic prophylaxis to prevent complications that may be caused by bacteremia have been defined very narrowly in corresponding guidelines.

For example, according to the European Society of Cardiology (ESC) guidelines, preinterventional single-shot antibiotics for endocarditis prophylaxis should be given only in high-risk patients (certain congenital heart defects, survived infective endocarditis, artificial valve prostheses, or reconstructed valves made of prosthetic material). Peripheral implants such as hip or knee replacements are also indicated for perioperative antibiotic administration only in the presence of additional risk factors such as ongoing immunosuppressive therapy or (inadequately controlled) diabetes mellitus.

In general, a prophylactic perioperative antibiotic prescription should consider procedure-specific and patient-specific risk factors. Procedure-specific factors include extensive flap preparations and osteotomies, foreign materials introduced in the course of tissue regeneration, and prolonged duration of surgery. Patient-specific factors include, above all, an infected surgical site, smoking, antiresorptive therapy and a condition after radiotherapy, diabetes mellitus, immunosuppression, and the abovementioned cardiac diseases (Table 14-3).

Considering the different intervention-related and patient-specific risk situations, one can speak of a local and a systemic indication for perioperative antibiotic prophylaxis. This must be distinguished from the therapeutic use of antibiotics, which is aimed at eliminating an already existing focus of infection. Since the majority of odontogenic and periodontal infections are mixed aerobic–anaerobic infections, preparations with a broad spectrum of activity and good tolerability are preferably used systemically in a calculated manner. The first-choice agents are the ß-lactam antibiotics, especially aminopenicillins (amoxicillin) and cephalosporins (cefalexin). Penicillin V is no longer recommended due to frequent resistance in anaerobes. In therapeutic use, the combination with a ß-lactamase inhibitor (e.g. clavulanic acid) has proven to be particularly effective. In cases of penicillin allergy, the use of lincosamides (clindamycin) – for which, however, resistance is increasing significantly, especially in the anaerobic region – or macrolides (clarithromycin) is indicated. Depending on the local or systemic risk situation, administration is performed as a preoperative single shot, short-term administration over 4 to 5 days or long-term antibiotic therapy until the completion of soft tissue healing (Table 14-3).

Table 14-3 Recommended perioperative antibiotic prophylaxis according to risk situation.

Risk situation	Prophylactic antibiotic administration
Local	
Procedure-related	
Extensive flap preparations/osteotomies/tissue regeneration Long duration of surgery	Short-term antibiotic administration for 4 to 5 days – Amoxicillin with clavulanic acid 1 g, 3x1 – Cefalexin 1 g, 3x1 – Clindamycin 300 mg, 4x1 (adult patient)
Patient-specific	
Smoking	Short-term antibiotic administration for 4 to 5 days (as above)
Infected surgical site	
Uncontrolled diabetes mellitus	
After local radiotherapy High risk of AR-ONJ	Long-term antibiotic administration for 10 to 14 days (as above)
Systemic	
High risk of endocarditis	Single-shot double dose 1 hour preoperatively, e.g. amoxicillin 2 g or clindamycin 600 mg
Immunosuppression	

Consideration of relevant ongoing medication

Interactions may occur when different drugs are taken concomitantly, resulting in enhancement, attenuation or even cancellation of the desired effect. It can even result in an adverse effect. NSAIDs are most commonly responsible for hospital admissions due to adverse effects. In addition, with increasing age, the average number of medications taken increases, which in turn leads to a higher percentage of undesirable side effects. Particularly in the case of existing anticoagulant medication, care must be taken to ensure that the perioperative use of analgesics and antibiotics is as neutral as possible in terms of coagulation. In pain prophylaxis, alternatives such as paracetamol and metamizole or, if necessary, low-potency opioids should be considered, although these preparations are not without influence on hemostasis. An overview of common interactions is provided in Table 14-4.

Table 14-4 The most important side effects and interactions for common analgesic agents and antibiotics.

Drug group	Interaction	Possible effect	Side effects
Paracetamol	Alcohol	Liver intoxication	Headache, sweating
	Coumarins	Gastrointestinal bleeding	Asthma
	Barbiturates	Liver damage	Liver damage, failure
	Phenytoin	Liver damage	Cardiac arrhythmias, blood count changes
	Chloramphenicol, Rifampicin	Increased level of action	Liver damage
Classic NSAIDs	Coumarin/heparin	Gastrointestinal bleeding	Mucosal ulcers
	Cortisone	Gastrointestinal bleeding	Stomatitis, glossitis
	SSRI	Gastrointestinal bleeding	Toxic-allergic skin lesions
	Acetylsalicylic acid	Gastrointestinal bleeding, myocardial infarction	Asthma (AIA)
	ACE inhibitors	Increase in blood pressure	Renal damage
	Loop diuretics	Loss of effect, increased water retention	Edema, cardiac arrhythmias
	Potassium-sparing diuretics	Hyperkalemia, cardiac arrhythmias	Anaphylaxis
	Lithium	Lithium intoxication	Blood count changes
Metamizole	Alcohol	Intoxication	Bronchospasm
	Cyclosporine	Level drop	Blood count changes, skin reactions, itching
Opioids	SSRI	Serotonin syndrome	Nausea, vomiting
	MAO inhibitors	Central dysfunction	Sedation, visual disturbance
	Benzodiazepines	Increased effect	Skin redness, itching, micturition disturbance
Penicillin	Oral anticoagulant (OAC)	Increased OAC effect, risk of bleeding	Allergic reaction, diarrhea
Clindamycin	Oral anticoagulant (OAC)	Increased OAC effect, risk of bleeding	Diarrhea
Metronidazole	Oral anticoagulant (OAC)	Metabolism of OAC, risk of bleeding	Nausea, vomiting
Tetracyclines	Digoxin	Increase in digitalis level	Photosensitivity
	Lithium	Increase in lithium level	
Erythromycin	Digoxin	Increase in digitalis level	Inappetence, diarrhea
	Lithium	Increase in lithium level	

Recommended literature

1. Acham S, Jakse N. Perioperative Medikation bei zahnärztlich-chirurgischen Eingriffen. Quintessenz 2012;63:917–929.
2. Acham S, Klampfl A, Truschnegg A, Kirmeier R, Sandner-Kiesling A, Jakse N. Beneficial effect of methylprednisolone after mandibular third molar surgery: a randomized, double-blind, placebo-controlled split-mouth trial. Clin Oral Investig 2013;17:1693–1700.
3. Deutscher Arbeitskreis für Hygiene in der Zahnmedizin (Hrsg). Hygieneleitfaden, 12. Ausgabe 2018. http://dahz.org/hygieneleitfaden. Abgerufen am 30.12.2019.
4. ESC. The 2015 ESC Guidelines for the management of infective endocarditis. Eur Heart J 2015;36:3036–3037. doi: 10.1093/eurheartj/ehv488.
5. Halling F. Zahnärztliche Antibiotika- und Analgetikaverordnungen. In: Glaeske G, Schicktanz C, Hrsg. BARMER GEK Arzneimittelreport 2012. St. Augustin: Asgard 2012:78–95.
6. Kongkaew C, Noyce PR, Ashcroft DM. Hospital admissions associated with adverse drug reactions: a systematic review of prospective observational studies. Ann Pharmacother 2008;42:1017–1025.
7. Koyuncuoglu CZ, Aydin M, Kirmizi NI, et al. Rational use of medicine in dentistry: do dentists prescribe antibiotics in appropriate indications? Eur J Clin Pharmacol 2017;73:1027–1032.
8. Nkenke E. Systemische Antibiotikaprophylaxe bei Patienten ohne Systemerkrankungen zur Vermeidung postoperativer Wundinfektionen: Stellungnahme der Deutschen Gesellschaft für Zahn-, Mund- und Kieferheilkunde (DGZMK). Dtsch Zahnärztl Z 2008;63:140–142.
9. Pirmohamed M, James S, Meakin S, et al. Adverse drug reactions as cause of admission to hospital: prospective analysis of 18820 patients. Br Med J 2004;329:15–19.
10. Poveda Roda R, Bagan JV, Sanchis Bielsa JM, Carbonell Pastor E. Antibiotic use in dental practice. A review. Med Oral Patol Oral Cirugia Bucal 2007;12:E186–E192.
11. Sollecito TP, Abt E, Lockhart PB, et al. The use of prophylactic antibiotics prior to dental procedures in patients with prosthetic joints: Evidence-based clinical practice guideline for dental practitioners – a report of the American Dental Association Council on Scientific Affairs. J Am Dent Assoc 2015;146:11–16. doi: 10.1016/j.adaj.2014.11.012. Epub 2014 Dec 18.
12. Stamer UM, Stammschulte T, Erlenwein J, et al. Empfehlungen zur perioperativen Anwendung von Metamizol - Expertenempfehlung des Arbeitskreises Akutschmerz der Deutschen Schmerzgesellschaft, des Wissenschaftlichen Arbeitskreises Schmerzmedizin der Deutschen Gesellschaft für Anästhesiologie und Intensivmedizin und der Chirurgischen Arbeitsgemeinschaft Akutschmerz der Deutschen Gesellschaft für Chirurgie unter Beteiligung von Vertretern der Arzneimittelkommission der deutschen Ärzteschaft. Anaesthesist 2019;68:520–529. https://doi.org/10.1007/s00101-019-0622-y.
13. Suda KJ, Henschel H, Patel U, Fitzpatrick MA, Evans CT. Use of antibiotic prophylaxis for tooth extractions, dental implants, and periodontal surgical procedures. Open Forum Infect Dis 2018;5:ofx250.
14. Wacha H, Hoyme U, Isenmann R, et al. Perioperative Antibiotikaprophylaxe: Empfehlungen einer Expertenkommission der Paul-Ehrlich-Gesellschaft für Chemotherapie e.V. Chemother J 2010;193:70–84.
15. World Health Organization. WHO draft interim guidelines: Handbook on relief of cancer pain. WHO technical document, CAN/84.2. Geneva: WHO 1984.

Behavior after oral surgery

15

Andreas Filippi

Behavior after oral surgery influences the healing process. How patients should behave after an operation is not self-explanatory and requires appropriate instruction. This should already take place preoperatively in the course of the explanatory consultation, but must be refreshed again immediately after the procedure. The latter applies in particular if the explanatory consultation took place weeks or even months before. In principle, this instruction should be given not only verbally but also in the form of written information (Figs 15-1 to 15-4). Experience shows that patients remember hardly more than half of the recommendations given once they get home. This applies not least to the dosage of postoperative medication such as analgesics or, in individual cases, antibiotics.

The instruction on how to behave after surgery serves to ensure that wound healing is not compromised, that the first postoperative days are not accompanied by any complaints, and that the risk of postoperative bleeding is kept to a minimum. However, this instruction also serves to help the patient be alert in case of general medical deterioration and to seek medical or dental help if needed. Last but not least, it serves to ensure that medications are taken as prescribed, and that the patient is not left to improvise self-medication.

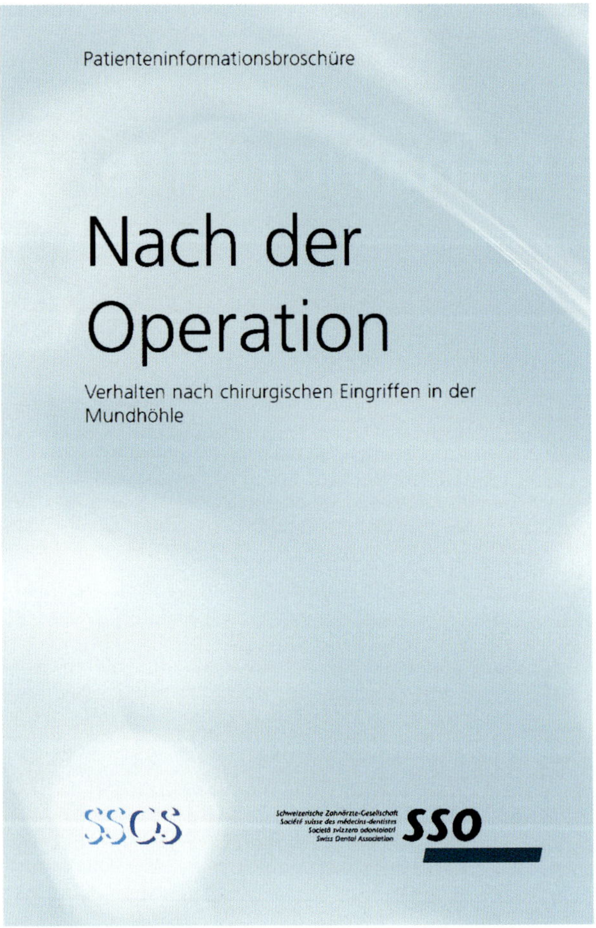

Fig 15-1 The jointly produced leaflet of the Swiss Society for Oral Surgery and Stomatology (SSOS) and the Swiss Dental Association (SSO) for distribution to patients after oral surgery: The outside...

Hemostasis and prevention of secondary bleeding

Immediately after the surgical procedure, the patient is given a bite block swab (preferably walnut-sized or at least 4 cm in diameter) (Fig 15-5). In the absence of antagonists, an additional swab may be required to build up appropriate pressure. Whether the bleeding has stopped in the process must be checked while the patient is still in the treatment chair or after any possible sutures have been performed. In non-anticoagulated patients, hemostasis takes 3 to 4 minutes. The patient is instructed to bite down on a bite swab with moderate pressure for 20 to 30 minutes. The patient should not talk during this entire time because the pumping effect of talking can make it more difficult for the bleeding to stop.

There are two typical times for the occurrence of postoperative secondary bleeding: the waning of the vasoconstrictor additive of the local anesthetic, and (on about the second/third day) the beginning of the remodeling of the granulation tissue into connective tissue. In order to prevent possible postoperative bleeding, the following additional recommendations are given:

You have undergone a surgical procedure. In order to achieve the most painless wound healing possible without complications, you should observe the following points:

1. Bite on the inserted cloth swab during the first 30 minutes after surgery, then remove the swab. This is to stop the bleeding.

2. If there is slight bleeding after the surgery, bite again on a cloth swab or a clean cloth handkerchief for half an hour. If the bleeding cannot be controlled with these measures, contact your dentist.

3. Apply cold compresses at least hourly for 1 to 2 days, changing them frequently. Avoid heat on the area in the first 2 to 3 days. Do not go out into the sun.

4. Do not rinse your mouth on the day of surgery. Use the prescribed irrigation solution the day after the surgery.

5. Take prescribed medication according to the dentist's instructions. Any antibiotics that are prescribed should usually be used up. In case of intolerance such as skin rashes, diarrhea, itching or similar symptoms, stop taking the medication and contact your dentist.

6. Clean your teeth as usual, gently in the wound area using a soft toothbrush. Do not touch the wound with your hands.

7. Speak little and avoid physical exertion for 1 to 2 days. Do not lie flat – keep your head elevated at night for the first 2 days after surgery. Do not put your head on the operated side when you are lying down.

8. Do not drink alcohol or coffee, and do not smoke for 2 to 3 days.

9. Soft food is preferable. Do not eat anything until the anesthesia has worn off.

10. During the first few days, the following symptoms are possible: soreness, swelling of the lip or cheek up to under the eyes, difficulty in opening the mouth, difficulty in swallowing, formation of a hematoma (bruise), hypersensitive tooth necks. From the third day after the surgery, the swelling should subside. If swallowing difficulties, fever or increasing mouth opening difficulties occur afterwards, contact your dentist.

11. An increase in temperature up to 38.5°C is possible. If your body temperature exceeds 38.5°C, contact your dentist.

Fig 15-2 ... and the inside of the leaflet.

Department of Oral Surgery
Mattenstrasse 40
CH-4058 Basel
Tel. 061 267 26 10
or central telephone number UZB:
Tel. 061 267 25 25

UZB
University Center for Dental Medicine Basel

Recommendations for behavior after surgical procedures in the oral cavity

You have undergone a surgical procedure at our clinic. In order to ensure that the healing process is as undisturbed and pain-free as possible, we would like to ask you to observe the following points.

Possible symptoms

- After surgical interventions in the oral cavity, the following are possible and typical: wound pain, swelling of the lips or cheeks, restriction of mouth opening, slight difficulty in swallowing, the formation of a hematoma (bruise), hypersensitive tooth necks in the surgical area, and an increase in body temperature up to 38.5°C. All this usually subsides slowly from the third day after surgery.

Immediately after the surgery

- You should bite down on the swab in your mouth for about 30 minutes and speak as little as possible. After that, the swab can be removed.
- Do not rinse your mouth, but at most spit out the saliva mixed with blood.
- If there is secondary bleeding after the swab is removed, bite down on a rolled-up, clean cloth handkerchief or another gauze swab.

Pain, swelling, and medication

- Moist, cold compresses (e.g. a cool pack or ice wrapped in a cloth) are helpful for pain. This will also reduce swelling at the same time.
- Avoid direct sunlight for the first 2 days.
- Take the recommended or prescribed painkillers as instructed by the dentist. Take them as needed.
- When you are no longer in pain, you may reduce or eliminate the pain medications.
- If you have been prescribed antibiotics, they usually need to be used up. If you have intolerances such as skin rashes, itching or similar symptoms, stop taking the medicine and contact us.

UZB
University Center for Dental Medicine Basel

Food and drink

- Do not eat or drink until the effects of the local anesthetic have worn off completely.
- Avoid hot foods and drinks and hard or spicy foods for the first 2 days after surgery.
- Abstain completely from alcohol and nicotine for the first 2 days, and use it sparingly between days 3 and 7.
- Refrain from caffeinated beverages such as coffee, black tea, cola or energy drinks for the first 2 days.

Brushing your teeth and oral hygiene

- Clean your teeth as usual from the day of surgery, but be more careful in the wound area.
- Do not touch the wound with your hands. This also applies to your relatives.

Exercise and sports

- No physical exertion or sports within the first 7 days.
- Do not go swimming within the first 7 days.

When do you need to call us or consult the emergency dental service?

- In case of prolonged postoperative bleeding, increase of body temperature to over 38.5°C or very severe pain, you can reach us Monday to Friday from 8:00 am to 6:00 pm at **061 267 26 10** or **061 267 25 25**.
- Outside these hours, please dial the number of the Medical Emergency Center: **061 261 15 15**.

We wish you as pain-free and speedy a recovery as possible.

Your team at the Department of Oral Surgery

Figs 15-3 and 15-4 Individual information sheet of the University Center for Dental Medicine Basel (UZB) on postoperative behavior: Pages 1 and 2.

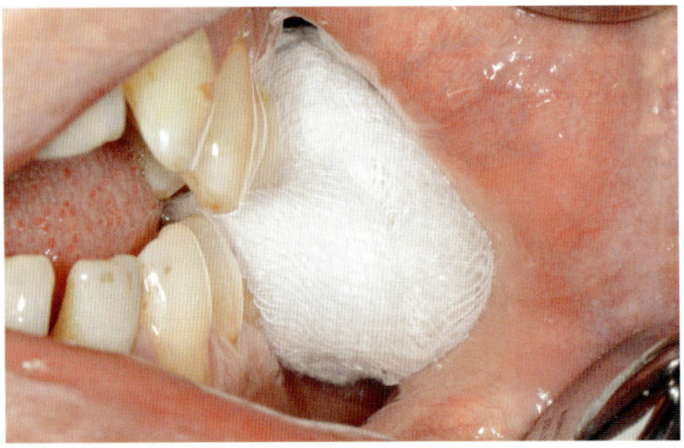

Fig 15-5 Bite block swab placed after tooth removal.

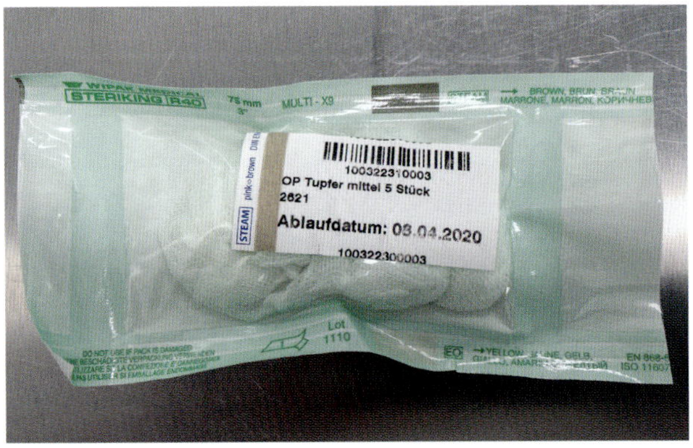

Fig 15-6 Additionally, sterilely packed bite block swabs are to be given to the patient.

Do not rinse the mouth vigorously within the first 72 hours after the procedure, do not drink beverages that stimulate blood circulation (alcohol, coffee, energy drinks), do not exercise heavily, and do not engage in sports. Depending on the professional orientation, the patient should be issued an appropriate doctor's certificate/sick note for this period. The patient should always be given additional swabs in case of possible slight postoperative bleeding (Fig 15-6). The instructions regarding bite pressure and duration correspond to those given on the day of surgery. If bleeding cannot be brought under control, the attending dentist or the emergency dental service should be consulted.

Intermittent extraoral cooling over 48 hours can additionally reduce the risk of postoperative bleeding by corresponding thermal vasoconstriction in the buccal soft tissue (see below: Extraoral cooling).

Eating and oral hygiene

The resumption of eating and drinking after oral surgery is not permitted until the local anesthetic has completely worn off because the risk of possible bite injuries to the lips, inner cheeks or tongue is too great. Since this period can be an hour or more, patients should always have eaten before oral surgery procedures are performed and should never present to the dental office fasting. During the first few days after the procedure, foods that are very hot in temperature or very spicy foods should be avoided.

Oral hygiene should be resumed as early as the day of surgery, including and especially in the operated area (see Section 16). This should be done with a soft toothbrush, with movements from gum to tooth. Plaque accumulation in the surgical area should be avoided because it can compromise wound healing. Accompanying chemical plaque control with disinfecting mouth rinses may be useful in individual cases (see Section 16). Chlorhexidine digluconate-based preparations are suitable for adults, but not for children. In this case, Meridol (Gaba, Therwil, Switzerland) can be used. Today, the standardized use of mouth rinses after oral surgery is no longer indicated.

Extraoral cooling

Postoperative cooling of the extraoral region for about 48 hours should always be recommended. This relieves postoperative pain and can prevent pronounced swelling, especially at high external temperatures. The medium that is used for cooling should be at refrigerator temperature, although it does not necessarily have to come from the refrigerator. Constant cooling with ice, in particular, carries the risk of throttling blood flow in the surgical area, with corresponding delayed or even compromised wound healing. In principle, cooling should be intermittent: Phases of cooling and non-cooling – approximately every 10 to 15 minutes – should be alternated. Preferably, patients should be given a cooling bag in the practice or clinic before they leave after the procedure (Fig 15-7).

Sun exposure should be avoided within the first 72 hours after surgery, as should sauna sessions or similar activities.

Antiphlogistic pain medication may also have a beneficial effect on swelling.

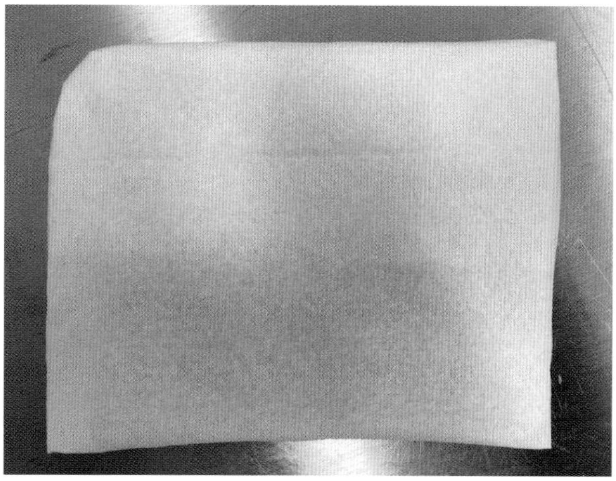

Fig 15-7 Cooling bag (wrapped in soft paper) to be handed out immediately after the procedure.

Postoperative medications

Most oral surgical procedures are accompanied by pain after the local anesthetic wears off. The perceived severity of this pain can vary widely depending on the procedure and the patient's constitution. Postoperative analgesic recommendations or prescriptions basically depend on body weight, general medical history, any allergies or intolerances that may be present, and the extent of the oral surgical procedure.

While paracetamol preparations are usually sufficient after simple tooth removal, more extensive surgical interventions require the prescription of nonsteroidal anti-inflammatory drugs (ibuprofen, diclofenac, mefenamic acid) or metamizole (see Section 14). The preparations should always be taken as required; the maximum daily dose or maximum quantity of tablets prescribed must be pointed out. If it turns out that appropriate analgesic medication is not sufficient, the patient must return to the practice. For gastric protection in sensitive normal-weight patients or prolonged use, pantoprazole should also be prescribed concomitantly (40 mg, 1-0-0).

In some general medical conditions or local osseous predispositions associated with an increased risk of postoperative wound infections, and also after very extensive and/or prolonged surgical procedures, postoperative antibiotic administration may be required. In most patients, preparations with a combination of amoxicillin and clavulanic acid are indicated. In normal-weight adults, the daily dosage of 3 x 625 mg (1-1-1) is preferable to 2 x 1 g (1-0-1) because of less pharmacologic variability. In children or overweight/underweight individuals, the dosage should be adjusted accordingly. In patients with penicillin allergy, clindamycin is favored (normal weight adults 3 x 300 mg, 1-1-1). It is important to note that clindamycin is not a first-line preparation and should be prescribed only when penicillin-based preparations are excluded. Usually, 5 to 7 days of postoperative antibiotic administration is sufficient; in individual cases, this may need to be extended. Administration of an antibiotic can and should be combined with that of a probiotic (e.g. Perenterol; Medice, Iserlohn, Germany) (1-1-1), especially in children and adolescents, but also in patients who suffer from significant gastrointestinal problems when taking antibiotics.

Other instructions

In principle, smoking should be avoided within the first week after oral surgery. The reality is that this is difficult in individual cases and often cannot really be implemented. However, it should be clearly pointed out that smoking increases the risk of postoperative wound infections.

In principle, patients can return to work when they feel able to do so. This can vary greatly in individual cases, so that in the case of predominantly sedentary work and simple tooth removals, work can be resumed on the same or the next day, whereas in the case of more extensive surgical interventions and heavy physical work, the patient should not work for several days. This should be communicated to the employer by a doctor's certificate/sick note.

Patients should not drive themselves home after oral surgical interventions, even though there are indications that they are significantly more agitated and unsafe driving to the intervention than driving back from it. This should already be communicated to the patient during the preoperative educational discussion.

All patients must also be made aware of possible accompanying symptoms that can typically (but not always) occur after surgical procedures: pain, swelling, restriction of mouth opening, reduced performance capacity, hematomas, and slight difficulty in swallowing. If they occur, these symptoms peak after about 48 hours, and from then on should improve successively each day. If the symptoms increase beyond this point, if the patient's general condition has noticeably deteriorated, if there are significant swallowing difficulties beyond the second day, and if the patient's body temperature rises above 38.5°C, the dentist in charge or the respective dental emergency service should be contacted (if outside office hours). After most oral surgical procedures, a postoperative check-up on the second or third postoperative day is in any case recommended.

Recommended literature

1. AWMF. S2k-Leitlinie Operative Entfernung von Weisheitszähnen (Stand August 2019).
2. Rueppell C, Meier R, Filippi A. Normale und gestörte Wundheilung nach Zahnentfernung. Quintessenz 2016;67:1225–1232.

Oral hygiene after oral surgical procedures

16

Cornelia Filippi

Biofilms play a crucial role in the contamination of surgical sutures and can be responsible for wound healing delays and chronic wounds[13]. Biofilms are formed by highly adhesive microorganisms (community of bacteria and possibly fungi). These are able to release extracellular polysaccharides (EPS) and form microcolonies within 2 to 4 hours. After only 6 hours, this protective community begins to become less sensitive to biocides such as antiseptics, disinfectants, and antibiotics. The complete maturation of a biofilm is completed after 2 to 4 days. The germs are then markedly resistant to bactericidal substances. Even after mechanical destruction of the biofilm, they can recover within 24 hours and form a new, mature biofilm[13]. However, in order to achieve the desired healing of an oral surgical procedure, dental hygiene and antiseptic mouth rinses are clinically relevant.

Tooth brushing after oral surgical procedures

Dental hygiene is a cultural achievement. There is no reflex to practice dental hygiene[12]. In contrast, there is an innate behavioral pattern of responding to pain with avoidance behavior. Avoidance behavior is also expected when pain is anticipated, e.g. brushing teeth after oral surgery. Cultural influences make themselves felt in the acquired knowledge of dental professionals and patients. There are differences in dental care recommendations regarding method, frequency and duration, auxiliaries, tongue and interdental space care, and mouth rinses. Previous habits are important for healing after oral surgery. Diseases caused by insufficient dental hygiene such as caries and periodontitis lead to local inflammation. If oral hygiene is insufficient before the planned surgery, it is less likely that dental care with toothbrush and toothpaste after the treatment will be qualitatively sufficient to contribute to an undisturbed healing phase. The germ-reducing effect of manual plaque removal at least twice daily should therefore be encouraged at an early stage.

It makes sense to assess the quality of dental care during the planning phase of the oral surgery, to ask about the daily dental care procedure, and to optimize it at least for the wound healing phase of 14 days. A hygiene phase may be useful preoperatively.

Wound infection after oral surgery and antiseptic rinsing solutions

Antiseptic treatment of the wound is becoming increasingly important. Current developments in multiresistant germs and antibiotic intolerance as well as cross-resistance between some antiseptic agents and antibiotics have prompted hygiene institutes in Germany, Austria, and Switzerland to issue joint consensus recommendations. They are valid for all medical fields, including oral wound treatment[10,11].

For practical application after oral surgery, the following questions arise:

- Which wounds require postoperative preventive antiseptic treatment?
- Which patients require antiseptic wound treatment?
- Which agents are indicated or contraindicated?

Wounds and antiseptic treatments

Microbial colonization of wounds is considered the norm and is classified as mostly irrelevant to the wound healing process[10]. The only exception is colonization with methicillin-resistant

Staphylococcus aureus (MRSA), which must be treated in any case when hospitalized patients are treated with germ carriers[10]. In principle, it is recommended to treat localized infections with antiseptics and to treat wound infections with incipient general infection as well as manifest systemic infections (sepsis) with systemic antibiotics (if necessary, in combination with antiseptics)[10]. In clinically manifest wound infection, antisepsis should only be performed as long as signs of wound infection are present. This is generally for no more than 2 to 6 days[10]. Wound antiseptics should only be used after careful indication, otherwise disturbances in wound healing may result[10]. To determine the risk of infection, the "Wounds at risk of infection" score is used, which in the original works with a point system[10]. Preventive antisepsis is indicated from 3 points. For the decision regarding which patient group presents with an increased risk of infection after oral surgery, the present article omits this in the listing[10]. This takes into account the fact that the risk of infection is fundamentally increased, and thus the use of a preventively prescribed antiseptic mouth rinse is justified (Table 16-1).

For the selection of antiseptic mouth rinses, the active substances must best meet the requirements for safe broad-spectrum action, rapid onset of action, efficacy in the presence of organic contamination, wound tolerance, absence of allergenicity, absence of the risk of anaphylactic reactions, absence of resorptive risk, and absence of development of resistance[10]. As chlorhexidine has been included in the list of obsolete or dispensable agents for wound antisepsis due to its inefficacy, cytotoxicity, mutagenicity, reversible premalignant alterations in the oral cavity in animal studies, anaphylaxis, neurotoxicity, and suspected resorption, alternatives are described below[10].

Table 16-1 Checklist for wounds at high risk of infection (modified from Dissemond et al[8]).

Diabetes mellitus
Wounds that are exposed to a high bacterial load due to their localization (e.g. after surgical removal of wisdom teeth in the mandible)
Difficult hygienic conditions due to social or occupational environment (e.g. farmer, truck driver) or insufficient oral hygiene prior to oral surgical intervention
Patient age > 80 years
An oral infection has existed for longer than 1 year (e.g. *periodontitis marginalis*)
Wound area > 10 cm^2
Chronic wounds of any etiology with a depth of > 1.5 cm
Severe immunodeficiency (e.g. HIV infection)
Heavily contaminated acute wound infections
Severe immunodeficiency such as agammaglobulinemia (treatment always in consultation with treating physician)
Acquired immunodeficiency due to pharmacotherapy such as cyclosporine, methotrexate, glucocorticoids, antibodies (treatment always in consultation with treating physician)
Solid tumor disease (treatment always in consultation with treating physician)
Systemic hematologic disease (treatment always in consultation with treating physician)

Povidone-iodine

The active ingredient has a reliable microbicidal effect against Gram-positive and Gram-negative bacteria, fungi, and protozoa. It also has a sporicidal effect with longer exposure times and an affect against a number of viruses[10]. The effect lasts approximately as long as the brown stain is present[10]. However, the patient should be given a rinse recommendation. To reliably prevent colonization with microorganisms, rinsing 2 or 3 times daily for 30 seconds with 10 ml rinsing solution is a proven standard recommendation. Iodophores are very well tolerated by tissue and can therefore also be used to rinse deep wounds, but then should be diluted 1:10[10]. Mouth rinses containing povidone-iodine are available on the market (e.g. Betadine disinfecting gargle concentrate; Mundipharma Medical Company, Basel, Switzerland). However, the formulation offered contains 36% ethanol, which fundamentally calls into question its use in the oral cavity and rules it out for children, adolescents, and dry alcoholics. A contraindication is declared by the manufacturer in case of hypersensitivity to the active ingredient iodine or the povidone-iodine complex or one of the excipients according to the composition; hyperthyroidism or other manifest thyroid diseases; *dermatitis herpetiformis* during, before, and after radio-iodine application (until the application is completed); and in children under 6 years of age[4].

Octenidine dihydrochloride

The microbicidal activity of octenidine dihydrochloride includes Gram-positive and Gram-negative bacteria and fungi as well as certain viral species but has no sporicidal or protozoal activity[10]. There is no evidence of carcinogenic, mutagenic, teratogenic, embryotoxic, and fertility impairing effects; systemic side effects; or neurotoxic reactions as well as no resorptions after application to wounds[10]. Cytotoxicity and tissue toxicity, on the other hand, are about the same as that of chlorhexidine and higher than that of iodophores and polyhexanide (PHMB). A randomized double-blind study needs to clarify whether the mechanism of action of octenidine dihydrochloride complexes with cells or proteins. This is thought to have a beneficial effect on tolerability in vivo, in that bacterial colonization may be impaired by such complexes[10]. However, evidence is still lacking. The application refers to skin and mucosal surfaces. Irrigation of deep wounds is strongly discouraged as this has been shown to cause tissue damage[3].

The use of Octenimed Gargle Solution is not recommended in children under 12 years of age because it has not been tested to date. This restriction is surprising; after all, the active ingredient octenidine is even used in infant care, infants, and children, and is considered safe when used superficially. Off-label use is sometimes the only way to treat children in this regard. In this case, parents must be informed about off-label use in addition to the application (mouth rinse in children who can spit or dabbing of the mucosa if spitting is not possible) and the frequency of use (standard recommendation 2 to 3 times daily with 10 ml mouth rinse for 30 seconds) – this is especially important in light of possible adverse effects. These include not precisely defined disturbances of the immune system and allergic reactions in individual cases (< 1/10,000)[5]. Taste disturbances, burning, and mild paresthesia (furry sensation) in the mouth and throat as well as a bitter aftertaste have been reported. In addition, tooth discoloration may occur[5]. During the application period, attention should also be paid to the possibility of interactions with anionic substances such as those contained in toothpastes[5]. Thorough rinsing of the mouth with water after brushing the teeth therefore appears necessary in combination with mouthwash containing octenidine. Alternatively, a toothpaste without anionic surfactants should be used. The antiseptic treatment is carried out after the teeth and tongue have been cleaned and after the toothpaste residues have been rinsed away with water. If dental hygiene is not possible or only possible to a reduced extent as a result of the surgical procedure (e.g. restricted mouth opening), the mouth rinse 2 or better 3 times daily completely replaces the reduction of the biofilm.

Polyhexanide

The active ingredient polyhexanide (PHMB) was discovered by the cosmetics industry as early as 1959 and may be added as a preservative in a concentration of up to 0.3%. Together with betaine, it forms an active ingredient complex that is finding increasing medical use. For this reason, a discussion of the two active ingredients in the context of oral surgery is necessary and is considered in more detail below.

PHMB is effective against Gram-positive and Gram-negative germs as well as multi-resistant pathogens. For use in the mouth, it is particularly important that plaque- and biofilm-forming bacteria as well as fungi are eliminated[9]. The antiseptic onset of action was observed in vitro after 5 to 20 minutes, but it is not virucidal and sporicidal[10]. For this reason, the antimicrobial efficacy of PHMB, both in clean and dirty wounds, is stronger than that of chlorhexidine. Maximum activity occurs at a pH between 5 and 69. Since PHMB is not absorbed systemically, but interactions between antibiotics and antiseptics may occur, the interaction was studied. When antibiotic is administered systemically, it is also washed up in the wound area via the blood and leads to a synergistic effect with PHMB in in vitro studies, unlike chlorhexidine[9]. PHMB is also transferred to the cytoplasm of the germs, where it leads to disruption of bacterial metabolism. Neutral phospholipids, on the other hand, are little affected or unaffected by PHMB. This is generally considered to be the main reason for its low toxicity to human cells and its wound-healing effect[9]. For prescribing purposes in dentistry, it is important to know that microbial attachment to tooth surfaces of plaque- and biofilm-forming bacteria as well as fungi is prevented by PHMB[9]. In a clinical study, four rinsing solutions were compared. Volunteers had their teeth cleaned and were given an appropriate mouth rinse. Plaque growth was determined on defined tooth surfaces and on defined mucosal areas by swabbing and counting bacteria. The subjects had received professional tooth cleaning at the beginning. They then discontinued home dental care and instead rinsed twice daily with a mouth rinse. The reduction in the number of bacteria on the tooth and mucosal surfaces resulting from 0.2% PHMB-containing rinsing solution was significant[14]. However, at the present time, there are no standard recommendations in this regard.

Betaine can react as an amphoteric surfactant in both acids and bases. It breaks through biofilm, but at the same time is compatible with the skin. Thus, according to cosmetic regulations, it may be added to baby shampoos in an amount up to 40%. In mouth rinsing solutions, betaine has the task of reducing surface tension, and contributes to a rinsing effect of infected wounds[1,2].

In a mouth rinse product that is available without prescription under the name ProntOral (B. Braun Medical AG, Sempach, Switzerland), 1.5 mg PHMB and 1 mg betaine are contained in 250 mg of the solution. This product is also suitable for children without age restriction. No statement is made regarding use during pregnancy. It is recommended to rinse 2 to 3 times daily with 10 ml for 30 seconds or for 60 seconds in case of multiresistant germs. When prescribing, it is up to the practitioner to also recommend that it be used 3 times daily for 60 seconds. This would give greater consideration to preventing biofilm formation on tooth and mucosal surfaces. Since anionic compounds such as those found in toothpastes cause PHMB to precipitate, a decision must be made on how to handle the dental care recommendation. One recommendation could be that the patient rinses the mouth thoroughly with water after brushing before starting the antiseptic mouth rinse. However, as shown by in vitro studies, cells remain firmly attached to detergents from toothpaste even when thoroughly washed under laboratory conditions[6,7]. An alternative could be to give a toothbrush dispensation for 2 to 6 days if adequate wetting of all tooth and mucosal surfaces with the rinse occurs at least twice daily.

References

1. Andriessen AE, Eberlein T. Assessment of a wound cleansing solution in the treatment of problem wounds. Wounds 2008;20:171–175.
2. Bester E, Kroukamp O, Wolfaardt GM, Boonzaaier L, Liss SN. Metabolic differentiation in biofilms as indicated by carbon dioxide production rates. Appl Environ Microbiol 2010;76: 1189–1197.
3. Bundesinstitut für Arzneimittel und Medizinprodukte (BfArM)/Paul-Ehrlich Institut (PEI): Octenisept®. Schwellungen und Gewebeschädigungen nach Spülung tiefer Wunden – weitere Maßnahmen zur Risikominimierung. Bulletin zur Arzneimittelsicherheit, Ausgabe 2 (2016).
4. Compendium Schweiz: Swiss-medic genehmigte Fachinfo Betadine® desinfizierendes Gurgelkonzentrat, Swissmedic Zulassungsnummer 34284 (2017).
5. Compendium Schweiz: Swiss-medic genehmigte Fachinfo Octenimed® Gurgellösung. Swissmedic Zulassungsnummer 62809 (2013).
6. Cvikl B, Lussi A, Gruber R. The in vitro impact of toothpaste extracts on cell viability. Eur J Oral Sci 2015;123:179–185.
7. Cvikl B, Lussi A, Moritz A, Gruber R. Dentifrices for children differentially affect cell viability in vitro. Clin Oral Investig 2017;21:453–461.
8. Dissemond J, Assadian O, Gerber V, et al. Classification of wounds at risk and their antimicrobial treatment with Polihexanide: A practice-oriented expert recommendation. Skin Pharmacol Physiol 2011;24:245–255.
9. Hübner N, Kramer A. Review on the efficacy, safety and clinical applications of Polihexanide, a modern wound antiseptic. Skin Pharmacol Physiol 2010;23:17–27.
10. Kramer A, Daeschlein G, Kammerlander G, et al. Konsensusempfehlungen zur Auswahl von Wirkstoffen für die Wundantiseptik. Zschr Wundheilung 2004;9:110–140.
11. Kramer A, Dissemond J, Kim S, et al. Consensus on wound antisepsis: Update 2018. Skin Pharmacol Physiol 2018;31:28–58.
12. Künkel A. Die Psychologie der zahnärztlichen Gruppenprophylaxe. Schlütersche, Hannover (2003).
13. Phillips PL, Wolcott RD, Fletcher J, Schultz GS. Biofilme einfach erklärt. Wounds International 2010;1:1–6. https://www.woundsinternational.com/uploads/resources/6e7fffcdeef76d-9d3e652be2854315a6.pdf (letzter Zugriff am 13.08.2020).
14. Rosin M, Welk A, Bernhardt O, et al. Effect of a polyhexamethylene biguanide mouthrinse on bacterial counts and plaque. J Clin Periodontol 2001;28:1121–1126.